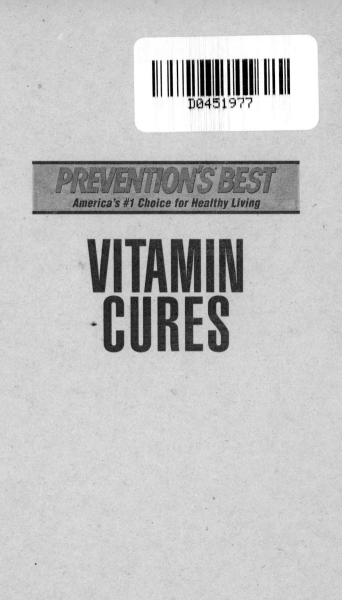

D0451977

PREVENTION'S BEST
America's #1 Choice for Healthy Living

VITAMIN CURES

PREVENTION'S BEST

America's #1 Choice for Healthy Living

VITAMIN CURES

The Ultimate Compendium of Vitamin and Mineral Cures with More than 500 Remedies for Whatever Ails You!

By the Editors of Prevention Health Books

RODALE

ST. MARTIN'S
PAPERBACKS

The information in this book is excerpted from *Food and You* (Rodale, 1996), *Prevention's Healing with Vitamins* (Rodale, 1996), and *Vitamin Vitality* (Rodale, 1997).

Prevention and *Prevention Health Books* are registered trademarks of Rodale Inc.

VITAMIN CURES

© 1998; 2000 by Rodale Inc.

Interior designer: Diane Ness Shaw
Cover designer: Anne Twomey

ISBN 0-312-97476-0   paperback

Printed in the United States of America

Rodale/St. Martin's Paperbacks edition published February 2000

St. Martin's Paperbacks are published by St. Martin's Press, 175 Fifth Avenue, New York, NY 10010.

10   9   8   7   6   5   4   3

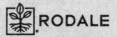

RODALE

WE INSPIRE AND ENABLE PEOPLE TO IMPROVE
THEIR LIVES AND THE WORLD AROUND THEM

Contents

Part 2: Know Your ABCs

Part 3: Making Mineral Deposits

Part 4: Therapeutic Prescriptions for Healing

Part 5: Everyday Vitality

Introduction

Tapping Into Nature's Vital Healing Power

Vitamins are not magic pills. But let's face it: It's really tempting to think of them that way. Anything that can help you live longer, look younger, stave off cancer and heart disease, enhance your immune system, fight off illness, and boost your energy certainly sounds pretty miraculous or magical.

A few decades ago, when word started to spread about the healing potential of vitamins and minerals, the general public went wild for bottled nutrients. So did health writers and even some doctors. For a while, it was starting to sound as though megadoses of vitamins could cure anything. Just take enough vitamins or the right combination of vitamins, and bingo! You were on your way to total health.

Well, that bubble burst soon enough. Of course, vitamins and minerals can't cure everything. But they can do a lot. Research breakthroughs over just the past few years are making interest in the topic heat up all over again. Some of the things that scientists have discovered about the healing power of these vital nutrients all but boggle the mind.

Let's take a brief look at just one study that didn't get all that much publicity. Researchers in London looked at 180 middle managers employed in the manufacturing industry in Britain. In a rigorous study, they gave one group a typical multivitamin/mineral supplement and another group a look-alike pill that did not contain nutrients. At the end of eight weeks, those receiving supplements revealed in tests that they perceived an improvement in their quality of life. The group not receiving supplements did not perceive a change. Researchers concluded that the supplements seemed to play a role in improving the managers' moods and reducing their stress levels. All of this from just a daily multivitamin pill with hard scientific data confirming that it works.

As more and more rigorous scientific studies accumulate showing spectacular health benefits from vitamins and minerals, we're all back where we were a few decades ago: eager to take advantage of all of this healing potential—and thoroughly confused. While the reasons for taking vitamins and minerals are now based on solid science, shopping for nutrients is still nothing less than overwhelming.

You know what happens when you make a trip to your local pharmacy or supermarket to buy nutrients. You're faced with overwhelming choices. Shelf after shelf in aisle after aisle offers nothing but confusion. Letters and numbers, single nutrients and combinations, capsules and tablets, bottles in different sizes and colors from different companies, covered with enticing claims that compete for your attention and your precious consumer dollar.

What's a person who wants to take vitamins and minerals in a safe and responsible manner supposed to do? All you really want to know, after all, is what really works.

Well, search no more. That's what this book is all about.

A staff of writers from *Prevention* Health Books interviewed hundreds of the nation's top doctors and researchers, asking exactly those questions that you want answered: Which vitamins and minerals can you take to prevent, cure, or ameliorate specific diseases? How much of the nutrients do you take? Are they safe? What kinds of results can you expect?

These writers also scanned computer databases and reviewed thousands of scientific studies to answer these questions. And in this fast-breaking, ever-changing, ever-expanding arena of nutritional therapy, they've put it all together in one easy-to-use volume. You're holding it in your hands right now. If you want to know which nutrients to take and in what amounts, simply look up the condition you want to know about.

Along with the scoop on how to use nutrients to fight disease, the writers made several important discoveries during the course of their research.

One is that supplements are not a substitute for good nutrition. It will come as no surprise to anyone who pays attention to natural healing and prevention that scientists can't beat nature when it comes to packaging healing therapies.

And that's why, so often in this book, you'll find doctors and researchers saying that you should get your healing vitamins and minerals from foods whenever you can. At the same time, doctors and researchers often recommend taking supplements—at least a multivitamin for what they call insurance. Why is that?

It's often not practical to get adequate therapeutic amounts of vitamins and minerals from foods. That's right, therapeutic. Large doses of some nutrients have such powerful effects on the body that they act like drugs.

That brings us to the second important discovery that the writers made: Vitamin and mineral supplements should be treated with the same care and concern for safety that you reserve for prescription and over-the-counter medications.

Large doses of certain nutrients can be toxic. They can cause side effects. They can interact with medications that you might be taking. So there are a few rules to follow when using this book.

Please take the Medical Alerts seriously. They are there for your safety. If you are under a doctor's care for a serious disease, you should talk to him or her about your interest in using nutrients as part of your treatment. With all of the scientific breakthroughs in this area, doctors are increasingly open to nutritional therapy. You may be pleasantly surprised to find that your doctor is willing to work with you to find the right dosages and monitor your progress.

If you're pregnant or nursing a baby, make sure that you mention any supplements you're taking, even a multivitamin, to your physician.

Finally, pay attention to the Daily Values of any vitamins and minerals that you're taking. Daily Values are a system from the Food and Drug Administration designed to help you keep track of your body's nutritional requirements.

Many researchers and doctors feel that the Daily Values for certain nutrients—vitamin C, for example—should be set much higher. They've also found that the body's need for nutrients goes way, way up when it's fighting disease. That's why you'll find that the recommendations in this book often go way beyond the Daily Values for many nutrients.

Here's wishing you all of the healing that nature's nutrients can supply.

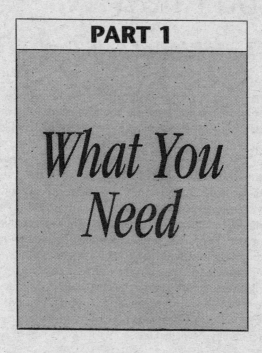

PART 1

What You Need

What Do You Know?

A Nutritional Self-Test

Every time you pick up the paper or turn on the news, it seems you hear about some new discovery relating to vitamins and minerals. It's tough to keep on top of all the changes.

For instance, it seems like hardly a week passes without some new study making some new claim about beta-carotene. But be honest: Do you really know what beta-carotene is? Do you know whether it is (a) a vitamin, (b) a mineral, or (c) neither? (The correct answer is neither.) Before you embark on our guided journey through the nutrient maze, take a few minutes to test your knowledge. Then, after you've read through the book, come back and take the test again. As your score soars, so will your health—provided that you put the nutritional power of your newfound knowledge into practice in your daily life.

Self-Test

1. The Daily Value for vitamin C is 60 milligrams. How many milligrams did early vitamin C pioneer Linus Pauling, Ph.D., the double Nobel prize–winning doctor who wrote *Vitamin C and the Common Cold*, take every day; and how old was he when he died?
   a. 18,000 milligrams and 62 years old
   b. 12,000 milligrams and 93 years old
   c. 250 milligrams and 81 years old
   d. 1,000 milligrams and 54 years old

2. Which mineral joins vitamins A, C, and E as an antioxidant?
   a. Selenium
   b. Magnesium
   c. Iron
   d. Chromium

3. Which mineral transports oxygen in the blood?
   a. Chromium
   b. Zinc
   c. Sulfur
   d. Iron

4. If you drink a little more than you should, what do you lose?
   a. Sodium
   b. Potassium
   c. B vitamins, particularly B_{12}
   d. Your balance

(continued)

Self-Test—Continued

5. Why were British sailors called Limeys?
  a. Their faces turned the color of limes when they got seasick.
  b. Someone once told them to eat citrus fruits, such as limes, to combat scurvy.
  c. Their uniforms were lime green.
  d. French sailors were called Lemonheads.

6. You're a Caucasian who lives in Alaska, and it's summertime. Should you take extra vitamin D or not?
  a. No, because your body will process vitamin D from the sun, and too much vitamin D can be dangerous.
  b. Yes, because there's no such thing as getting too many vitamins.

7. Folic acid, a member of the B vitamin family, has been known by many names, including:
  a. Popular vitamin, factor vitamin, vitamin B_3, and leaf vitamin
  b. Pteroylglutamic acid, Wills' factor, factor U, and vitamin M
  c. Vitamin B_4, skin factor H, and Preparation H

8. Table salt. You know it; you probably use too much of it. What two minerals are in it?
  a. Sodium and phosphorus
  b. Sodium and chloride
  c. Sodium and potassium

9. Which diseases are caused by vitamin and/or mineral deficiencies?
   a. Pellagra
   b. Beriberi
   c. Cretinism
   d. Goiter
   e. Night blindness
   f. All of the above

10. What's the difference between vitamins and minerals?
   a. Vitamins are needed in larger amounts.
   b. Vitamins come from organic things; minerals come from inorganic things.
   c. Vitamins don't have names, just letters and numbers.
   d. All of the above

11. RDA is an acronym for:
   a. Rural Delivery Association
   b. Registered Dietitians Association
   c. Recommended Dietary Allowance
   d. Recommended Daily Amount

12. Is beta-carotene added to processed food for coloring?
   a. Yes, because it's a pigment that can make foods more yellow-orange.
   b. No, because it's found in green, leafy vegetables.

Correct answers: 1. b, 2. a, 3. d, 4. c, 5. b, 6. a, 7. b, 8. b, 9. f, 10. b, 11. c, 12. a

What Are Vitamins and Minerals?

Better Living through Chemistry

Iᵉn their quest to create a more tasty and attractive dish, cereal makers in the Far East began to refine rice in the mid-1800s. At the same time, a disease called beriberi, also known as polyneuritis, spread like wildfire through countries where rice made up a huge part of the average diet. The Philippine word *beriberi* translates to "I can't, I can't." Or, more descriptively, "I'm so sick, I don't have the energy to get up and move around." The disease causes inflamed nerves, which lead to paralysis.

At the turn of the twentieth century, Filipino and Indonesian physicians came up with a reliable cure for beriberi: a drink called tikitiki. And what was tikitiki made from? Rice bran extract. The same part that was removed from rice during the refining process. An important connection between food and health was made. Clearly, some substance in rice bran was the key to curing beriberi. But it would be more than two decades before scientists figured out that the substance was thiamin, also known as vitamin B_1.

Of course, you can't really blame them for taking so long. When they started looking for the cure, vitamins didn't even exist.

Vital Facts

To be precise, vitamins have always been around. We just didn't have a clue what they were. That all changed in 1912, when a Polish biochemist named Casimir Funk coined the word *vitamines*. Funk believed that there was just one substance in our diets necessary for life, so he combined *vita*, Latin for "life," with *amine* because he thought that the one substance contained nitrogen. Later research showed that there were many "vitamines," but few were nitrogen-based. So the final "e" was dropped. Funk's word, however, endured. As they used to say on *Laugh-In*, you can look *that* up in your Funk and Wagnall's.

Funk's concept also has endured. Vitamins are tiny, organic substances necessary for at least one metabolic function. In other words, necessary for life. They are essential micronutrients, which means precisely what it sounds like: very small things that your body absolutely must have for nourishment. Miss out on any of them and you risk contracting diseases. If you don't have vitamin C, you get scurvy; no vitamin A and you'll suffer from night blindness. A shortage of niacin and you'll come down with pellagra, an ugly little syndrome that leaves you with cracks and sores around your mouth; scales on the back of your hands, neck, and chest; vomiting; and diarrhea. A nutrient is a substance that you must consume because your body can't produce it.

A, B, C, D, E, . . . K?

There is only one vitamin A, but there are eight B vitamins. There is a C, D, E, and K but no F, G, or H. What's the story behind these out-of-order letters? International research and lots of backtracking.

Many scientists work on the same compounds and questions at the same time, often without knowing it. That was the case even more so 50 to 100 years ago, when much of the groundbreaking vitamin research was done. So, each person discovered one or more uses for a compound and then gave it a name relating to that use.

Letters were picked often just to distinguish the unstudied compounds from other more researched ones. But earning a vitamin letter is much tougher than getting a varsity letter in college. Consider poor vitamin G. Never heard of it? That's because what was originally tagged as an exciting new discovery turned out to be just another member of the B-complex brood. It's now known as riboflavin, or vitamin B_2.

So how did we jump to vitamin K? It's necessary for coagulation, spelled with a "K" in Dutch, the nationality of its discoverers.

Just because vitamins are small doesn't mean that they aren't as important as other nutrients like water, carbohydrates, fat, and protein. Vitamins act as catalysts for vital processes in the body. For example, your body converts thiamin into a coenzyme called thiamin pyrophosphate, which aids in metabolizing carbohydrates and sugars. Without thiamin, your body wouldn't be able to turn the spaghetti you eat into the energy you burn during aerobics.

"We often think of the body as a machine analogous to a car," says Cathy Kapica, R.D., Ph.D., associate professor of nutrition and clinical dietetics at Finch University of Health Sciences/Chicago Medical School. "Food with lots of nutrients is like gasoline: The higher the quality of the gasoline, the better the car runs. The same is true of your body. The higher and more varied the amount of vitamins and minerals in your food, the more likely it is that your body will run better."

Meet the Minerals

Like vitamins, some minerals are necessary for life. They are composed of various arrangements of the naturally occurring elements found in the periodic table, which most of us haven't looked at since high school. Where vitamins are organic, meaning that they contain carbon atoms, minerals are inorganic, meaning that they don't contain carbon.

Minerals come in two sizes: macronutrients and micronutrients. We need large amounts of 7 minerals, including calcium, magnesium, and potassium. But we require only trace amounts of 9 others, including zinc and iron. And there are 29 other minerals inside our bodies that scientists can't account for. Why do we need lead, mercury, and lithium? No one knows.

When it comes to minerals, size truly doesn't matter. Just because one mineral comes in trace amounts and another in huge quantities doesn't mean that the bigger one is more important. For example, calcium makes up about 2 percent of your body weight, while iodine represents only 0.00004 percent of that same weight. But almost all of that iodine is concentrated in the thyroid gland, where it becomes part of the hormones that promote growth and regulate energy. If you don't get enough iodine, you'll develop a goiter, or enlarged thyroid gland.

While 16 minerals (both macro and micro) currently meet the "essential" criteria, researchers don't discount the importance of the other minerals in the body. Fluoride is not considered essential, even though it's a generally accepted practice to use it as protection against tooth decay. Is it essential for life, growth, or reproduction? No. But it certainly is responsible for a lot more smiles in your life.

While scientists have, during the past two centuries, isolated the numerous vitamins and minerals in your body, they also have found that your diet, genetic history, exercise habits, age, and geographical location impact on your intake and absorption of these same vitamins and minerals, says Shari Lieberman, Ph.D., certified nutrition specialist and co-author of *The Real Vitamin and Mineral Book*.

Antioxidants and Free Radicals

The Battle for Your Body

Welcome to your bloodstream, which even as you read this, is happily transporting oxygen from the air to various sites in your body. Feels good, doesn't it? There's just one small problem. Some of that oxygen is damaged. Pollution, sunlight, cigarette smoke, and other environmental factors can damage the oxygen molecule by increasing or decreasing the number of electrons it holds. This damage can occur before you breathe the oxygen in, or it can occur inside your body.

An oxygen molecule wants to keep its number of electrons stable, so if one is missing or a new one appears, the molecule attempts to restabilize its electron supply. It will pick up an electron from a nearby molecule. That sets off a chain reaction of electron grabbing. From there, it's like a pinball free-for-all inside your body. Everybody's grabbing an electron, the cells are going crazy, the radical molecules are free!

Free radicals—the name that scientists came up with for these altered oxygen molecules—can cause a lot of trouble in your body. For example, they are a big contributor to the clogging of arteries. Free radicals like to steal electrons from a type of cholesterol in your blood called low-density lipoproteins, or LDLs. This damages the LDL and causes it to stick to an artery wall, which, in turn, clogs the artery.

Truth be told, some free radicals have a positive impact on your body. The immune system sometimes produces free radicals to fight infections and viruses, for instance. However, there is much more evidence pointing to the damage that free radicals can do than the reverse.

The best way to protect yourself against the damage done by free radicals is to discourage their replication in the first place. The experts agree: Don't smoke, do try to breathe in lots of clean air, get a good amount of moderate exercise, and stay away from processed foods. And now doctors recommend that you eat—and possibly supplement your diet with—antioxidants. These include vitamins C and E and beta-carotene, the best-known of the carotenoid compounds that the body converts into vitamin A.

Meet Your Allies

When an antioxidant vitamin meets up with a free radical, it happily donates an electron to the damaged molecule. This not only restores one molecule to health but also cuts short the free radical chain reaction. Consume enough antioxidants to counteract the oxidization process and you will age more slowly and in better health. Think of a swing set that sits in the backyard year after year. If you cover it with a tarp during the winter, chances are the snow won't cause as much damage and it'll be in better condition come next spring when it's time to play. Similarly, free radicals cause rust in your body.

According to a 1994 study done by the U.S. Department of Agriculture, many people actually consume 100 percent or more of the recommended amounts of vitamins E, C, and A. But that may not be enough to fight free radicals. "The Recommended Dietary Allowances (RDAs) weren't created to combat diseases such as cancer and heart disease," says Alan Gaby, M.D., endowed chairman of therapeutic nutrition at Bastyr University in Seattle. "Now we know that antioxidants can help prevent these problems."

For example, the Cambridge Heart Antioxidant Study (CHAOS) found that people with arteriosclerosis (blocked arteries) who took 400 to 800 international units (IU) of vitamin E a day had a 47 percent decrease in their risk of heart attack and death from heart attack. However, the Daily Value for vitamin E in the United States is 30 IU, a much smaller amount than the subjects in the CHAOS study took. Be advised, though, if you're considering taking more than 600 IU of vitamin E, you should first consult your doctor.

A good diet will provide you with the vitamin E that you need, says David Meyers, M.D., professor of internal medicine and preventive medicine at the University of Kansas School of Medicine in Kansas City. Many people choose supplements, however, because vitamin E is found mainly in high-fat foods. "But a prudent use of olive oil and other monounsaturated fats is very reasonable," he adds.

Dr. Meyers believes that supplementing with vitamin E makes sense, provided it's just part of a healthy lifestyle. "Along with eating a well-balanced diet and exercising, I take vitamin E. I figure that it's a low-risk investment that is easily affordable, so why not?"

While vitamin E's sole purpose is to act as an antioxidant, the same is not true for vitamins A and C.

Another Antioxidant Ally

Vitamins are not the only antioxidants. The mineral selenium also protects against free radical cell damage. In fact, selenium and vitamin E, another antioxidant, work so well together that they often substitute for each other.

Selenium may also play a pivotal role in helping to prevent AIDS. In fact, studies at the University of Georgia in Athens indicate that a selenium deficiency may be the switch that turns HIV into AIDS.

Selenium seems to protect the eyes from cataracts and the heart from muscle damage, just like vitamin E. In fact, if you're deficient in vitamin E, your body may use its store of selenium to make up for the vitamin E loss, and vice versa.

That's why it is important to get most of those two vitamins from food, says Dr. Meyers. "Vitamin A comprises about 1,000 different compounds, including beta-carotene. All of these carotenoids are present in a well-balanced diet, but a beta-carotene supplement contains only one type of carotenoid," Dr. Meyers says. "How are we to know it's the most important one?"

Similarly, fruits high in vitamin C, such as oranges, contain many other healthy compounds, including fiber and bioflavonoids, which may help relieve inflammation and allergy symptoms, among other things.

Researchers are still learning about the various ways that each of the antioxidants work. Vitamin C, for example, seems to be particularly effective in fighting the damage caused by cigarettes. If you smoke and then take a vitamin C supplement, you won't "cure" the damage, but the vitamin C will lessen it. But if you quit smoking, you may not need the high doses of vitamin C anymore. In other words, vitamin C—unlike vitamin E—may not counteract free radicals in people who already take pretty good care of themselves, Dr. Meyers says.

In fact, cautions Dr. Meyers, all the vitamins and minerals in the world can't undo the effects of smoking, a sedentary lifestyle, or bad food choices. "The effect of vitamin E is dwarfed by cigarette smoking," he says. "Vitamin E is much less powerful than daily exercise, and its effect is much smaller than achieving optimal weight and normalizing blood pressure."

In other words, no pill in the world—vitamin or not, antioxidant or not—can take the place of a healthy lifestyle.

What the Government Says You Need

Understanding RDAs and Daily Values

At the start of World War II, the Department of Defense began calling up young men to fight but found that many American guys just didn't have what it takes to go to war. Their stores of vitamins and minerals were way down, which left them with a number of deficiency diseases, such as rickets, pellagra, and anemia. To get the weakened would-be soldiers into fighting form, a number of scientists got together to form the Food and Nutrition Board of the National Research Council. The group published the first set of Recommended Dietary Allowances—immediately shortened to RDAs—in 1943. The goal was to help ensure that all citizens got the minimum amounts of nutrients necessary to stay alive and maintain satisfactory health.

And so it remains today. The RDAs are formulated to maintain good health. These are the nutrient values that are absolutely essential for healthy living.

The Food and Nutrition Board is a nongovernmental agency, but the government uses its numbers to set official labeling and dietary standards. These are the numbers and percentages that you see on the sides of cereal boxes and other food products.

The idea is that if you consume the levels of vitamins and minerals set by the board, you'll be protected from deficiency diseases. For example, if you get the RDA for vitamin C, you won't contract scurvy. The board even pads the number to ensure that, even if you just barely meet its recommendation, you will still consume enough of any given nutrient. You need only 10 to 12 milligrams a day of vitamin C to ward off scurvy, but the RDA is 60 milligrams because that amount keeps blood levels of vitamin C in balance. In other words, the board factors in absorption levels and nutrient losses through cooking and other factors when it makes an RDA recommendation.

When setting the RDAs, the Food and Nutrition Board also takes a person's size and diet into account. Since, for example, infants do not need the same amount of nutrients as adult men, the board divides the RDAs along age and sex lines. In fact, 17 different groups of people can find RDAs for 26 different nutrients.

Give Us This Day Our Daily Value

Sounds way too complicated, doesn't it? Well, the Food and Drug Administration agrees with you. So around 1994, it simplified matters. Rather than slicing up the population into so many sex and age categories, it came up with just a few categories based on a person's daily caloric needs. The typical food label today lists either one or two sets of Daily Values (DVs), as these new amounts are called: the daily nutrient needs for a person needing 2,000 calories a day and the needs for a person needing 2,500 calories a day.

Daily Values are reported two ways. One is the actual amount of the nutrient needed, in micrograms, milligrams, or whatever. This is often the same as or very close to the RDA. But the big innovation was the other, newer reporting method. This was to give a percentage of your day's needs that a food provides for each nutrient. Here's an example: An average adult man should consume 2,500 calories a day to fuel his body properly. His DV for vitamin C is 60 milligrams. If the man eats an orange, he gets 69.7 milligrams of vitamin C, which is 116 percent of the DV. Meanwhile, a serving of marinara sauce has 16 milligrams of vitamin C, and thus meets 27 percent of his Daily Value.

Daily Values are listed as percentages on the labels of vitamin and mineral bottles and all packaged foods instead of RDAs because it is easier to deal with percentages than having to remember actual amounts for all those nutrients.

The Food and Nutrition Board continues to meet every five to six years to review the studies and publish new RDAs, which then have an impact on the DVs, since scientists, doctors, and researchers are always finding out new things about vitamins and minerals. In fact, we are now on our tenth set of RDA guidelines.

The Daily Values are set at a level that you should be able to achieve through eating a balanced diet. So if you basically follow the Food Guide Pyramid—eating more grains, fruits, and vegetables than dairy foods, meats, and sweets—you probably fulfill the Daily Values. But if you smoke cigarettes (which can deplete your stores of vitamin C), drink alcohol (which can impair the use of vitamins and minerals), or spend much

Reading the Label

Take off your thinking cap. This chart makes it easy for you to figure out how to understand all that stuff you see on vitamin and food nutrition labels.

Milligram. $\frac{1}{1,000}$ gram (1,000 milligrams equal 1 gram). Abbreviated as mg.

Microgram. $\frac{1}{1,000,000}$ gram (1,000,000 micrograms equal 1 gram). Abbreviated as mcg.

International unit. An arbitrary standard of measurement used for vitamins A, D, and E. It has no obvious equivalents in milligrams or micrograms. Abbreviated as IU.

Recommended Dietary Allowance. The amount of a vitamin or mineral that a healthy person should get in one day. Broken down by age groups and gender. Abbreviated as RDA.

Daily Value. A simpler government standard that lets you know what percentage of recommended nutrients are in foods and supplements. It's always listed in the right-hand column of a product's nutrition label. Abbreviated as DV.

of your life in the fast-food lane of your local burger joint, then there's a good chance that you don't always get the minimum levels that you need.

And that's an important point to keep in mind: These numbers are intended only as guidelines for what the average person should consume in a day. Government agencies use the RDAs and their corresponding DVs as nutritional guidelines to provide adequate intakes for large groups of people, such as prisoners, schoolchildren, and the armed forces.

For example, while the DV for vitamin C is 60 milligrams, early vitamin C pioneer Linus Pauling, Ph.D., took 12,000 milligrams of C daily. That's 200 times the amount that most Americans are told to consume.

Dr. Pauling thought that vitamin C and other nutrients can be used to fight a large spectrum of health problems, not just deficiency diseases. He believed that vitamins and minerals can help prevent illnesses such as cancer and the common cold. Considering that he lived to be 93, he may have been on to something.

The question then becomes: Do you need to supplement your healthy diet with vitamin and mineral tablets? And if so, how can you do it safely?

What You Really Need

The Keys to the Health and Happiness Club

Among the nation's top killers are heart disease, cancer, stroke, and motor vehicle accidents, according to the National Center for Health Statistics. All of these, including accidents, can be affected by the foods you eat and the liquids you drink. While the relationship of fatty foods to heart disease and of alcohol to car accidents has been well-documented, good nutrition alters health in many less obvious, but equally important, ways. You need good nutrition to live long and live well.

For instance, researchers have found that if two people have oral surgery on the same day, the one who eats a balanced, healthy diet will heal more quickly. And it comes down to something as simple as eating an orange instead of a candy bar.

If you've turned the corner on 40 and noticed that your eyesight isn't what it used to be, don't blame age. Look at what's on your plate. When researchers looked at the possible causes of age-related macular degeneration (ARMD)—which, in layman's terms, means starting to have blurred vision as you get older—they found that those who increased their levels of the antioxidants selenium, beta-carotene, and vitamins C and E halted the progression of ARMD.

The point is that while vitamins and minerals were first thought only to fight off deficiency diseases such as anemia and rickets, we now know that they improve our quality of life as well. The appropriate use of vitamins and minerals can improve many health characteristics, such as energy, mental sharpness, and some everyday aches and pains, says Cathy Kapica, R.D., Ph.D., associate professor of nutrition and clinical dietetics at Finch University of Health Sciences/Chicago Medical School.

Making Smart Choices

A healthy lifestyle is really nothing more than a composite of the dozens of small, seemingly insignificant choices that you make each day. We're not about to tell you that no cheeseburger will ever again cross your lips or that you can't enjoy a cold beer on a hot summer day. If you gag at the mere whiff of Brussels sprouts, we sure aren't going to tell you to hold your nose and choke them down anyway. The key is to arm yourself with nutritional knowledge and then make smart choices so that your body gets what it needs. If you do, when you and your best friend are standing around the shuffleboard court in 30 to 40 years, you might be the one without glasses and the one who can follow the bingo game without asking, "What number did they just call?"

Not only that, but you may also be happier and healthier starting today. Here's how.

Trust Mother Nature. There's a good reason why they call vitamin pills supplements and not replacements. "People want to know if they can eat whatever they want and just take a supplement to get their vitamins and minerals. But the answer is no. You have to eat right," says Dr. Kapica.

Your best source of nutrients is always food. "We know we need certain vitamins, but there are other nutrients out there that are necessary for good health that scientists don't know about yet," Dr. Kapica says. "Relying on a supplement that has been created by researchers is only as good as the most current study, and that's not nearly as smart as relying on Mother Nature."

That's because science is still figuring out all the amazing things that vitamins and minerals do for you. For example, manganese is now considered an essential mineral because of the role it plays in numerous bodily functions. Your body uses manganese to release energy from mitochondria, part of what makes up your fast-twitch and slow-twitch muscle fibers. So even if you eat sufficient amounts of protein and fatty acids, without manganese, your body would struggle to run and jump.

Keep your balance. You have no problem popping some antacid tablets to get calcium. You even buy the orange juice with added antioxidants. But eat a tomato? No way. Broccoli? Forget about it. And you just can't seem to remember to take that mineral supplement to make sure that you get your magnesium. The problem is that missing one nutrient can have a domino effect on others.

For example, vitamin D is added to milk because its presence can increase calcium absorption by up to 30 percent. Without vitamin D, the calcium you absorb would just be chalk in your intestines. It isn't enough to simply get most of your vitamins and minerals; you have to get all of them.

And you have to get them in the right amounts. Like calories, vitamins and minerals must be used in balance. Just as too many calories will make you gain weight and too few will cause fatigue, too many vitamins can cause just as much of a problem as too few.

For example, getting your Daily Value (DV) of magnesium may ease allergic reactions because magnesium relieves bronchospasms, or constricted airways. But don't think that loading up on magnesium will leave you wheeze-free. It's more likely to leave you with diarrhea. The moral: Just because a little of a vitamin or mineral is good doesn't mean that a lot is better.

Balance doesn't have to be as complicated as it sounds. Besides eating a well-balanced diet, you can get added insurance by taking the right multivitamin/mineral supplement, says Joanne Curran-Celentano, R.D., Ph.D., associate professor of nutrition and food sciences at the University of New Hampshire in Durham. But

Terms of Confusion

Okay, you understand Daily Values, micrograms, milligrams, international units, and the other standard information relating to vitamins and minerals. Then, you pick up a supplement bottle and are confronted by a bunch of terms that you've never heard before. Here's a quick glossary defining some of the most common terms that you're likely to encounter.

d-alpha-tocopherol. The natural form of vitamin E.

dl-alpha-tocopherol. Synthetic form of vitamin E.

Dietary supplement. A pill, capsule, tablet, or liquid that contains at least one of the following: a vitamin, a mineral, an herb, or similar nutritional substances. Includes such products as ginseng, garlic, fish oils, and psyllium.

Potency. Any vitamin or mineral in a nutritional supplement at levels well above the 100 percent Recommended Dietary Allowance.

Provitamin. A substance that can be converted into a vitamin by the body. Beta-carotene is a provitamin, or precursor, of vitamin A.

Retinol equivalent (RE). A unit of measurement for vitamin A and its various forms (1 RE equals 1 microgram of retinol or 6 micrograms of beta-carotene).

Tocopherol equivalent (TE). A unit of measurement for the vitamin E content of food (1 TE equals 1 milligram of d-alpha-tocopherol).

USP. Stands for the U.S. Pharmacopeia, an independent nonprofit and nongovernmental organization that establishes legally enforceable standards for drugs and supplements.

supplements should be just a form of insurance for days when you don't eat well or if you're under a lot of stress, she says. Although they're easy, cost very little money, and have little risk, the best form of insurance, says Dr. Curran-Celentano, is just eating right most days and reducing overall stress.

Most multivitamin/mineral supplements should have 100 percent of the DV for most of the nutrients, plus extra E and C. Although most men should not take a supplement with iron, says Dr. Curran-Celentano, women should.

Living Right

Just as vitamin and mineral supplements are no substitute for a healthy diet, they can't make up for unhealthy lifestyle habits. "Since the turn of the century, we've seen a decline in the incidences of heart disease in this country. But that may not have anything to do with an increased use of supplements," says Christopher Gardner, Ph.D., a nutrition researcher at Stanford University's Center for Research in Disease Prevention. "It reflects changes in our lifestyles and the environment."

In other words, the top killers these days cannot be stopped by popping a magic dose of vitamins and minerals. While vitamin C may help the body mitigate the effects of cigarette smoking, it can't undo much of the damage that smoke in your lungs can generate. Likewise, people have been taking beta-carotene supplements to help prevent heart disease, and research is now showing that at best, they haven't helped at all, Dr. Gardner says.

There still are a lot of experts who don't believe in the use of vitamin and mineral supplements, including Dr. Gardner, who advocates a balanced diet and lots of

The Future

Some nutrition researchers think that the current Daily Values (DVs) should be bumped up because the numbers tell us only how much we need to maintain nutritional health, not how much we need for maximum benefits. The Food and Nutrition Board has been considering whether to present the idea of chronic disease into the equations of the Recommended Dietary Allowances (RDAs).

In fact, a special subcommittee of the Food and Nutrition Board began meeting in 1993 to review the studies on vitamin and mineral intake. "The committee may come out with new values that would help a health-conscious consumer make better food choices," says Mona Calvo, Ph.D., a member of the clinical research and review staff for the Food and Drug Administration in Washington, D.C.

The board is moving to create three categories: Estimated Average Requirement, Daily Recommended Intakes, and a number that reflects the Upper Level of Safety, or the amount that could possibly prove toxic, Dr. Calvo says. These terms, regardless of whether they are finally adopted by the board, should prove valuable.

■ The Estimated Average Requirement would reflect the average amount a person needs to consume in order to avoid any deficiency disease. In the case of vi-

exercise. "I'm totally opposed to using supplements in place of a nutritious diet," he says. Although Dr. Gardner cautions that no vitamin can replace a prescribed drug, he admits, "If I had a choice between taking a medicine tamin C, for example, that would most likely be lower than its current DV of 60 milligrams.

■ The Daily Recommended Intake would reflect the amounts that have been shown to fight other illnesses. For example, research has found that vitamin C may help prevent shortness of breath caused by asthma and bronchitis. Likewise, another study found that taking 2,000 milligrams (or about 33 times the DV) helps open blocked arteries. The Daily Recommended Intake would reflect the highest level at which a vitamin or mineral has been safely shown to provide disease protection.

■ The Upper Level of Safety would caution consumers against the amount of each vitamin and mineral that is considered dangerous to consume. For example, taking more than 1,200 milligrams of vitamin C at any given time may lead to diarrhea and possibly kidney stone problems.

The committee looking at the changes has divided the nutrients into nine subcategories. The first group to be reviewed and revised includes calcium, vitamin D, phosphorus, magnesium, and fluoride—all bone-building materials. These vitamins and minerals are being studied together so that the board can organize a nutritional fight against osteoporosis, a disease that afflicts both men and women.

to fight heart disease and a vitamin that did the same thing, I would choose the vitamin."

For one thing, says Dr. Gardner, there are a lot of side effects to drugs that vitamins don't have. And second, there is often less risk associated with taking supplements. "In most cases, you're wasting your money by taking a supplement if you aren't lacking in it because extra doesn't do you any good," he says. In a few cases, overdoing it with supplements can even have severe consequences. For instance, regularly taking large quantities of vitamin A (more than 50,000 international units a day) could cause blurred vision, hair loss, enlarged liver and spleen, or even death.

So do your homework. If heart disease runs in your family, ask your physician if a vitamin E supplement will help. If you're in recovery from alcohol or drug addiction, ask about including antioxidants and a multimineral supplement. If you have diabetes, talk to your doctor about chromium.

"Unfortunately, some doctors and pharmacists aren't well-trained in nutrition," says Dr. Curran-Celentano. In general, dietitians will tell you to eat better before they will recommend supplementation. "Ask questions and do research into your illness to see which diets best helped other sufferers and if there is a record of supplementation use associated with it. Then ask your physician if any changes that you'd like to make will interfere with the actions that you're already taking or with your medication."

On the flip side, if you're on medication, find out if it interferes with your body's use of certain vitamins and minerals. Both over-the-counter and prescription drugs, including antacids, antibiotics, and tranquilizers, can diminish your body's ability to utilize certain nutrients. If that's the case, a supplement might be in order while you're on the medicine.

Are Supplements for You?

Take a Look at Your Diet and Lifestyle

With food, as with so many other good things in life, much is lost in imitation. Food offers an enticing aroma, sensuous textures, an intoxicating array of flavors and, if you make the right choices, all the nutrients you need for good health. Dietary supplements offer whatever is listed on the label—no more, no less.

A supplement is just that: an addition to a diet, not the sole source of nutrients. If your food choices lean heavily in the direction of buffalo wings and ice cream, you can't expect a pill to provide the wherewithal to keep you going, say nutrition experts.

You need more than 20 different vitamins and minerals each day. (Daily requirements established by the government are expressed as Daily Values, or DVs.) For some nutrients, women's needs vary from those of men. Since women are generally smaller-boned, they're at higher risk for osteoporosis and need more calcium. If you're menstruating, you need extra iron. If you're trying to conceive, you need extra folate. And if you're pregnant or nursing, you need higher amounts of almost everything.

Food is the best source of the nutrients we need. While most multivitamin/mineral supplements contain essentials like folic acid (the supplement form of folate), calcium, and iron, they offer no protein, fiber, or carbohydrates, which are major building blocks of nutrition. What's more, most supplements can't possibly offer the hundreds of other protective substances (collectively known as phytochemicals) that are found in fruits, vegetables, and grains and are now believed to be just as vital to health as vitamins and minerals, notes Martha L. Rew, R.D., assistant clinical professor of nutrition at Texas Woman's University in Denton. Some studies suggest that phytochemicals can help protect us against bone loss, heart disease, and even cancer.

That said, surveys indicate that a gap exists between what we eat and what we need. Women, in particular, are coming up short. According to one study conducted by the U.S. Department of Agriculture, only about 1 out of 10 women eats even one nutrient-dense dark green or deep yellow vegetable daily, let alone three to five, as authorities recommend. And most eat only a quarter of the calcium-rich foods they should.

If women have a hard time getting the nutrients that they need from food, it's not entirely for lack of trying. Since women tend to be smaller, they don't have as many calories to work with as men do. Women who cut back on calories intentionally to lose weight or avoid gaining weight cut back on good and bad foods alike, and they lose out on nutrients in the bargain.

When dietitians at Utah State University in Logan tried to design menus that supplied the Recommended Dietary Allowances of the vitamins and minerals women need, they were hard-pressed to keep the calorie count below 2,200. That's as many as 700 calories more than many women can enjoy without gaining weight.

Vitamins: À la Carte or a Multi?

You can go about getting your nutritional insurance in one of two ways, say experts. One is to supplement only the individual nutrients you need. The other approach is to take a multivitamin/mineral supplement.

Both approaches have merit, say researchers. If you're trying to eat better but aren't there yet, your best bet is to analyze your diet, see where you have a deficiency, and choose the supplements that are necessary to take up the slack, says Mark Levine, M.D., senior investigator at the Cell Biology and Genetics Laboratory at the National Institutes of Health (NIH) and director of the Nutrition Program of the National Institute for Diabetes and Digestive and Kidney Diseases of the NIH in Bethesda, Maryland.

If you don't or can't drink much milk, for instance, it's likely that you could use a calcium supplement, says Dr. Levine. If you eat fewer than three to five servings of fruits and vegetables a day, your folate, beta-carotene, and vitamin C intake could be flagging. If you limit meat intake to avoid the fat and calories, your iron stores might be low—and so on.

If, on the other hand, your dietary stock-taking shows that you're missing the boat on several vitamins and minerals, you should consider a multivitamin/mineral supplement, says Dr. Levine.

Some people are better off with a multi in the first place. For one thing, multis usually pack the right combination of vitamins and minerals, says John Pinto, Ph.D., associate professor of biochemistry in medicine at Cornell University Medical College and director of the Nutrition Research Laboratory at Memorial Sloan-Kettering Cancer Center, both in New York City. Most multis that offer calcium, for instance, also include vitamin D, which is needed to absorb calcium, he says.

"Nutrients work in a coordinated fashion," says Dr. Pinto. "They depend on one another for their activities." And, he adds, most multivitamins won't give you megadoses of isolated nutrients—more than three times the DV. For some nutrients, like vitamins A and D, excessive doses can be dangerous, say experts.

The balanced nutritional insurance that multivitamins provide can pay off. A study conducted in Hungary, for example, found that women who took multis prior to conception and early in pregnancy were less likely to deliver babies with neurological defects than those who took a supplement containing only copper, manganese, zinc, and a low dose of vitamin C. Studying people over age 65, scientists in Canada found that those who took a multi were sick only half as many days per year as those who took a placebo (an inactive look-alike pill). The supplemented group had only 23 days of infection-related illnesses, compared with 48 days for the placebo group.

Supplements Tailor-Made for You

To get on a supplement program that's most beneficial to your health, you should consult your doctor or a qualified nutrition expert. Be prepared to answer the following questions.

Do you regularly eat carrots and other rich sources of beta-carotene? If you're not averaging two to three servings of fruits and vegetables rich in beta-carotene (like carrots, apricots, papayas, tomatoes, pumpkins, and mangoes) a day, take 10 milligrams of beta-carotene in supplement form, suggests Jeffrey Blumberg, Ph.D., associate director and chief of the antioxidants research laboratory at the Jean Mayer U.S. Department of Agriculture Human Nutrition Research Center on Aging at Tufts University in Boston. If your multi doesn't supply that much or if you're not taking one, pick up a separate beta-carotene supplement. If your eating habits are erratic—you eat two servings each of tomatoes and carrots one day but no trace of beta-carotene the next—it's still perfectly safe to take that supplement every day, says Dr. Blumberg.

Do you regularly drink vitamin C–rich juice or eat citrus fruits, peppers, and other good sources of vitamin C? Unless you're averaging two large glasses of orange juice or two large servings of cantaloupe or other foods high in C each day, you'll need some extra C, says Dr. Blumberg. He recommends a daily intake of 250 to 1,000 milligrams—more than four times the DV.

Research suggests that higher-than-DV doses of vitamin C reduce the risks of cancer, heart disease, and cataracts. One study of 50,000 American women found a 45 percent lower risk of cataracts among those who took 250- to 500-milligram supplements of vitamin C daily for 10 or more years.

Again, if you're not taking a multi or yours doesn't supply 250 milligrams of C, add an individual vitamin C supplement. And yes, it's safe to take it even on those days when you're getting C from your diet, Dr. Blumberg says.

Do you smoke cigarettes (or have you quit recently)? Smokers in particular should make a point of getting more than the DV of vitamin C, says Howerde Sauberlich, Ph.D., professor in the nutrition department of the University of Alabama in Birmingham. Smoking appears to deplete the body's antioxidant stores, Dr. Sauberlich explains.

Are you at high risk for heart disease? Like C, vitamin E may help protect you from heart disease.

The Harvard University Nurses' Health Study found that, among more than 87,000 women, those taking 100 international units (IU) of vitamin E each day were 34 percent less likely to have heart attacks than those who weren't taking E. This suggests the vitamin could be particularly important for older women who face a higher risk of heart disease.

Researchers like Dr. Blumberg suggest 100 to 400 IU of vitamin E daily. Unfortunately, most foods rich in E—like oils and nuts—are also rich in fat. "You'd have to have lots of fat to get protective amounts of E in your diet," notes Dr. Blumberg. To get 100 IU of E, for instance, you'd need to eat 1½ cups of peanut butter. So Dr. Blumberg recommends supplements. If your multi doesn't give you 100 IU or if you're not taking one, make up the difference with individual E capsules, he says.

Do you drink milk and eat yogurt, cheese, ice milk, frozen yogurt, broccoli, spinach, or canned salmon with the bones? Your bones need a minimum of 1,000 milligrams of calcium every day to ward off osteoporosis. Good sources of calcium include skim milk (300 milligrams per serving), nonfat yogurt (450 milligrams), and part-skim ricotta cheese (335 milligrams). But even if you ate a serving of each of these foods each and every day, you'd still have a calcium shortfall. And let's face it, most of us don't eat that well every day.

"In my mind, there's no doubt—you have to take a calcium supplement every day," Dr. Blumberg says.

If you drink a glass of milk every morning at breakfast (and get the accompanying 300 milligrams of calcium), take another 700 to 1,200 milligrams in supplement form, advises Dr. Blumberg. If you never eat dairy foods or if your milk-drinking habits are erratic, he recommends upping the dose to 1,000 to 1,500 milligrams. It's safe to take that much even on those days when you do remember to drink your milk and eat your broccoli, Dr. Blumberg says.

Since most multis give you only 200 milligrams of calcium, you'll need individual supplements to reach your goal. Choose a brand that gives you the mineral as calcium citrate or calcium carbonate, the most easily absorbed forms, advises Neva Cochran, R.D., a nutritionist in Dallas and spokesperson for the American Dietetic Association.

Do you get vitamin D in your diet? Your body needs D to use calcium effectively. Good dietary sources include milk, herring, sardines, and salmon. And your skin will produce the vitamin when exposed to sunlight; just 5 to 10 minutes in the morning or late-afternoon sun three times a week will do it.

If you're running a deficit of D from either food or sunlight, make a habit of taking a multi that provides 100 percent of the DV, says Walter Willett, M.D., Dr.Ph., professor of epidemiology and nutrition and chairman of the department of nutrition at the Harvard University School of Public Health. It's safe, even when you get your sun and drink your milk. But vitamin D tablets are not recommended. They come in doses much higher than those in a multiple, and vitamin D can be toxic in large amounts.

Is meat on your menu? The DV for iron is 18 milligrams. Red meat is a particularly good source. Soybeans, lentils, and enriched cereal grains, including

A Supplementation Self-Test

Here is a list of questions to identify people who could most benefit from increasing their intakes of certain nutrients. It was developed by Alexander Schauss, Ph.D., director of the life sciences division of the American Institute for Biosocial Research in Tacoma, Washington, and author of *Minerals, Trace Elements, and Human Health.*

■ Are you at high risk due to family history or lifestyle for illnesses such as cancer, cardiovascular disease, or diabetes?

■ Do you exercise at least three times a week?

■ Are you under a lot of stress?

■ Do you have skin problems?

■ Do you want to strengthen your immune system?

■ Do you frequently drink alcohol?

Cream of Wheat, also contain a fair amount of iron. But your body can make better use of the type of iron found in meat than of the form found in plant foods, says Mary Frances Picciano, Ph.D., professor of nutrition at Pennsylvania State University in University Park. If you don't eat three servings of red meat a week (averaging three ounces per serving), you may need an iron supplement, she says. To be sure, ask your doctor.

For women, an iron-fortified multi supplying 18 milligrams is the best bet, Dr. Willett says. And yes, it's also safe to take it even on those days when you're eating iron-rich food, he says.

Do you plan to get pregnant? Orange juice is

- Do you smoke or are you exposed to secondhand smoke at home or work?
- Do you live in an area with high pollution rates?
- Did a diet or nutritional analysis indicate a deficiency of any nutrients?
- Do you have a diagnosed degenerative disease?
- Do you drink more than three cups of coffee or five to six cups of tea (all types) a day?
- Are you over 50?

If you answered yes to at least one of these questions, you may need additional vitamin or mineral supplementation. Discuss with your doctor which vitamins and minerals could be helpful to you and your health, and always check with your doctor before supplementing, says Dr. Schauss.

probably the best source of folate around, Dr. Willett says. Even then, you'd have to drink three to four eight-ounce glasses to get the folate you need if you're trying to conceive or are expecting a baby. Numerous studies suggest that an adequate supply of folate during the first month of pregnancy can help prevent birth defects like spina bifida.

Since it's so hard to get enough folate in your diet, Dr. Willett suggests taking a multi that provides 400 micrograms of folic acid (the supplemental form of folate), even on days when you've downed a few glasses of OJ.

Are you past menopause? After menopause, you still need folate. Folate may help lower the risk of cardiovascular disease, cancer of the cervix, and cancer of the colon, says Joel B. Mason, M.D., assistant professor of medicine and nutrition at Tufts University School of Medicine in Boston.

Are you age 70 or over? Those over 70 should get slightly higher doses of certain B vitamins, calcium, and vitamin D, Dr. Blumberg says. As we age, we absorb calcium and the B vitamins less efficiently, he explains. Our skin, which produces vitamin D when exposed to sunlight, also starts doing its job less efficiently.

Dr. Blumberg suggests one of the special-formula multivitamin supplements that are geared toward older people, one that provides two to three times the DV for vitamins B_6, B_{12}, and folate.

Make the Most of Supplements

If you find that supplements are warranted, nutrition experts offer the following tips for optimal safety and effectiveness.

Maximize your multi. When shopping for a multi, choose one that supplies 100 percent of the DVs of most vitamins and minerals, suggests Joanne Curran-Celentano, R.D., Ph.D., associate professor of nutrition and food sciences at the University of New Hampshire in Durham. Remember, though, no multi will include all the calcium you need.

Look for selenium and chromium. There are no official DVs for these nutrients, but it's a good idea to include them in your supplement program, says Dr. Blumberg. Deaths from heart disease rose dramatically among residents of an Italian village after their public water supply was switched from wells that supplied water high in selenium to those whose water was low in the mineral. And preliminary studies suggest that chromium may lower cholesterol levels. Dr. Blumberg suggests a multi with 25 to 70 micrograms of selenium and 50 to 200 micrograms of chromium.

Be cautious. There's a big difference between the supplement levels used in medical studies and what doctors recommend for general good health. No matter how old you are, you want to avoid taking potentially harmful megadoses of vitamins and minerals. For most nutrients, two or three times the DV should be the limit, according to Dr. Blumberg.

Separate calcium and iron. Your body can't absorb certain nutrients in the presence of others. Calcium and iron are a case in point, says Dr. Pinto, so try to take calcium supplements and multivitamin-with-iron preparations at different times of the day.

Pair your iron with orange juice. Your body does a better job of absorbing iron when vitamin C is around, says Dr. Pinto. So consider taking your multivitamin with iron with your orange juice or other vitamin C-rich juice, he says.

Swallow with food. "Vitamins are more efficiently absorbed in the presence of food," Dr. Pinto explains. "There's increased blood flow through the intestines, and the absorption mechanism is more effective."

Cork the bottle. If you have wine or cocktails with dinner, wait a couple of hours after your last drink before taking your vitamins, Cochran says. Alcohol can interfere with absorption. By the same token, you shouldn't wash down your supplements with any form of alcohol.

Enrichment and Fortification

Understanding the Jelly Bean Rule

There's vitamin D in your milk, niacin in your bread, and iodine in your salt. And have you looked at orange juice lately? You can now choose among juices with extra calcium, a cocktail of vitamins A, C, and E, or just plain old no pulp.

These are all examples of enrichment and fortification, two of the reasons why the United States has such a healthy and nutritious food supply. While the words are used interchangeably, they both refer to the addition of specific nutrients to food.

Enrichment and fortification are inexpensive and efficient ways to ensure that people get at least the minimum amount of necessary vitamins and minerals. Some nutrients are added to food because they are lost in processing (such as the B vitamins in white bread), while others are added because they aid the absorption of other nutrients already found in a food (such as adding vitamin D to milk, which helps the absorption of calcium).

"Fortification of foods generates controversy among food technologists," says James Giese, associate editor of *Food Technology* magazine. One problem is that manufacturers could add vitamins and minerals to nutritionally insignificant foods—such as jelly beans—so that people who live on junk food would think that they are getting at least some nutrients. But U.S. Food and Drug Administration guidelines discourage adding nutrients to foods of little nutritional value. This conundrum is known informally as the jelly bean rule, says Giese.

The Prize in the Cereal Box

The easiest place to see the impact of fortification is to look at the nutritional information on the side of a cereal box.

"Breakfast provides about 25 percent of daily calories for most Americans," says Joanne Curran-Celentano, R.D., Ph.D., associate professor of nutrition and food sciences at the University of New Hampshire in Durham. Therefore, most cereals are fortified at those levels. "Eating a fortified cereal is one way to help reach your Daily Values for some nutrients," she says.

The vitamins used in cereal are the same vitamins you get in a supplement. For example, look on the side of a box of Kellogg's All-Bran and you'll see, listed among the ingredients, pyridoxine hydrochloride, or vitamin B_6, just as you will on a bottle of Centrum.

"Fortified breakfast cereals provide a more nutrient-dense breakfast than many other breakfast foods, including home fries and eggs," Dr. Curran-Celentano says. "Eating a high-fiber cereal will make the meal even more healthful."

There is a catch, though: The presence of fiber inhibits the absorption of some vitamins and minerals. On top of this problem is the addition of sugar and salt to

The Wonders of Wonder Bread

The number one selling bread in the United States is Wonder bread, a fortified product famous for "helping to build strong bodies 12 ways." Wonder bread, owned by the Interstate Bakeries Corporation, has been fortified since 1941, when it joined the government-supported bread-enrichment program. But Wonder bread is no more enriched than any enriched white flour or white bread.

Talk to some nutritionists and they may let you in on the secret of enriched white bread. Yes, it has added vitamins and minerals but not nearly enough to equal the nutritional strength of a whole-wheat product. Processing removes several key nutrients from whole-wheat flour, including zinc, folate (the natural form of folic acid), magnesium, and vitamin E. But the enrichment of white bread adds only five nutrients back in: thiamin, niacin, riboflavin, iron, and folic acid.

"Half of all bread sold in the country is white bread," says Mark Dirkes, senior vice president of marketing for Interstate Bakeries Corporation, in Kansas City, Missouri. "And we think that the question of which is more nutritious is almost irrelevant. We offer a whole-wheat bread wherever we sell Wonder, but only 25 percent of breads sold are whole-wheat. People, especially kids, prefer white."

almost all fortified cereals. All-Bran's second ingredient is sugar, followed by corn syrup and malt flavoring—all sweetening agents. Some cereals are high in sodium, too (it's All-Bran's fifth ingredient).

In some ways, cereals look more like a dessert than an entrée, but Dr. Curran-Celentano says that could be a good thing. "A lot of people are inclined to overeat after dinner," she says. "And what they eat are tradition- ally snack foods, which are low in nutrients but high in calories. Cereals, especially high-fiber ones, can be a good replacement for an evening snack. If you're careful about which cereal you choose and eat the proper serving size, eating cereal as a snack rather than potato chips or ice cream will cut down your calorie intake but still give you a rich amount of vitamins and minerals."

While a fortified cereal boasts a long list of vita- mins and minerals, it is only part of a healthy diet. It's true that you'll get a well-rounded amount of nutrients in a fortified cereal, but you won't get the phytochemi- cals found in whole foods. Even cereal companies sug- gest that you complement their foods with at least a glass of orange juice or some fruit. Foods like these that come by their nutrients naturally contain components other than vitamins and minerals that are important for your body's nutritional needs.

The New Wave

"The government used to order fortification solely to fight deficiency diseases," says Liz Applegate, Ph.D., nu- trition columnist for *Runner's World* magazine and au- thor of *Power Foods*. "But the Food and Drug Adminis- tration ordered many manufacturers to fortify their foods with folic acid, and that isn't to prevent a defi- ciency disease but to optimize the health of newborns, whose mothers need more folic acid." Men should ben- efit, too, she says, because folic acid seems to play a role in fighting heart disease. Folic acid is now being added to all enriched grain products.

Enriched and fortified foods are a good dietary supplement for people who know that they don't get enough of certain vitamins and minerals, says Dr. Applegate. Athletes and vegetarians often don't get enough calcium and B_{12} in their diets. They would benefit from eating one meal or snack with a fortified food, such as cereal. Another good group of candidates is people who don't eat milk products, either because they are lactose-intolerant or because they just don't like milk. If you don't drink milk on a regular basis, says Dr. Applegate, then calcium-fortified orange juice is a good option.

Make the Most of What You Get

Enter the Theater of the Absorb

File this under the category "Life Isn't Fair." You can swallow all the vitamins and minerals—either from food or supplements or both—that the government says you need and still miss out on the health benefits. Because the real question is not how much you consume but how much of the nutrients are absorbed by your body.

Absorption is a multistep process. Your mouth chews the food (or swallows the supplement) and the small pieces travel down, eventually settling in your small intestine. Covering the 20 feet or so of your small intestine are small cells that absorb nutrients. These cells, called microvilli, regulate the passage of each nutrient into the bloodstream.

The microvilli have enzymes in them that digest the nutrients and allow them to be absorbed by other cells within the intestines. In a sense, the microvilli are your bloodstream's traffic cops, deciding whether to wave the nutrients on to travel through the blood or to detour them along the digestive tract for excretion.

"The Recommended Dietary Allowances (RDAs) don't take absorption issues into account," says J. Cecil Smith, Ph.D., a research chemist at the U.S. Department of Agriculture's phytonutrients laboratory in Beltsville, Maryland. In other words, the present RDAs don't tell us how readily a nutrient can be absorbed from different foods. For example, iron is more readily absorbed—more bioavailable—from steak than from spinach. There is a push to incorporate this knowledge in future editions of the RDAs, Dr. Smith adds. That already has been done in some other countries, including the United Kingdom.

They'll Melt with You

If you're a vitamin, it all comes down to one question: What does it take to break you down? Four vitamins— A, D, E, and K—can be absorbed only with help from dietary fat, so they're known as fat-soluble. They are stored in fatty tissues and in the liver, hanging around the body until they're needed. That means you're less likely to run short of them, but it also means you run the risk of stockpiling too many, which can be dangerous—especially with vitamins A and D. Adults who get too much vitamin A have been known to suffer from a number of symptoms ranging from headaches to hair loss. Getting too much vitamin D can cause appetite loss, weight loss, and nausea.

The B-complex and C vitamins dissolve in water, earning them the moniker—you guessed it—water-soluble. Only small amounts of these vitamins get stored in the body, so the odds of toxic side effects are much slimmer. However, the chances of not getting enough are that much greater.

It's the B vitamins that change the color of urine. If you have adequate stores of the vitamin in your body, then you'll excrete what you don't need. Depending on how hydrated you are, this could take anywhere from a half-hour to 4 to 6 hours.

But all of this really means one thing to you: Water-soluble vitamins have to be replenished daily. Fat-soluble vitamins don't. Just be aware that large doses of fat-soluble vitamins can cause trouble because they won't be excreted as easily as their water-soluble cousins.

The Gatekeeper

In some cases, your body will hold on to a particular nutrient if it needs it and let it go if it doesn't. In fact, the rate of absorption of some nutrients can vary from one meal to the next. So if you've eaten iron-rich Cream of Wheat cereal for breakfast, your body may decide to forgo some of the iron found in the tofu on your salad at lunchtime.

"Each individual apparently has genetic components for absorption that he doesn't have much control over," Dr. Smith says. "But there is flexibility and a desire for homeostasis within that level. It's almost as if there's a gatekeeper within your gut who allows an appropriate level of nutrients to pass through depending on the nutritional needs of the person."

For instance, if you're deficient in iron, or anemic, your absorption level may be as high as 80 percent; but it can also be as low as 5 percent if your iron stores are high.

Bioavailability: What the Body Keeps

"Researchers are much more interested in the bioavailability of vitamins and minerals, which is not synonymous with the total amount found in the food by chemical analysis," says Dr. Smith. Bioavailability measures how much of any given nutrient the body is able to absorb from a single food or supplement. For instance, growing children absorb 75 percent of the dietary calcium in foods such as milk. But as people age, they begin to absorb less, in amounts as low as 10 percent.

Likewise, the calcium in milk is more bioavailable than the calcium in broccoli. Several factors play into that, including the presence of protein, the type of calcium found in each food, and the amount of vitamin D added to milk.

"We know that there are often large differences in the bioavailability of minerals from plant-derived foods compared with foods from animal products," Dr. Smith says. "For instance, zinc from wheat germ is less bioavailable than from flesh or seafood sources." A number of things can affect bioavailability.

♦ Phytates and oxalates. These two plant fibers bind to calcium and iron, among other minerals, and carry them out of the body. Oxalates are one reason why only about 5 percent of the iron in spinach·is bioavailable.

"Phytic acid is in a plant because it's a source of phosphorus required for the germinating seed," Dr. Smith says. "But phytic acid also binds zinc and inhibits its absorption." Another word for this binding process is chelation, pronounced "kee-LAY-shun."

◆ **Prescription and over-the-counter drugs.** For a variety of reasons, antacids, antibiotics, laxatives, and other medications can affect the body's ability to absorb certain minerals. Talk to a doctor or pharmacist about possible absorption side effects from both over-the-counter and prescription medications. Also ask if you should use a vitamin or mineral supplement while using a medication.

◆ **Food additives.** Some of the products added to foods, both natural and synthetic, affect the body's ability to use minerals. For instance, gums used to thicken processed foods bind with iron and copper, creating a nonabsorbable complex. Processed and refined foods usually have fewer nutrients than unprocessed foods. For example, table sugar has a markedly lower mineral content than the molasses from which it is refined.

◆ **Fiber.** We're all for a high-fiber diet, but think about it. The point of that extra fiber is to get stuff out of your body. Bran is rich in phytates, for example, which bind to minerals. On the other hand, bran has much higher levels of minerals overall than bleached or white flour, so it's still a better food choice than processed grains, says Cathy Kapica, R.D., Ph.D., associate professor of nutrition and clinical dietetics at Finch University of Health Sciences/Chicago Medical School.

◆ **Metabolism problems.** Diabetes, high blood pressure, anemia, and other illnesses can alter the body's balance of vitamins and minerals. Diabetes, for example, can lead to depletion of bone calcium and muscle potassium. Once again, talk to a nutritionist or physician about any illness, including temporary problems such as the flu or a cold. He may be able to advise you on dietary additions that will decrease the likelihood of deficiency problems.

♦ Age. As you get older, the hydrochloric acid levels in your stomach begin to decrease, and this can impair absorption levels. At the same time, older people need to eat fewer calories because their metabolism has slowed, yet they need the same amount of nutrients. It's hard for them to get those nutrients if they're eating less. The RDA levels do not reflect these changes, but some nutritionists believe that supplementation is important for people over the age of 50.

Increasing Absorption

There is a direct correlation between the richness of soil and the nutrient density of the food that it yields. Selenium, iodine, and other minerals, for example, are found in varying levels throughout the world. Some regions in the United States have rich levels of selenium, while others have almost none.

In addition, overgrazing and intense farming as well as the use of pesticides and other chemicals in agriculture can alter the levels of nutrients in our foods. Some studies suggest that organic farming, which strives to maintain the health of the soil by building up its organic matter, rotating crops, and minimizing the use of pesticides, may produce higher yields as well as plants with higher mineral levels. One study done by a Swiss researcher found that organically grown spinach

Get Dense

Overcooking broccoli in a big pot of boiling water renders its nutrient powers as limp as the soggy stalks that you pull out of the pot. Most of the water-soluble vitamins are left in the pot of water.

Statistics show that most of us don't get anywhere near the number of vegetables that we should each day. So it certainly makes no sense to boil the vital vitamins and minerals out of the precious few we do get. Here's how to keep your vegetables dense—nutrient-dense, that is.

Watch the time. "The best way to cook vegetables is with a minimum amount of water for the shortest period of time possible," says Barbara Klein, Ph.D., professor of food science and human nutrition at the University of Illinois in Urbana-Champaign. "Microwaving and steaming are ideal. But if you prefer the color and texture of vegetables that are boiled in water, the critical thing is to boil them for the shortest time possible."

The shortest time possible, in this case, translates to 3 to 7 minutes, because that's long enough to extract the water-soluble vitamins (all the Bs and C) from the food. The key is to aim for a texture known as crisp-tender, says Dr. Klein. That means the broccoli or carrots or zucchini should be just soft—not too crunchy but not soggy.

had twice as much B_{12} as conventionally grown spinach. Barley was found to have three times more B_{12}. Organically grown foods also have been found to have lower moisture content than those grown conventionally,

Avoid the thaw. If you buy frozen vegetables, don't let them thaw before cooking them. Freezing food weakens the cell walls, and that allows nutrients to escape during thawing. Just place the still-frozen vegetables in the microwave, adding only a little bit of water.

Soak the spinach. Before cooking your spinach, let it soak in water for a few minutes. This removes the oxalates that bind with calcium, iron, and other minerals, whisking them out of your body before they can do much good.

Scrub it. Of course, while it's always a good idea to wash produce before you cook it, think twice about peeling edible skins. Carrots and potatoes, for example, are two vegetables that benefit from scrubbing rather than scraping. That's because their skins are richer in minerals than the rest of the vegetable.

Buy small. If you prefer the taste of fresh fruits and vegetables to canned or frozen, cut down the time the produce will need to stay in the refrigerator. Wilting and brown spots are signs of oxidation, which means that the nutrients are slowly leaving the food. Refrigeration increases the time that fruits and vegetables stay fresh, but only by a day or so.

which could mean that the nutrients in organic foods might not break down as quickly during storage.

But the question of whether organically grown foods have higher nutrient levels than conventionally grown plants has been debated by scientists for decades. They've been unable to reach a clear conclusion on the issue because hard-to-control variables such as climate and crop variety make it difficult to accurately compare the two farming practices.

But it still may be worth spending a few extra cents to buy organic fruits and vegetables. The U.S. Department of Agriculture recognized more than a decade ago that organic produce contains lower levels of pesticide residue and nitrates. Organic farming is also better for the environment, as it conserves natural resources and cuts down on air, water, and soil pollution.

So how a plant is grown may help determine its nutrient density and its level of pesticide residue, but what's done with the plant after harvesting is what can really make the difference between a limp stalk of broccoli that has lost many of its nutrients and a crisp stalk that's rich in vitamins and minerals.

Getting Fresh

Pop quiz: Which of these has the most nutrients?

    a. Canned vegetables

    b. Frozen vegetables

    c. Fresh vegetables

It has to be c. A no-brainer, right? Wrong.

"We did a comparison of the data that are out there, including what's on the cans and packages, and we found that vitamin content is comparable regardless of how you get your vegetables and fruits," says Barbara Klein, Ph.D., professor of food science and human nutrition at the University of Illinois in Urbana-Champaign.

Supermarket fresh translates to produce that is about two weeks old, Dr. Klein says. "So you do just as well using a processed product that has been canned or frozen within hours of being picked."

For instance, vitamin C in the form of ascorbic acid is an extremely unstable compound. A just-picked orange has about 70 milligrams of vitamin C (nearly 117 percent of the Daily Value). But cook that orange or store it at room temperature and the orange rapidly loses high amounts of its number one nutrient. In fact, orange juice concentrate made immediately after an orange is picked may have more vitamin C than an orange that has traveled from Florida to Idaho in a nonrefrigerated truck.

So it all comes down to this: It doesn't make much difference if you choose fresh, frozen, or canned produce—as long as you eat your fruits and vegetables.

How Vitamin Pills Are Made

From Tons of Raw Materials to a Tablet

Start with a half ton each of calcium, phosphorus, and magnesium. Mix them with about two tons' worth of 14 or 15 other vitamins and minerals. Divide the whole shebang into a million or so servings, each about ½ inch long and ¼ inch wide. And keep each serving fresh and healthy for three years. That's the challenge vitamin tablet makers face each day.

"It's not easy," says Barry Cason, manager of research and development for Perrigo Company's vitamin and mineral supplement manufacturing facility in Greenville, South Carolina. "And yes, it does involve getting truckloads of vitamins and minerals and finding a way to squish them down into a tablet." Perrigo is one of the largest private-label nutritional supplement manufacturers. Its products are similar to Centrum, Theragran-M, and One-a-Day. But Perrigo sells them to drugstores, for example, who then put their own names on the formulations.

A supplement manufacturer's first step is to research raw materials. "We have to learn what forms the nutrients are available in and what each one's price and effectiveness is," says Cason. Calcium carbonate, for example, can come from oyster shells from the ocean or mined limestone purified for humans as well as other sources.

Supplement sources come from all around the world, but there are only a handful of raw material suppliers. And most are used by both the pharmaceutical and food industries. So the thiamin in your vitamin supplement may well come from the same place as the thiamin in your Wonder bread.

Putting It to the Test

After doing research on each source, Cason and his team begin to assemble very small experimental batches of their formulations. "We have to see what will happen to the formulations at various humidities and temperatures," Cason says. "We examine the supplement's reaction at one-, two-, and three-month intervals and extrapolate those findings out to one-year, two-year, and three-year findings." Researchers look for physical and chemical changes as well as potential problems with dissolution.

Dissolution is how the supplement divides into nutrient parts that the body can absorb. In general, vitamins are absorbed in the upper part of the intestine, and minerals mostly in the lower intestine. Water-soluble vitamins are absorbed quickly, while fat-soluble vitamins take longer.

Vitamin manufacturers also sample their products throughout the real shelf-life period at 3, 6, 12, 18, 24, and 36 months, says Cason. Eventually, a performance trial goes to the pilot stage of manufacturing.

One of the greatest challenges for a supplement manufacturer is figuring out how to guarantee that each tablet will deliver its promised amount of every ingredient. Since the master blend of a supplement can weigh a couple of tons, a manufacturer must evenly distribute each ingredient throughout the master blend of a supplement. For instance, if a multivitamin/mineral supplement label claims to have a certain amount of calcium, then controls must be in place to assure that the amount of calcium in the tablet falls within a specified range prescribed by regulation.

"We have to deal with a tremendous amount of weight variations," Cason says. "For example, 162 milligrams of calcium might have to be in the same tablet with 2 milligrams of copper, 400 international units of vitamin D, and 150 micrograms of boron, among 20 other ingredients."

Perrigo and most other manufacturers use a specially designed, "twin-shell" blender to mix their nutri-

Tuning In for Good Health

Most consumers get their information about nutrition from television, but only 17 percent say they find that information valuable, according to *Nutrition Trends Survey 1995*, a study conducted by the American Dietetic Association.

Why? Because one study seems to come to one conclusion and then, a week later, another one contradicts the first report. And let's not forget that the evidence is often "not conclusive."

"The media rarely gives you the bigger picture," says Bonnie Liebman, licensed nutritionist and director of nutrition for the Center for Science in the Public Interest in Washington, D.C. "They say that a new study came out with one finding, but they don't tell you that 20 other studies found no link between a vitamin and a disease."

Here are some questions to ask if you want to figure out whether a study is relevant to you: How much of one vitamin or mineral was studied? Did the researchers look at vitamin and mineral amounts that are found in the diet or in supplements? Once you know the number, compare it with the amount found in your supplement. Also, if you know the amount, try to find out how much of it is found in food. If 500 milligrams of mineral X seems to make a difference in an illness, is there a way to get that solely from food?

ents. "It's two huge cylinders that form a V," explains Cason. "Each cylinder spins or tumbles the ingredients. It's almost a kneading action that continuously halves and remixes the dry blend of ingredients, keeping everything evenly distributed."

One process that assists in the blending is called geometric dilution. "There's a sequence to the addition of ingredients," Cason says. "Some of the lighter ingredients are preblended, and we graduate up to heavier ingredients."

Holding It Together

Once the ingredients are mixed together, the trick is to get them to stay together. "A tablet filled with so many ingredients wants to do a lot of things except stay together," says Cason. "It wants to split or fall apart or break up. Or it wants to get so hard that it won't dissolve properly."

A multivitamin/mineral tablet has more than just its active ingredients. It's also filled with excipients, or nonactive ingredients. Each formulation requires a variety of additives to make the nutrients bind together and dissolve properly. Vitamin and mineral supplements come in tablets, liquids, soft gels, and two-piece hard-gelatin capsules. "Tablets are not only the most popular form for supplements but also the most cost-effective formulation to make," Cason says.

Finally, thousands of tablets are dropped into thousands of bottles and sent to thousands of cities throughout the country. "And we start all over again," says Cason. "New research is always being published, and people want to try different nutrients, like more vitamin E and more antioxidants. Me? I try them all."

The Ultimate Program for Men

For Those Who Live to the Max

While the Daily Values (DVs) are designed to keep everyone healthy at the most basic level, people now want their vitamins and minerals to go beyond the minimum requirement. We want our nutrients to help us be active, work hard, combat stress, and prevent illnesses such as cancer and heart disease.

So we asked two of the leading experts in the field—Shari Lieberman, Ph.D., certified nutrition specialist and co-author of *The Real Vitamin and Mineral Book*, and Alexander Schauss, Ph.D., director of the life sciences division of the American Institute for Biosocial Research in Tacoma, Washington, and author of *Minerals, Trace Elements, and Human Health*—to come up with recommendations that will help men live life to the fullest.

"Scientific literature has consistently demonstrated a protective effect for people using supplements," Dr. Lieberman says. "Reports of toxicity problems have been very rare."

The information that follows, which lists optimal vitamin and mineral intakes, is divided into three sections: one for nutrients that you can easily get from food; one for nutrients that you probably need to supplement; and one for nutrients that you may want to consider supplementing. The goal is to devise a sensible vitamin and mineral program for men that offers optimal but safe levels to bestow maximum disease protection and health benefits.

The category "Toxicity and symptoms" lists the levels at which harmful side effects occur. However, some people will experience problems at significantly lower levels. That's why you'll notice cautions in chapters throughout this book advising that you consult a physician before exceeding certain levels, even though they fall below the amounts in the "Toxicity and symptoms" category. Also, pay careful attention to the abbreviated amounts for each vitamin and mineral. "Mg." is short for milligrams, which are $\frac{1}{1,000}$ gram. "Mcg." stands for micrograms, or $\frac{1}{1,000,000}$ gram. That's a big difference, so take the time to be sure.

The Food and Nutrition Board (which sets the Daily Values and Recommended Dietary Allowances) doesn't use the word *optimal*, perhaps because it's not an easily definable term and is somewhat relative. However, the National Institutes of Health used the term in a 1994 paper on calcium and osteoporosis. That was one of the first times an official paper has used it.

Does this mean that everyone should start popping vitamins at the highest dosage they can find? Absolutely not. The difference between the government recommendations and the optimal levels varies tremendously depending on the vitamin or mineral involved. Some, like vitamin K, remain the same. But others, like vitamins C and E, increase dramatically. So it's important to understand that megadosing and optimal levels are not one and the same. "Megadosing technically means 10 or more times the Recommended Dietary Allowance," says Joanne Curran-Celentano, R.D., Ph.D., associate professor of nutrition and food sciences at the University of New Hampshire in Durham.

Buyer Beware

Here are some key things to look for when you're considering a supplement.

Check the expiration date. Supplements have a shelf life of about three years, and there's a good chance that you'll happen upon a bargain that offers you 100 tablets with an extra 60 thrown in. That's a five-month supply of vitamins and minerals. Check the date on that package. If it expires soon, it's not worth the money.

Forget about being Mr. Natural. Vitamins and minerals that boast of their "natural" ingredients are usually just money-wasters, says Bonnie Liebman, licensed nutritionist and director of nutrition for the Center for Science in the Public Interest in Washington, D.C. In most cases, your body doesn't distinguish between a synthetic vitamin and a natural one.

Form an opinion. Ask yourself, "What form of supplement do I prefer?" If you don't want to swallow tablets, look for a chewable (yes, children's supplements are okay here) or a liquid.

Also, your options will expand if you don't mind taking more than one tablet a day. Many companies offer divided dose supplements to optimize blood levels of nutrients throughout the day. But be honest: Will you really take more than one tablet a day? If you can't remember where your keys are in the morning or you've had trouble being consistent with vitamin taking in the past, stick with one tablet. Don't make things tough on yourself.

Make sure that the price is right. "There's no reason to spend more than $4 to $5 a month on a multi," Liebman says. "Generally, supplements sold at health food stores cost more than brand names, while generic supplements from large supermarkets or drugstore chains are the cheapest." There is often little difference between the effectiveness of a brand-name and a generic supplement. In fact, they're often made by the same companies. Only the labels change.

"We have to meet the same quality standards as a brand-name company," says Barry Cason, manager of research and development for Perrigo Company's vitamin and mineral supplement manufacturing facility in Greenville, South Carolina. "We get the national brand and test it. Then we back it up with independent testing laboratories. In every case, our quality meets or exceeds the brand-name product. The only difference is that we don't pay millions of dollars for advertising."

And in reality, that means you don't pay for those advertising costs every time you pop a pill. But lots of people prefer the security of a brand name, and that's okay, considering the price is only about a dime a day, says Leon Ellenbogen, Ph.D., assistant vice president for Lederle, the makers of Centrum. "Although there are some good generic companies out there, you know exactly what you're buying with a name you recognize. For example, we clinically tested our calcium product, Caltrate, in humans to be certain that it's well-absorbed."

Can the iron. There should be something missing from your multivitamin/mineral supplement: iron. "Men don't need added iron," Liebman says. So make sure that you choose one without it.

No Supplementation Necessary
Vitamin A

Daily value (DV) for men: 5,000 IU.

Suggested optimal amount: 10,000 IU.

Toxicity and symptoms: 50,000 IU. Dry skin, nausea, headaches, fatigue, irritability, liver damage.

Uses: Helps maintain good vision and healthy skin. Supports the immune system and promotes growth.

Food sources: Carrots, fortified skim milk, pumpkin, sweet potatoes, dark green leafy vegetables (like spinach and kale), winter squash, tuna, halibut, cantaloupe, mangoes, apricots, broccoli, and watermelon.

Beta-Carotene

Daily value (DV) for men: Not established.

Suggested optimal amount: 25,000 IU.

Toxicity and symptoms: None known.

Uses: Helps protect against cancer, cardiovascular disease, and cataracts.

Food sources: Carrots, sweet potatoes, spinach, fresh parsley.

Vitamin D

Daily value (DV) for men: 400 IU.

Suggested optimal amount: 400 IU.

Toxicity and symptoms: 1,000 IU. Loss of appetite, headache, excessive thirst.

Uses: Helps absorption of calcium and phosphorus for strong bones.

Food sources: Fortified skim milk, tuna, salmon, sardines, and fortified cereals, plus sunlight.

Vitamin K

Daily value (DV) for men: 80 mcg.

Suggested optimal amount: 80 mcg.

Toxicity and symptoms: In rare instances toxicity can result when water-soluble substitutes are prescribed. Can result in jaundice or brain damage.

Uses: Plays major role in blood clotting.

Food sources: Green tea, spinach, broccoli, Brussels sprouts, cabbage, asparagus, parsley, chickpeas, cauliflower, lentils, carrots, avocados, and tomatoes.

Biotin

Daily value (DV) for men: 300 mcg.

Suggested optimal amount: 300 mcg.

Toxicity and symptoms: None known.

Uses: Helps metabolize fat, protein, and carbohydrates.

Food sources: Peanut butter, oatmeal, wheat germ, poultry, cauliflower, nuts, legumes, fat-free or low-fat cheese, and mushrooms.

Boron

Daily value (DV) for men: Not established.

Suggested optimal amount: 3 mg.

Toxicity and symptoms: None known.

Uses: Helps metabolize calcium and magnesium. Enhances mental alertness.

Food sources: Apples, pears.

Copper

Daily value (DV) for men: 2 mg.

Suggested optimal amount: 2 mg.

Toxicity and symptoms: 10 mg. Vomiting, diarrhea.

Uses: Works with iron to make hemoglobin.

Food sources: Oysters and other shellfish, nuts, cherries, cocoa, mushrooms, gelatin, whole-grain cereals, fish, and legumes.

Fluoride

Daily value (DV) for men: Not established.

Suggested optimal amount: 4 mg.

Toxicity and symptoms: 20 mg. per day over many years. Teeth discoloration, nausea, chest pain, vomiting.

Uses: Helps form bones and teeth. Helps prevent tooth decay.

Food sources: Fluoridated water, fish, and tea.

Iodine

Daily value (DV) for men: 150 mcg.

Suggested optimal amount: 150 mcg.

Toxicity and symptoms: 2,000 mcg. Enlargement of thyroid gland.

Uses: Helps regulate growth, development, and metabolic rate.

Food sources: Spinach, lobster, shrimp, oysters, skim milk, and iodized salt.

Iron

Daily value (DV) for men: 10 mg.

Suggested optimal amount: 15 mg.

Toxicity and symptoms: 75 mg. Loss of body hair, lethargy, impotence.

Uses: Transports and stores oxygen in red blood cells. Helps with hormone production. Assists the immune system. Enhances thinking abilities.

Food sources: Clams, asparagus, lean meat, chicken, prunes, raisins, spinach, pumpkin seeds, soybeans, and tofu.

Manganese

> *Daily value (DV) for men:* 2 mg.
> *Suggested optimal amount:* 10 mg.
> *Toxicity and symptoms:* Usually occurs from inhalation of pollutants, not dietary intake.
> *Uses:* Development of the skeleton and connective tissue. Crucial to normal brain function.
> *Food sources:* Nuts, whole-grain cereals, legumes, tea, dried fruits, and spinach and other green leafy vegetables.

Molybdenum

> *Daily value (DV) for men:* 75 mcg.
> *Suggested optimal amount:* 75 mcg.
> *Toxicity and symptoms:* 250 mcg. Diarrhea, anemia.
> *Uses:* Moderates excretion of uric acid and sulfate.
> *Food sources:* Legumes, lean meats, whole-grain cereals, breads, and skim milk.

Phosphorus

> *Daily value (DV) for men:* 1,000 mg.
> *Suggested optimal amount:* 1,000 mg.
> *Toxicity and symptoms:* A calcium-to-phosphorus ratio lower than 1 to 2; lowering of blood calcium levels to detriment of teeth and bones.
> *Uses:* Numerous bone, muscle, and energy functions.
> *Food sources:* Lean meats, fish, poultry, fat-free or low-fat dairy products, and cereals.

Sodium

> *Daily value (DV) for men:* 2,400 mg.
> *Suggested optimal amount:* 2,400 mg.

Toxicity and symptoms: None because kidneys excrete excess.

Uses: Essential to nerve transmission and muscle contraction.

Food sources: Salt, soy sauce, processed foods.

Special considerations: Sodium is prevalent in many commonly eaten foods, especially processed foods, so there is no need to pay special attention to intake.

Supplementation Strongly Recommended

Vitamin B₆

Daily value (DV) for men: 2 mg.

Suggested optimal amount: 15 mg.

Toxicity and symptoms: 100 mg. per day over extended time period. Depression, fatigue, numbness of feet, hands, mouth.

Uses: Helps maintain healthy hair, skin, eyes, nerves, and digestion.

Food sources: Fish, soybeans, avocados, lima beans, poultry, bananas, cauliflower, green peppers, potatoes, spinach, and raisins.

Vitamin C

Daily value (DV) for men: 60 mg.

Suggested optimal amount: 1,000 mg.

Toxicity and symptoms: 2,000 mg. Headache, insomnia, rashes, diarrhea.

Uses: Helps form collagen, which strengthens blood vessel walls and forms scar tissue. Also strengthens resistance against infection.

Food sources: Oranges, grapefruit, bell peppers,

strawberries, tomatoes, spinach, cabbage, melons, broccoli, kiwifruit, raspberries, and Brussels sprouts.

Vitamin E

Daily value (DV) for men: 30 IU.

Suggested optimal amount: 400 IU.

Toxicity and symptoms: 900 IU: Digestive tract discomfort.

Uses: Fights heart disease and some cancers.

Food sources: Nut and vegetable oils, wheat germ, mangoes, blackberries, apples, broccoli, peanuts, spinach, and whole-wheat breads.

Calcium

Daily value (DV) for men: 1,000 mg.

Suggested optimal amount: 1,000 mg. up to age 65; 1,500 mg. age 65 and up.

Toxicity and symptoms: None known.

Uses: Builds strong teeth and bones. Promotes healthy growth.

Food sources: Skim milk, fat-free or low-fat cheese, fat-free yogurt, salmon and sardines with bones, broccoli, green beans, almonds, turnip greens, and fortified orange juice.

Chromium

Daily value (DV) for men: 120 mcg.

Suggested optimal amount: 200 mcg.

Toxicity and symptoms: Unknown as a nutrition disorder.

Uses: May help prevent adult-onset diabetes. Metabolizes glucose.

Food sources: Blackstrap molasses, whole grains, broccoli, grape juice, orange juice, lean meat, black pepper, brewer's yeast, and fat-free or low-fat cheese.

Folic acid

Daily value (DV) for men: 400 mcg.

Suggested optimal amount: 400 mcg.

Toxicity and symptoms: Levels of more than 400 mcg can mask B_{12} deficiencies.

Uses: Helps make DNA. Assists in cell reproduction. Reduces elevated homocysteine.

Food sources: Legumes, poultry, tuna, wheat germ, mushrooms, oranges, asparagus, broccoli, spinach, bananas, strawberries, and cantaloupe.

Magnesium

Daily value (DV) for men: 400 mg.

Suggested optimal amount: 500 mg.

Toxicity and symptoms: None known in people with normal renal function.

Uses: Works in metabolism and nerve functions.

Food sources: Molasses, nuts, spinach, wheat germ, pumpkin seeds, sesame seeds, seafood, fat-free or low-fat cheese, baked potatoes, broccoli, and bananas.

Niacin

Daily value (DV) for men: 20 mg.

Suggested optimal amount: 30 mg.

Toxicity and symptoms: 200 mg. Diarrhea, heartburn, dizziness, fainting, itching, sweating.

Uses: Used in energy metabolism. Supports health of skin, nervous system, and digestive system.

Food sources: Lean meat, poultry, fish, peanut butter, legumes, soybeans, whole-grain cereals and breads, broccoli, asparagus, baked potatoes. (Also, skim milk is high in tryptophan, which converts to niacin in the body.)

Potassium

Daily value (DV) for men: 3,500 mg.

Suggested optimal amount: 3,500 mg.

Toxicity and symptoms: 18,000 mg. Results from overuse of potassium salts, not overeating foods high in potassium. Can result in muscle weakness, vomiting, heart failure.

Uses: Balances electrolyte levels. Keeps nerves firing and muscles contracting.

Food sources: Baked potatoes, avocados, dried fruits, fat-free or low-fat yogurt, cantaloupe, spinach, bananas, mushrooms, skim milk, and tomatoes.

Riboflavin

Daily value (DV) for men: 1.7 mg.

Suggested optimal amount: 2.5 mg.

Toxicity and symptoms: None known.

Uses: Supports vision and skin health. Helps with energy conversion.

Food sources: Skim milk, fat-free or low-fat cottage cheese, enriched cereals, avocados, tangerines, prunes, asparagus, broccoli, mushrooms, lean beef, salmon, and chicken.

Selenium

Daily value (DV) for men: 70 mcg.

Suggested optimal amount: 200 mcg.

Toxicity and symptoms: 1,000 mcg. per day over extended period of time. Loss of hair and nails, skin lesions, tooth decay, nervous system disorders.

Uses: May fight cancer and heart disease.

Food sources: Lean meats, whole-grain cereals, fat-free or low-fat dairy products, fish, shellfish, mushrooms, and Brazil nuts.

Thiamin

    Daily value (DV) for men: 1.5 mg.

    Suggested optimal amount: 10 mg.

    Toxicity and symptoms: None known.

    Uses: Supports appetite and nerve function.

    Food sources: Lean pork, sunflower seeds, wheat germ, pasta, peanuts, legumes, watermelon, oranges, brown rice, and oatmeal.

Zinc

    Daily value (DV) for men: 15 mg.

    Suggested optimal amount: 15 mg.

    Toxicity and symptoms: 100 mg. Raised cholesterol, diarrhea, fever, fatigue, dizziness, reproductive failure.

    Uses: Strengthens immune system. Involved in taste perception, wound healing, and sperm production. Essential for brain function.

    Food sources: Oysters, lean beef, wheat germ, seafood, lima beans, legumes, nuts, poultry, skim milk, and low-fat Cheddar cheese.

Supplementation Should Be Considered

Vitamin B$_{12}$

    Daily value (DV) for men: 6 mcg.

    Suggested optimal amount: 6 mcg.

    Toxicity and symptoms: None known.

    Uses: Involved in DNA production. Protects nerve fibers.

    Food sources: Salmon, low-fat cottage cheese, swordfish, tuna, clams, crab, mussels, oysters, and lean beef or pork.

The Ultimate Program for Women

The Nutrients Women Need

Does your diet provide all the nutrients you need? Do you need to take supplements? If so, which ones? To find out what vitamins and minerals you should be getting—and how much you need for optimal health—consult the following information, which is designed for today's active women. If you feel that the condition of your health or your lifestyle might cause nutritional deficiencies, talk with your doctor about tailoring a personal supplement program.

The Daily Value (DV) is based on the levels of intake established by the National Research Council that are judged to provide adequate nutrition for a healthy person. The optimal amount gives you added benefit, based on available scientific research as interpreted by Jeffrey Blumberg, Ph.D., associate director and chief of the antioxidants research laboratory at the Jean Mayer U.S. Department of Agriculture Human Nutrition Research Center on Aging at Tufts University in Boston. Food sources were reviewed by Joanne Curran-Celentano, R.D., Ph.D., associate professor of nutrition and

71

food sciences at the University of New Hampshire in Durham.

Pay careful attention to the abbreviated amounts for each vitamin and mineral. "Mg." is short for milligrams, which are $\frac{1}{1,000}$ gram. "Mcg." stands for micrograms, or $\frac{1}{1,000,000}$ gram. That's a big difference, so take the time to be sure.

Vitamins
Vitamin A

Action in body: Helps maintain normal vision in dim light. Forms and maintains normal structure and functions of mucous membranes to assure healthy eyes, skin, hair, gums, and various glands. Helps build bones and teeth. Maintains strong immunity.

Daily value (DV) for women: 5,000 IU.

Optimal amount: 5,000 IU.

Especially important if you: Are a smoker, have diabetes, eat lots of junk food, are fighting an infection, are recovering from surgery, or are exposed to high levels of pollutants.

Food sources: Carrots, fortified skim milk, pumpkin, sweet potatoes, dark green leafy vegetables (like spinach and kale), winter squash, tuna, halibut, cantaloupe, mangoes, apricots, broccoli, and watermelon.

Thiamin

Action in body: Critical for energy. Important for carbohydrate metabolism. Maintains nerve function, muscle tone, normal appetite, and a healthy mental attitude.

Daily value (DV) for women: 1.5 mg.

Optimal amount: Not established.

Especially important if you: Drink alcohol heavily, drink lots of coffee or tea, or are on a weight-loss diet. Women over age 70 who eat poor diets or are recovering from surgery may be at risk for a thiamin deficiency.

Food sources: Lean pork, sunflower seeds, wheat germ, pasta, peanuts, legumes, watermelon, oranges, brown rice, and oatmeal.

Riboflavin

Action in body: Essential for growth and tissue repair. Important for carbohydrate, fat, and protein metabolism; aids in the formation of red blood cells in bone marrow and in the functioning of the adrenal gland.

Daily value (DV) for women: 1.7 mg.

Optimal amount: Not established.

Especially important if you: Exercise daily or strenuously (or both), fail to eat a variety of nutritious foods, are pregnant or nursing, or drink alcohol heavily. Women over age 70 with poor diets may be at risk for riboflavin deficiency.

Food sources: Skim milk, fat-free or low-fat cottage cheese, enriched cereals, avocados, tangerines, prunes, asparagus, broccoli, mushrooms, lean beef, salmon, and chicken.

Niacin

Action in body: Important for carbohydrate, fat, and protein metabolism. Needed for oxygen use by cells.

Daily value (DV) for women: 20 mg.

Optimal amount: Not established.

Especially important if you: Have high cholesterol or a history of cardiovascular disease (or both).

Food sources: Lean meat, poultry, fish, peanut butter, legumes, soybeans, whole-grain cereals and breads, broccoli, asparagus, and baked potatoes. (Also, skim milk is high in tryptophan, which converts to niacin in the body.)

Vitamin B₆

Action in body: Important for carbohydrate, fat, and protein metabolism. Aids in production of red blood cells; maintains integrity of the central nervous system. Of all the B vitamins, vitamin B_6 is the most important for maintaining a healthy immune system.

Daily value (DV) for women: 2 mg.

Optimal amount: 3 to 5 mg.

Especially important if you: Are on the Pill, are pregnant, have symptoms of premenstrual tension, or are over age 70.

Food sources: Fish, soybeans, avocados, lima beans, poultry, bananas, cauliflower, green peppers, potatoes, spinach, and raisins.

Folic acid

Action in body: Important for synthesis of DNA and RNA, which make up the genetic code vital to all cells in the body; aids in red blood cell development.

Daily value (DV) for women: 400 mcg.

Optimal amount: 400 mcg.

Especially important if you: Drink alcohol heavily, are pregnant, are on a low-calorie diet, have sickle cell disease, are trying to conceive a child, are past menopause, or are over age 70.

Food sources: Legumes, poultry, tuna, wheat germ, mushrooms, oranges, asparagus, broccoli, spinach, bananas, strawberries, and cantaloupe.

Vitamin B$_{12}$

Action in body: Important for red blood cell formation. Maintains nerve tissue. Aids in carbohydrate, fat, and protein metabolism.

Daily value (DV) for women: 6 mcg.

Optimal amount: 10 to 20 mcg.

Especially important if you: Smoke, are on a vegetarian or macrobiotic diet, or are over age 70.

Food sources: Salmon, low-fat cottage cheese, swordfish, tuna, clams, crab, mussels, oysters, and lean beef or pork.

Biotin

Action in body: Important for carbohydrate, fat, and protein metabolism.

Daily value (DV) for women: 300 mcg.

Optimal amount: Not established.

Especially important if you: Are on long-term oral antibiotics, eat poorly, or are on a very low calorie weight-loss diet.

Food sources: Peanut butter, oatmeal, wheat germ, poultry, cauliflower, nuts, legumes, fat-free or low-fat cheese, and mushrooms.

Pantothenic acid

Action in body: Important for carbohydrate, fat, and protein metabolism. Aids in formation of red blood cells, hormones, and nerve transmission substances. Helps maintain normal blood sugar levels.

Daily value (DV) for women: 10 mg.

Optimal amount: Not established.

Especially important if you: Have rheumatoid arthritis.

Food sources: Fish, whole-grain cereals, mushrooms, avocados, broccoli, peanuts, cashews, lentils, and soybeans.

Vitamin C

Action in body: Antioxidant—protects cells from damage by seeking out and neutralizing free radicals that cause oxidation in the body. Builds and maintains collagen, the substance that binds body cells together. Promotes healing of wounds and burns. Maintains healthy gums, teeth, bones, and blood vessels. Increases absorption of iron.

Daily value (DV) for women: 60 mg.

Optimal amount: 500 to 1,000 mg.

Especially important if you: Smoke or are exposed to tobacco smoke, have diabetes, are recovering from surgery, drink alcohol heavily, or are pregnant.

Food sources: Oranges, grapefruit, bell peppers, strawberries, tomatoes, spinach, cabbage, melons, broccoli, kiwifruit, raspberries, and Brussels sprouts.

Vitamin D

Action in body: Increases calcium absorption. Helps build bones and teeth.

Daily value (DV) for women: 400 IU.

Optimal amount: 400 IU.

Especially important if you: Drink alcohol heavily, do not drink milk, do not receive adequate exposure to sunlight, or are over age 70.

Food sources: Fortified skim milk, tuna, salmon, sardines, and fortified cereals, plus sunlight.

Vitamin E

Action in body: Antioxidant—protects cells from damage by seeking out and neutralizing free radicals that cause oxidation in the body. Important for stabilizing cell membranes. Protects lung tissue from air pollution.

Daily value (DV) for women: 30 IU.

Optimal amount: 100 to 400 IU.

Especially important if you: Are exposed to pollution.

Food sources: Nut and vegetable oils, wheat germ, mangoes, blackberries, apples, broccoli, peanuts, spinach, and whole-wheat breads.

Vitamin K

Action in body: Controls blood clotting. Helps maintain normal bones and aids in the healing of fractures.

Daily value (DV) for women: 80 mcg.

Optimal amount: 70 mcg.

Especially important if you: Are on a very low calorie diet or are on a long-term oral antibiotic therapy.

Food sources: Green tea, spinach, broccoli, Brussels sprouts, cabbage, asparagus, parsley, chickpeas, cauliflower, lentils, carrots, avocados, and tomatoes.

Minerals
Calcium

Action in body: Builds bones and teeth. Maintains bones. Aids in nerve transmission, muscle function, and blood clotting. Maintains strong immunity.

Daily value (DV) for women: 1,000 mg.

Optimal amount: 1,200 to 1,500 mg.

Especially important if you: Are a post-menopausal woman not on hormone replacement therapy, drink alcohol, are inactive, are on a low-calorie, high-protein or high-fiber diet, are lactose intolerant, or are pregnant or nursing. Postmenopausal women not on hormone replacement therapy and all women over age 65 should get 1,500 mg.

Food sources: Skim milk, fat-free or low-fat cheese, fat-free yogurt, salmon and sardines with bones, broccoli, green beans, almonds, turnip greens, and fortified orange juice.

Chromium

Action in body: Aids carbohydrate, fat, and protein metabolism. Contributes to the effectiveness of insulin.

Daily value (DV) for women: 120 mcg.

Optimal amount: 125 to 200 mcg.

Especially important if you: Are pregnant, engage in regular strenuous exercise (like running), or are over age 70.

Food sources: Blackstrap molasses, whole grains, broccoli, grape juice, orange juice, lean meat, black pepper, brewer's yeast, and fat-free or low-fat cheese.

Copper

Action in body: Facilitates absorption of iron; helps form red blood cells. Develops and maintains blood vessels, tendons, and bones. Aids in the functioning of the central nervous system. Required for normal hair color. Important for fertility.

Daily value (DV) for women: 2 mg.

Optimal amount: Not established.

Especially important if you: Are taking zinc supplements (zinc and copper should be balanced at a 10:1 ratio) or are over age 70.

Food sources: Oysters and other shellfish, nuts, cherries, cocoa, mushrooms, gelatin, whole-grain cereals, fish, and legumes.

Fluoride

Action in body: Maintains bones and teeth. Helps prevent tooth decay.

Daily value (DV) for women: Not established.

Optimal amount: Usually obtained from fluoridated drinking water.

Especially important if you: Live where the water is not fluoridated.

Food sources: Fluoridated water, fish, and tea.

Iodine

Action in body: Makes up thyroid hormones, which are involved in energy production, growth, nerve and muscle function, and circulation.

Daily value (DV) for women: 150 mcg.

Optimal amount: Not established.

Especially important if you: Have fibrocystic breasts.

Food sources: Spinach, lobster, shrimp, oysters, skim milk, and iodized salt.

Iron

Action in body: Carries oxygen in blood; contributes to energy metabolism.

Daily value (DV) for women: 18 mg.

Optimal amount: 10 to 18 mg.

Especially important if you: Are premeno-

pausal, are on a low-calorie diet, are pregnant or
nursing, are a vegetarian, or are over age 70 with poor
long-term dietary habits.

Food sources: Clams, asparagus, lean meat,
chicken, prunes, raisins, spinach, pumpkin seeds, soybeans, and tofu.

Magnesium

Action in body: Essential for every major body
process, including glucose metabolism, cellular energy,
muscle contraction, and nerve function. Helps build
bones and teeth.

Daily value (DV) for women: 400 mg.

Optimal amount: 400 to 800 mg.

Especially important if you: Are on a low-
calorie diet, have diabetes, drink alcohol, are pregnant,
take diuretics, exercise regularly and strenuously, or are
over age 70.

Food sources: Molasses, nuts, spinach, wheat
germ, pumpkin seeds, sesame seeds, seafood, fat-free
or low-fat cheese, baked potatoes, broccoli, and bananas.

Manganese

Action in body: Helps form bone. Aids growth of
connective tissue. Contributes to blood clotting. Aids in
carbohydrate, fat, and protein metabolism.

Daily value (DV) for women: 2 mg.

Optimal amount: Not established.

Especially important if you: Are taking large
doses of calcium or iron supplements, are on a low-
calorie diet, or are being fed intravenously.

Food sources: Nuts, whole-grain cereals,
legumes, tea, dried fruits, and spinach and other green
leafy vegetables.

Molybdenum

Action in body: Aids in carbohydrate, fat, and protein metabolism; a component of tooth enamel.

Daily value (DV) for women: 75 mcg.

Optimal amount: 75 to 250 mcg.

Especially important if you: Are on a low-calorie diet or are being fed intravenously.

Food sources: Legumes, lean meats, whole-grain cereals, breads, and skim milk.

Phosphorus

Action in body: Helps build bones and teeth. Maintains bones. Builds muscle tissue. Aids in carbohydrate, fat, and protein metabolism. Is a component of DNA and RNA, which make up the genetic code vital to all cells in the body.

Daily value (DV) for women: 1,000 mg.

Optimal amount: Not established.

Especially important if you: Drink alcohol heavily or use magnesium-containing or aluminum-containing antacids regularly.

Food sources: Lean meats, fish, poultry, fat-free or low-fat dairy products, and cereals.

Potassium

Action in body: Maintains acid/base balance in the body; involved in muscle function, energy production, and protein synthesis. Required for the release of insulin by the pancreas. Maintains normal blood pressure. Works with sodium to maintain fluid balance.

Daily value (DV) for women: 3,500 mg.

Optimal amount: Not established.

Especially important if you: Have high blood pressure or take prescription diuretics.

Food sources: Baked potatoes, avocados, dried fruits, fat-free or low-fat yogurt, cantaloupe, spinach, bananas, mushrooms, skim milk, and tomatoes.

Selenium

Action in body: Contributes to certain antioxidant functions. Maintains strong immunity.

Daily value (DV) for women: 70 mcg.

Optimal amount: 100 mcg.

Especially important if you: No special considerations.

Food sources: Lean meats, whole-grain cereals, fat-free or low-fat dairy products, fish, shellfish, mushrooms, and Brazil nuts.

Sodium

Action in body: Maintains water and acid/base balance in the body. Helps make up bile, sweat, and tears. Involved in muscle contraction. Contributes to nervous system function.

Daily value (DV) for women: 2,400 mg.

Optimal amount: Not established.

Special considerations: Sodium is prevalent in many commonly eaten foods, especially processed foods, so there is no need to pay special attention to intake.

Zinc

Action in body: Maintains strong immunity. Helps fight disease. Maintains normal skin, bones, and hair. Aids in digestion and respiration. Important for the development and functioning of reproductive organs. Involved in wound healing. Maintains normal sense of taste.

Daily value (DV) for women: 15 mg.

Optimal amount: 15 mg.

Especially important if you: Are a vegetarian, are on a low-calorie diet, are taking diuretics, have diabetes, drink alcohol heavily, sweat excessively, or are over age 70.

Food sources: Oysters, lean beef, wheat germ, seafood, lima beans, legumes, nuts, poultry, skim milk, and low-fat Cheddar cheese.

A Guide to Unusual Supplements

How to Extend Your Shelf Life

By all means, tune out the crank talk shows and their wild-eyed guests who subsist on organic bean sprouts and boiled tofu. But when an herb makes the front page of the venerable *Wall Street Journal*, it's probably time to take notice.

The "other" nutritional supplements have arrived. We're not talking about that alphabet of nutrients that you're beginning to know and love—the ABCs of vitamins—or their brethren in healing, those magnificent minerals.

Rather, it's that assortment of herbs, oils, and dietary preparations—once relegated to the back of your neighborhood health food store—that are now front and center in the health spotlight. And at your corner drugstore.

The question before the house: Do they work? Answer: A definite maybe, depending on what you choose. "Lots of herbal products definitely have an effect," says William J. Keller, Ph.D., professor and chairman of the department of pharmaceutical sciences at Samford University in Birmingham, Alabama. "They may not have the same striking effect that modern drugs have, but they can be helpful, depending on the condition."

Some supplements, like amino acids, glucosamine sulfate, and hormone replacements, will require more research before we know. But one thing is certain: You're bound to encounter more and more of them. Here's a guide to what you'll see along the way. If you think one of these might be right for you, see what your doctor says. In fact, always check with your doctor before taking any herbal products, especially if taking medication, because there can be harmful interactions, says Dr. Keller.

Amino acids. Used by Arnold Schwarzenegger wanna-bes, amino acids are frequently featured in bodybuilding magazines. While research shows that you need to eat more protein when you're trying to pack on lean body mass, the evidence for amino acids is tougher to come by—if you're already getting adequate protein. Originally used to prevent protein loss in folks recovering from surgery, amino acids are simply protein building blocks such as l-isoleucine, l-leucine, and l-glutamine. Although there are some small studies showing that amino acid supplements help burn fat and build muscle, more needs to be done. There are also some side effects, such as nausea and diarrhea, that you may want to do without.

Brewer's yeast. With a name like that, it has to be good, right? If you're looking for a mother lode of vitamins and minerals in one tablet, brewer's yeast delivers. Most contain thiamin, riboflavin, niacin, pyridoxine, pantothenic acid, biotin, and folic acid, not to mention chromium and selenium. Two studies note that it may also contain chemicals that speed wound healing. And yes, it's the actual stuff that's needed to make beer— without the alcohol, of course, says Dr. Keller. And although brewer's yeast is rich in various relatively non-toxic nutrients, follow the label's instructions because dosage can vary widely among products.

Capsaicin. Applying this red-pepper derivative topically has been found to reduce aches and pains by what might be called the "lights are on but nobody's home" mechanism—simply helping thwart the transmission of pain signals to your brain.

This same principle apparently came in handy during at least one study of people with arthritis who had hand pain. Those who rubbed on capsaicin cream for nine weeks had 22 percent less pain than the folks who got fake pills. You may also see capsaicin in candy, capsule, or cream form to treat mouth sores in cancer patients, bellyaches, psoriasis, and even the mysterious burning in the legs and feet of people with AIDS. Capsaicin cream is available without a prescription. Make sure to clean your hands thoroughly after you apply capsaicin though; it will burn your eyes and just about anything else that's tender.

Echinacea. The subject of a front-page *Wall Street Journal* article, echinacea is one of the best-selling herbal remedies on the market. The reason why the cash register is ringing is because regular folks swear that it can help ward off a cold and flu—or at least shorten the length and severity. What do doctors say? "Echinacea definitely stimulates the nonspecific immune system," says Dr. Keller. "In other words, it stimulates the cells that eliminate cold viruses and other harmful cells. It's probably one of the most viable herbal treatments around." For a two-fisted, cold-fighting punch, consider taking vitamin C and echinacea. Take echinacea according to package directions at the first sign of cold or flu symptoms, says Dr. Keller. And don't take it for long periods of time, as it could begin to depress your immune system. Be warned that echinacea tastes lousy in its most potent form: liquid.

Feverfew. Arthritis and migraine sufferers have turned to this herb in droves for relief. The active ingredient has been identified as parthenolide, but you may not be getting what you expect in pill form. Feverfew supplements are notoriously unreliable in their quality and potency. If you have a green thumb, try growing some yourself and chewing on one or two leaves. Discontinue use immediately if feverfew leaves irritate your mouth.

Fish oil. A review of 10 studies found that folks with arthritis who took 3 to 6 grams of fish oil a day had a modest benefit—without apparent side effects. Not only that, but fish oil figures to be heart-healthy: lowering blood pressure, reducing blood fat levels, and increasing clotting times. One British study showed that heart attack survivors who ate more fish, the best source of fish oil, were 29 percent less likely to die within the next few years than those who hadn't added fish to their dish. The American Heart Association prefers that you get your fish oil from fish because you're less likely to overdose, which can lead to excessive bleeding, drug interactions, and possibly high cholesterol.

Flaxseed oil. We're just beginning to get the facts on flax, but here's what we know so far: Like fish, it contains omega-6 fatty acids but actually has more omega-3 fatty acids—both considered heart-healthy. It's also one of the best sources of what's called gamma-linolenic acid, a substance that may help arthritis sufferers. What's more, flax may ease asthma and allergic reactions and boost your immune system. Add the oil to yogurt, or grind up and sprinkle the seeds the next time you bake—it's a grain, after all.

Garlic. There's a growing body of evidence suggesting that garlic will do more than ruin your chances for a smooch on your first date. In an analysis of several studies, taking dried garlic seemed to be of some benefit for people with mildly elevated blood pressure. The same research also found that 600 to 900 milligrams of dried garlic a day reduced bad cholesterol and blood fat. But more trials should be done before anyone can wholeheartedly promote garlic. Available in deodorized form, garlic has also been found to have a mild immune-boosting effect, says Dr. Keller, which might help ward off colds.

Ginger. Not only has ginger been found to reduce motion sickness and upset stomach, but it naturally aids digestion. How well? In one study, 940 milligrams of ginger outperformed 100 milligrams of dimenhydrinate (Dramamine) for motion sickness. And although a study funded by the National Aeronautics and Space Administration didn't find any benefit, 1 gram of ginger helped keep green Navy cadets from turning green when they were exposed to choppy seas.

Ginkgo. Considered a conventional drug in Europe, ginkgo has been shown to improve circulation problems, leading some to use it for conditions ranging from intermittent claudication (slowed blood flow in the legs) to tinnitus (ringing in the ears). You'll also see it in various formulations suggesting improved brain functions, such as boosting short-term memory, relieving headaches, and even combating vertigo.

If you choose to try ginkgo, make sure that it is a standardized formula. The recommended dosage is a 40-milligram tablet or capsule three times a day, according to Dr. Keller. Ginkgo is generally regarded as safe, but since it affects the body's clotting mechanism, use caution if taking aspirin or anticlotting medications. Some people may experience mild side effects, such as restlessness and digestive upset and should discontinue use.

Ginseng. Don't be surprised if you see the cartoon character Dilbert giving this Chinese herb to his boss someday. In a study of 95 British middle managers, those who had a poor diet and took a multivitamin containing 40 milligrams of ginseng reported less anxiety, anger, and confusion and more vigor than those who were given a placebo (dummy pill). Long touted by the Chinese as an aphrodisiac, ginseng is thought to be what's called an adaptogen, which means that it's supposed to help you better cope with stress. Ginseng has also been used successfully on conditions ranging from diabetes to clogged arteries. Some side effects of ginseng include insomnia and possibly diarrhea. However, since quality control is extremely difficult to maintain, you may not be getting quality ginseng or any ginseng at all in that supplement.

Glucosamine sulfate. As you age, you produce less glucosamine, a substance that helps keep your cartilage strong and rigid. So your cartilage breaks down, causing one form of the familiar joint pain and stiffness known as arthritis. The question is, can swallowing synthetic glucosamine sulfate capsules replace that lost glucosamine and save your joints? By the looks of health food store and drugstore shelves that stock the stuff, you'd think so. There have been several promising small, controlled trials done overseas testing glucosamine sulfate as an effective treatment for arthritis. And although some short-term pain relief was found, studies have yet to determine any long-term benefits. The Arthritis Foundation does not recommend the use of glucosamine sulfate in the treatment of arthritis and cautions that since it is considered a dietary supplement, it is not regulated by the Food and Drug Administration (FDA).

If you choose to take glucosamine sulfate, the dosage is a 500-milligram capsule three times a day, says Dr. Keller. There are virtually no side effects, but some people do complain of nausea.

Goldenseal root. Goldenseal is thought to make a nifty tea for soothing canker sores, chapped lips, and an otherwise sore mouth. It also comes in capsules, but its effects when taken internally are unreliable. Check with your doctor before taking goldenseal internally, as it may increase blood pressure.

Hawthorn. Keep your eye on this herb. Research has shown that hawthorn can help open coronary blood vessels, often lowering blood pressure. Not only that, but hawthorn is thought to "reduce the tendency to angina attacks," according to Varro E. Tyler, Ph.D., in his book *The Honest Herbal*, and even to aid the heart after injury from an attack.

If you think that hawthorn may help you, consult a doctor familiar with it. Don't try to self-diagnose heart problems, says Dr. Keller. They require a doctor's expertise.

Pycnogenol. You'll probably be hearing a lot about pycnogenol in the future. Made from the bark of the European coastal pine tree, pycnogenol contains chemicals called bioflavonoids that are thought to protect your cardiovascular system from free-radical damage. Much of the advertising information promoting pycnogenol is based on the tale of a French explorer and his crew who were given pine tea brewed by an Indian. This tea cured the crew members of scurvy. An interesting bedtime story for the kids, but until some serious studies of pycnogenol's antioxidant qualities are done, stick with reliable and cheaper forms of bioflavonoids, such as citrus fruits, blueberries, tea, onions, and apples. You could also have a reaction if you are allergic to pine.

Saw palmetto. This extract of the saw palmetto berry has been found in some studies to relieve symptoms caused by nonmalignant enlargement of the prostate. In one study of 500 men suffering from benign prostatic hyperplasia (BPH), 88 percent experienced reduction in their symptoms. Because the active chemicals of saw palmetto are fat-soluble, not water-soluble, drinking a tea made from the berries won't help. Also, you won't see saw palmetto advertising that it is beneficial for BPH. The FDA has not approved it for sale for BPH in the United States. You may find it, however, in some over-the-counter male potency supplements.

Valerian. Valerian has long been known for its mild tranquilizing effect. As a result, it's often recommended in Germany as a sleep aid or for restlessness. "It doesn't have the same potency as a prescription sleep aid, but it will definitely make you drowsy," Dr. Keller says. Be sure to follow label instructions and cautions. Check with your doctor before taking valerian if you are taking central nervous system depressants such as diazepam (Valium), and as with any product that causes drowsiness, don't operate a car or heavy machinery.

Getting What You Need from Food

Tapping Into Nature's Nutrient Storehouse

Want to give less money to your doctor next year? Then give more money to your grocer. Economic research has revealed that if Americans ate more foods high in vitamins C and E and beta-carotene, our national health care costs would decrease by 25 percent—for cardiovascular disease alone. Cancer costs would drop by 16 to 30 percent, and cataract costs would plummet by 50 percent. It's an alchemist's dream: turning carrots into dollars.

"You can fulfill the Recommended Dietary Allowances for vitamins and minerals by following the Food Guide Pyramid," says Keith-Thomas Ayoob, R.D., Ed.D., spokesman for the American Dietetic Association in Chicago, director of nutrition services at the Rose F. Kennedy Children's Evaluation and Rehabilitation Center, and assistant professor of pediatric medicine at Albert Einstein College of Medicine, both in New York City. "There are times when vitamin supplementation can be necessary and appropriate, but if you eat a proper diet, not only will you meet your nutrient needs but you'll probably also exceed them."

That's because vitamins and minerals are only the tip of the iceberg, nutritionally speaking. No amount of supplementation can replace a good diet, nor can it fix the damage that an unhealthy diet can do, in both the short and long term. In fact, trying to replace food with supplements can actually do more harm than good. Throughout the rest of this chapter, we'll discuss the variety of foods that you need to eat every day—fruits and vegetables, whole grains, dairy products, meats, and fats, sweets, and oils. If that list sounds familiar, it should: It's on the official Food Guide Pyramid.

Fruits and Vegetables

Scientists have discovered that plant foods—fruits and vegetables—seem to be as important for what we don't know about them as for what we do. "A natural food is much more than the sum of its known nutrients," says Barbara Klein, Ph.D., professor of food science and human nutrition at the University of Illinois in Urbana-Champaign. "We know a lot about vitamins and minerals, but we don't know a lot about the other compounds that are present in plants. Our knowledge is not sufficient to warrant taking supplements and not eating well."

In fact, researchers have found that vegetables and fruits contain chemicals, dubbed phytochemicals, that help protect against cancer and other diseases. Among the handful of phytochemicals that have been isolated so far are capsaicin (found in peppers), flavonoids (berries, citrus fruits, and yams), allylic sulfide (onions and garlic), and indole-3-carbinol (cauliflower and cabbage).

Like vitamins and minerals, phytochemicals lose some of their protective powers when they're isolated from the foods they come in.

For example, just a few years ago, researchers found that men with cancer had less beta-carotene in their blood than those without cancer. At first it seemed that beta-carotene alone could block the development of cancer, but when researchers looked further into the issue, they found something else entirely.

"It turned out that taking beta-carotene supplements actually had an adverse effect, because when you isolate beta-carotene down to a pill, something important that appears in the food is removed. But we're still not completely sure about what it is," says Christopher Gardner, Ph.D., a nutrition researcher at Stanford University's Center for Research in Disease Prevention.

Researchers are still learning how various chemicals work together to offer protection against disease. And their discoveries spark a sense of awe.

Nature packages foods in a miraculous way. For instance, while a mineral pill might contain more iron than a tomato, the tomato has vitamin C, which aids the body's absorption of that iron.

Likewise, the tomato will have other nutrients that can help your health. For instance, a study found that a carotenoid called lycopene has a more protective effect against prostate cancer than both vitamin A and beta-carotene. Lycopene is most commonly found in tomatoes and tomato-based foods, such as tomato sauce—a food, not a vitamin or mineral supplement. So, you'd have to take at least three supplements—vitamin C, iron, and lycopene—to equal just the known protective nutrients found in tomatoes and tomato products.

Even nutritionists who endorse supplementation agree that people taking vitamin and mineral tablets should do so in addition to a low-fat diet that features the recommended servings of fruits and vegetables. "A vitamin pill can't compensate for a diet that's loaded with fat or low in fruits and vegetables, because there are thousands of plant compounds that may help reduce the risk of cancer and heart disease," says Bonnie Liebman, licensed nutritionist and director of nutrition for the Center for Science in the Public Interest in Washington, D.C.

Federal surveys have consistently shown, however, that 60 percent of what Americans eat comes from animal-based foods, with the remaining 40 percent coming from plant sources. The ratio should be precisely the opposite, experts say.

Whole Grains

Talk to any nutritionist and she'll sing the praises of plants, but not just fruits and vegetables. The next group of foods to add to your shopping cart is whole grains.

"Whole wheat, oats, barley, rye, millet, brown rice, and corn are all whole grains," Dr. Klein says. "During processing, they have as little removed as possible to make them palatable." In other words, while the wheat no longer has those fuzzy things on the top, all that's taken off during processing is the hull. What's left (after processing) is the grain with the bran or the germ attached.

So, while oatmeal is a whole grain, traditional spaghetti isn't. (In fact, spaghetti, as we know it, contains all of the starch but little of the vitamins and minerals in the grain.) Rye bread contains whole grains, but white bread doesn't. Wheatena is a whole grain, but farina isn't. The more refined the flour, the less nutritious the food, Dr. Klein says.

Dairy Products

Americans don't drink enough milk, and that's bad because it's an extremely nutrient-dense food. In fact, all the vitamins as well as six minerals have been detected in cows' milk. Of course, the most obvious nutrient identified with milk is calcium.

Two glasses (8 ounces each) of milk provide about 60 percent of the Daily Value for calcium. About 95 percent of the milk supply in the United States is fortified with vitamin D, which helps the body absorb the calcium found in the milk. However, even though it's great to get calcium through milk, it's only worth it, calorically speaking, if you're drinking low-fat or skim milk. Whole milk is just too high in fat.

The ways in which milk is made into other dairy products also affects the food's level of calcium. For instance, one serving of Cheddar cheese has more than as much calcium as a serving of cottage cheese. The drawback is that it also has four times the calories. However, it is still more nutrient-smart to consume a small amount of Cheddar.

Meat

Unless you're following a vegetarian diet, low-fat meats can still have an honored place on your plate—though probably not quite as large—because many of the vitamins and minerals in meat are more bioavailable than those in plant food. That means that your body absorbs them better.

"It's not an issue of never eating meat," Liebman says. "It's about how often you eat it. Your diet should be largely plant-based." A plant-based diet can cut your risk of cancer, heart disease, stroke, and diabetes, she adds.

Surveys show that only half of all Americans eat fruit every day and more than 20 percent consume no milk products. But 25 percent of all Americans eat fried potatoes on any given day. "The problem is that a meat-and-potatoes diet usually means that you aren't eating fruits and vegetables," Liebman says. "If you want your steak, you should think of the salad as the main course and the meat as a side dish."

Or think of meat as what you eat when you go out to dinner on the weekends rather than your everyday evening meal. If you generally have meat for lunch and dinner, cut back to once a day, Liebman advises.

Fats

Hopefully, there's hardly any room left in your stomach. But if there is, you get to have a treat. And most people choose fat-laden treats.

The Food Guide Pyramid recommends that you eat fat "sparingly," says Dr. Klein, which means that if you eat any animal products, such as meats, you don't need to add much fat to anything during the day. "That source alone probably fills your recommended intake," she says.

So put down the butter knife. If you must, lean toward oils rather than margarine or butter. "We have a lot of hidden fat in our diets, particularly with fast food," Dr. Klein says. "It's not the hamburger that's killing us; it's the 'special sauce,' to say nothing of the french fries."

Aim for 2 tablespoons or less a day of oils (preferably those high in monounsaturates, such as olive oil), which translates into a serving of salad dressing. "If you have a choice, don't use fat," Dr. Klein says.

Smart Eating

If you focus on getting all your vitamins and minerals, not to mention your carotenoids and phytochemicals, you'll have a full plate as well as a full tummy. There might not be a lot of room left for nonnutritious items.

When it comes to food, Dr. Klein says, variety is indeed the spice of life. "There's no single food or group of foods that by itself is perfect," she says. "We have many nutritional needs that we know of and some that we don't know. Eating a balanced diet means that you should eat a wide variety of foods." So while there's tons of proof that fruits and vegetables can help prevent cancer, they're not the only foods that provide vitamins and minerals.

"Remember that you can eat a pizza or hamburger for breakfast and still have a balanced diet," says Dr. Klein. "You just want to make sure that there's a large distribution among the kinds of food you eat."

In fact, you could take a tip from the Japanese. Their government recommends that its citizens eat 30 "foodstuffs" each day, which roughly corresponds to the highest number of recommended servings in the Food Guide Pyramid.

And don't think that all this eating means that you'll never take supplements. In fact, just the opposite is true. Studies have shown that people who take supplements eat more servings of fruits and vegetables than those who don't eat well. And you know what other group you'll join? Those with higher personal incomes and more education. They, too, eat better and take more supplements.

The Perfect Eating Plan

Putting It All Together

A hot fudge sundae is an essential part of a nutritious diet.

Well, okay—it's not true. Chances are it got your attention, though.

The truth is, nutrition is a lot more interesting than those lectures on the four basic food groups that you heard in high school health class.

All told, you need about two dozen nutrients every single day, says Cheryl Rock, Ph.D., professor of nutrition at the University of Michigan at Ann Arbor. But don't worry—you don't have to memorize food groups in order to eat right. What follows is a detailed, meal-by-meal guide to what you need—and how to get it.

Breakfast—You Gotta Have It

Don't wait until noon to lay in provisions for the day. And remember that not just any breakfast will do.

Figure on fruit. Dr. Rock's number one rule is, "Every meal should include a fruit or vegetable."

That includes breakfast. Since few people can face broccoli first thing in the morning, Dr. Rock says that fruit is the logical choice. Concentrate on deep yellow fruits like cantaloupe, which provide beta-carotene and other carotenoids, along with vitamin C. Together, these antioxidant compounds help protect against cancer, heart disease, and stroke.

Or, suggests Pittsburgh dietitian Pat Harper, R.D., a spokesperson for the American Dietetic Association, try a peach, a mango, or a half cup of berries. Other options include half a banana or half a grapefruit, a quarter cup of raisins, or if you like, a half cup of stewed prunes.

Drink some juice. Six ounces of orange, cranberry, or strawberry-kiwi juice will also do the trick, says Dr. Rock. They supply vitamin C. When researchers in Spain compared women who had developed breast cancer with others who were cancer-free, they found that the latter ate far more fruits and vegetables than the former. What's more, the women with breast cancer included less vitamin C in their overall diets. Juice is also a rich source of beta-carotene, which is similarly protective.

Pour yourself some milk. You should also get some protein at breakfast, says Dr. Rock. Calcium-rich dairy products like milk are good choices. Calcium is one of the nutrients that women rarely get enough of, says Dr. Rock. And since their bones are often more fragile than men's, they're at greater risk for osteoporosis than men. The best defense against this bone-thinning disease is, of course, to build strong bones while you can. Unfortunately, our bodies get out of the bone-building business after age 35. From then on, the best you can do is preserve what you have, says Gail Frank, R.D., Dr. P.H., professor of nutrition at California State University in Long Beach and a nutritional epidemiologist.

Think yogurt. Low-fat and nonfat yogurt are other good choices because they also offer both protein and calcium, Dr. Rock explains. Low-fat yogurt tends to be higher in calcium than regular or nonfat (since low-fat yogurt is often fortified with powdered skim milk), so it's the best choice, says Dr. Rock.

Consider lactase. To use calcium, your body also needs vitamin D. Milk is a terrific source of both. It's such a good deal for your bones that you should include it in your diet even if you have lactose intolerance and can't digest milk sugar, says Mary Frances Picciano, Ph.D., professor of nutrition at Pennsylvania State University in University Park. If you have trouble tolerating lactose, simply add a few liquid lactase drops (Lactaid Drops) to the carton of milk about an hour before you have a glass. The drops, available at most pharmacies, will digest the milk sugar for you.

You can also find relief with lactase tablets (Lactaid Caplets) taken with milk or dairy products (or immediately afterward).

Buy lactose-friendly dairy products. Try yogurt, frozen yogurt, and sweet acidophilus milk. They contain no lactose. But keep in mind that yogurts and cheeses don't contain vitamin D.

Chill that milk. If you don't much like the taste of milk, make your relationship even chillier. Drinking milk from a thick, frosty glass mug improves its flavor.

Remember cereal and milk—they're not just for kids. With your fruit, protein, and calcium you need a serving or two of grains. That makes cereal and milk the perfect centerpiece for breakfast, says Dr. Rock.

Most breakfast cereals are fortified, so they're good sources of many vitamins and minerals, Dr. Rock says. If you're troubled by constipation (more common during pregnancy and after age 50), a high-fiber bran cereal is probably a good idea every day, she says. Sprinkle on some plump raisins (more fruit) or a sliced peach.

Or you can add a quarter cup of chopped dried fruit or a half cup of fresh fruit (like apricots or strawberries) to your cereal, suggests Chris Rosenbloom, R.D., Ph.D., a Georgia nutritionist and spokesperson for the American Dietetic Association.

Whole grains are also reputable sources of zinc, a mineral with many functions, one of which is to maintain your immune system. Your body needs 15 milligrams of this mineral per day to stay up to snuff, according to the government's Daily Value. If the stresses of academics, work, and family leave you vulnerable to frequent bouts with colds or other infections, your immune system may need a boost.

Grill a cheesy English muffin. Another quick way to combine dairy and grains, says Dr. Rock, is to melt two ounces of low-fat cheese over a hot, crusty English muffin.

Toast up a peanut butter bagel. For variety, spread two tablespoons of peanut butter on toast or a bagel, says Dr. Rock. Serve with milk.

Peanut butter is a fairly good source of vitamin E,

Real Food versus Instant Breakfasts and Energy Bars

It's one of those mornings: If you're going to have breakfast, it's gotta be fast.

In emergencies, there's nothing wrong with relying on fortified instant breakfast mixes, says Cheryl Rock, Ph.D., professor of nutrition at the University of Michigan at Ann Arbor. All you have to do is add milk. But there's a caveat.

"With instant breakfasts, you get certain vitamins but none of the fiber or protective nutrients (called phytochemicals) offered by real food," says Dr. Rock. Adding a piece of fresh fruit to your instant breakfast makes for a more nutritious meal, she says. You add fiber, vitamins (especially beta-carotene and vitamin C if you choose yellow fruit like cantaloupe or citrus fruit like oranges). Adding fruit also assures that you're getting protective phytochemicals, hundreds of which scientists are just beginning to study but which don't necessarily show up in factory-formulated foods.

What about lunch on the run? Will an energy bar do?

"If you're really strapped for time, they're okay," says Dr. Rock. But add an apple, peach, or other nutritious fruit that's easily consumed out of hand, she says, to get the phytochemicals, vitamins, and minerals that energy bars don't provide.

another antioxidant. Yes, peanut butter is high in fat, but it's unsaturated fat, which is less likely to raise the level of cholesterol in your blood.

When it comes to breads, muffins, and bagels, Dr.

Rock suggests that you alternate between white and whole-grain choices. Like fortified cereals, refined breads are enriched with iron. But whole-grain breads offer more fiber. Studies suggest that a diet high in fiber will spare you from constipation and lower both your blood cholesterol and your risk of heart disease and colon cancer. We all need at least 20 to 30 grams of fiber daily.

"If you're eating a minimum of five fruits and vegetables and choosing some whole grains every day, you really don't need to count fiber grams," Dr. Rock says. "Chances are, you'll hit your quota."

Select apple butter and fat-free cream cheese. "A lot of people still think that grains are fattening, but the truth is, it's what you put on top of them, like butter, that's fattening," Dr. Rosenbloom adds.

Try nonfat or low-fat cream cheese on your bagel. Spread fruit butter on your toast, suggests Dr. Rock.

The Art of the Mid-Morning Snack

Snacking is an opportunity to bolster your nutritional intake, provided you go about it methodically.

Borrow from breakfast. If you're not especially hungry when you first wake up, eat your raisins or drink your juice as a mid-morning snack, says Dr. Rock.

Crackers and fruit beat a Danish. The ideal mid-morning snack, says Dr. Rock, might consist of fruit and whole-wheat crackers. You get carbohydrates (for quick energy), fiber, and—as a bonus—folate, an essential B vitamin.

Make the Most of Lunch

Your stomach empties out and trips the hunger alarm every four hours or so. So by lunchtime, you'll be ready for more food.

Think beyond cold cuts. A tuna or chicken salad sandwich gives you protein and grain, says Dr. Rock. Use lots of celery and carrots for added fiber and beta-carotene.

Adding a couple of tablespoons of low-fat mayonnaise to your chicken salad or roast beef sandwich will make it tastier and help you absorb the vitamins in your diet, Dr. Rock explains.

Fat carries vitamins A, D, E, and K through your body and performs other essential tasks, explains Dr. Rosenbloom. And because fat is a natural component of body tissues, you need some fat in your diet, she says. And it makes food taste better all around. The trick is to keep the amount of fat that you eat to a minimum.

Otherwise, there's nothing wrong with a lean roast beef sandwich—a couple of ounces of meat between slices of whole-grain or even white bread, says Dr. Rock. In moderation, red meat is a perfectly fine addition to your menu. In fact, three ounces of lean red meat three times a week will give you a significant percentage of the iron that you need to keep going, Dr. Picciano explains.

Red meat is a particularly good dining companion for premenopausal women, who lose iron via menstrual flow. To make up for the loss, you need 18 milligrams of iron in your diet daily, one and a half times as much as you need after menopause.

Nutritionists suggest just three ounces of meat a day. Men and women alike eat more protein than they need, says Philadelphia nutritionist Mona Sutnick, R.D., Ed.D., a spokesperson for the American Dietetic Association. When you eat excess protein, your body excretes calcium, so you risk doing your bones harm. Get only the amount of protein that you actually need. A three-ounce serving is about the size of a deck of cards.

Fortified breads also add needed iron, adds Dr. Rock, as do dark green leafy vegetables, chickpeas (garbanzo beans), tomato juice, and raisins. If you're a vegetarian, though, you should know that the iron you get from vegetable sources isn't as easily utilized by the body. If you don't eat meat, ask your doctor whether you should be taking a multivitamin that includes iron, suggests Jodie Shield, R.D., adjunct instructor of nutrition communication at Rush University in Chicago and a nutritionist in Kildeer, Illinois.

Rendezvous with fruits and vegetables. Dr. Rock recommends including a vegetable or two with lunch. Carrot sticks are tops—they're rich in beta-carotene and other cancer-fighting carotenoids. Tomatoes, cantaloupe, and other deep yellow and orange fruits and vegetables are also rich in these key nutrients. Or have a frosty glass of tomato juice or some tomato soup, both loaded with vitamin C.

Diversify your vegetable portfolio. The more varied your vegetable repertoire, the better, say dietitians. No single food will give you all the nutrients that your body needs, notes Harper. Some carotenoids (there are about 400 different kinds), for instance, occur in certain fruits and vegetables but not others. Yet these nutrients, close cousins of beta-carotene, may help ward off illness.

Broaden your lunchtime palate. Pasta (like shells stuffed with ricotta or other low-fat cheese) gives you two servings of grain, two or three ounces of protein, and little fat, says Dr. Rock. Chicken breast strips and vegetables stir-fried in a few drops of vegetable oil and served over rice are fine, too, Dr. Rock says.

Maxi-Nutrients, Mini-Calories

Nutritionally, some foods are far superior to others, offering lots of nutrients without a lot of high-calorie baggage. According to Janis Jibrin, R.D., a nutrition consultant in Washington, D.C., a diet based primarily on fruits, vegetables, nonfat dairy foods, and whole-grain complex carbohydrates like pasta and brown rice is a balanced approach to healthy eating. Since most Americans are getting too much protein in their diets, limit your meat to three-ounce portions, or better yet, says Jibrin, substitute beans for meat whenever you can. To make sure that you're getting maximum nutrition for your caloric intake, Jibrin recommends that you focus on these nutrition-packed standouts.

Nutrient	Look for
Antioxidants, other vitamins	Broccoli, carrots, collards, Swiss chard, citrus fruits, papaya, cantaloupe
Folate	Oranges, orange juice, dark green leafy vegetables
Calcium	Nonfat yogurt, most dark leafy greens, calcium-fortified orange juice (calcium and folate), skim milk, sardines

Mid-Afternoon Delight

Even on a waist-watching plan, you can afford a mid-afternoon snack, says Dr. Rock. Here are some of your options.

Iron	Fortified cereal, beans, especially chickpeas, pinto beans, and white beans; most dark green leafy vegetables
Magnesium	Dark green leafy vegetables, whole grains, nuts, and beans such as black beans and chickpeas

Protein Source	Look for
Meat	Select (extra-lean) cuts, particularly flank steak and top round
Fish	White fish, flounder, red snapper, most other fish
Poultry	Chicken (skinless), turkey (skinless), ground turkey (ground without the skin)
Legumes (beans)	Dried beans such as chickpeas, kidney beans, black beans, soybeans, and soy-based foods such as tofu, tempeh, and soy milk

Carry over from lunch. Save the vegetable juice or banana or a piece of bread from lunch and eat it at mid-afternoon, suggests Dr. Rock.

Fruit and crackers make a fine pick-me-up. If you like, have an orange or some whole-grain

crackers with a dab of jelly at mid-afternoon, Dr. Rock
suggests.

Just-Right Dinners

Call it dinner, supper, whatever you prefer, the evening
meal is your last chance to pack in essential nutrients
and have some gustatory fun before toddling off to bed
for the night. Dr. Rock's second rule about a nutritious
menu is, "Enjoy what you eat." Her suggestions, which
follow, reflect that advice.

Your dinner plans should include two servings of
grains, a little bit of fat, and a modest amount of high-
protein food.

Beef? Make it lean. If you didn't have roast beef
for lunch, consider a couple of ounces of red meat, like
an extra-lean hamburger patty, beef kabobs, or thinly
sliced flank steak, says Dr. Rock.

Serve soup as an entrée. Lots of vegetables and
delicious broth make a little meat go a long way, says
Diane Woznicki, R.D., a nutritionist at Albright College
in Reading, Pennsylvania.

Make a pasta or rice dish. And garnish it with
thinly sliced beef or chicken, says Woznicki. That way,
you can stretch two or three ounces of meat into an
entire meal.

Veg-e-size your fajitas. Use lots of peppers and
onions but only three strips or so of meat.

Catch some fish. Tuna, mackerel, herring, oysters, clams, and halibut are good sources of B vitamins,
making fish a valuable option. Birth control pills can deplete the body's B vitamin stores, including folate, says
Dr. Rosenbloom. So if you take the Pill, watch your B vitamin intake. For most people over age 65, the body is
less efficient at absorbing vitamins B_6 and B_{12} and folate,

says Jeffrey Blumberg, associate director and chief of the antioxidants research laboratory at the Jean Mayer U.S. Department of Agriculture Human Nutrition Research Center on Aging at Tufts University in Boston. That's another time to eat more B-rich foods.

Seafood is also a good source of zinc, needed for immunity.

Befriend beans. Beans are a good protein choice, since they're low in fat and cholesterol, not to mention price. A cup of black beans will give you as much protein as two ounces of lean ground beef.

The fiber in beans can help lower your risk of colon cancer as well. Comparing people who got roughly 30 grams of fiber in their diets with those who consumed around 12 grams daily, researchers at the Harvard School of Public Health found that the first group had a 50 percent lower risk of developing colon tumors.

Finally, beans—like so many other plant foods— contain various protective substances collectively known as phytochemicals. Studies have found that women who eat diets rich in these plant chemicals have a lower risk of breast cancer than those who don't.

You can cook red beans into vegetarian chili, roll black beans in tortillas, dip pita shells in mashed chickpeas, or simmer beans into a beautiful dinnertime soup served with crusty French bread.

Cheese and pasta, the perfect mates. If you haven't had two servings of milk, yogurt, or cheese yet, serve yourself a dinner of pasta primavera sprinkled with two ounces of shredded nonfat mozzarella, says Dr. Rock.

If it's Friday, this must be pizza. Homemade pizza—a low-fat crust topped with low-fat cheese and steamed vegetables—can go a long way toward meeting your remaining nutritional requirements for the day, says Dr. Rock.

Calling all vegetables. Speaking of vegetables, you should invite at least one vegetable over to your dinner plate, two if you didn't have two at lunch. At least one should be dark green or deep yellow. Small and round but intriguing—truly the Danny DeVito of vegetables—Brussels sprouts are a good choice. They're a respectable source of both calcium and iron. Kale, Swiss chard, beet greens, and broccoli are top picks, too. You can add broccoli to your stir-fry, toss greens in a salad with dressing, or sauté them in a couple tablespoons of olive oil and some garlic. That way, you'll get the fat you need to absorb all those good vitamins, plus a lot of great taste.

Garnish your entrées with a couple of apple slices. It's half a serving, says Dr. Rosenbloom, but it counts.

Put dessert to work for you, not against you. Few things taste as refreshing as fresh seasonal fruit. Have some. If you're lagging in the calcium category, a frosty dish of frozen yogurt topped with fruit (and maybe a dab of chocolate syrup) would be ideal.

Make fruit sorbet. Puree fresh fruits like strawberries, then pour the mixture into ice-cube trays and freeze, says Dr. Rosenbloom.

Shake it up. Make an exquisitely delicious fruit shake by mixing sliced banana, skim milk, cinnamon, and vanilla in the blender, says Dr. Rosenbloom.

As you can see, with these pointers, good nutrition doesn't have to be a chore. You can choose and prepare deprivation-free, good-for-you meals—without a fuss.

PART 2

Know Your ABCs

Vitamin A and Beta-Carotene

Where you get it: Liver and carrots (richest sources), dark green leafy vegetables (spinach, collards, mustard greens), yellow vegetables (squash, pumpkins, sweet potatoes), yellow fruits (peaches, apricots).

What it does for you: Keeps your eyes healthy; prevents night blindness; is essential for body growth and normal tooth development; protects and maintains linings of the throat and respiratory, digestive, and urinary systems; helps with protein and glycogen synthesis.

What you need: Daily Value of 5,000 international units (IU).

Cautions: Too little can cause night blindness, stunt growth in children, promote tooth pitting and decay, create rough, dry, scaly skin, and cause reproductive disorders. Taking more than 50,000 IU per day over a long period of time can lead to headaches, blurred vision, loss of hair, dry skin (with flaking and itching), drowsiness, diarrhea, nausea, and enlargement of the liver and spleen. Acute toxicity, and even death, may occur in massive doses of 2,000,000 to 5,000,000 IU daily.

Vitamin A is probably the most important vitamin to your body. That certainly qualifies it as interesting. But more astounding is this: You need vitamin A to live but can't make it on your own, so you eat plants. And here's the rub: Plants don't have any vitamin A either.

Confused? Don't be. This little chemical conundrum is what makes vitamin A so exciting—and so important.

Three Blind Mice

Every living animal, including man, the wildest animal of all, needs vitamin A to live. Vitamin A, as a scientist would say, is the product of animal metabolism, which means that your body—and the body of every species of mammal, bird, and fish—manufactures vitamin A internally through the physiology of life and living.

Most of the vitamin A you need comes from the food you eat, particularly plants. Yet, plants themselves don't have any vitamin A. Their chemical counterpart is a similar substance called carotene, a yellow-colored, fat-soluble substance that gives the characteristic yellow-orange color to carrots. (Carotene got its name because it was first isolated from carrots more than 100 years ago.) As a result, the ultimate source of man's vitamin A comes from carotene synthesized by plants. Our bodies, and the bodies of other animals, take the carotene—also called a vitamin A precursor—and, through the wonders of our metabolic chemistry sets, turn it into vitamin A. In other words, plants have the ingredients for vitamin A, but it's your body that mixes the batter.

"To put it another way, vitamin A really isn't a true vitamin at all. Your body can make it from carotene," says Michael Janson, M.D., president of the American Preventive Medicine Association and director of the Center for Preventive Medicine in Barnstable, Massachusetts, and author of *The Vitamin Revolution in Health Care*.

As for the history of vitamin A, it is—like a

carrot—long and colorful, in part because vitamin A is older than Methuselah. Early remedies using vitamin A surfaced in ancient China, where the Chinese made vitamin A–rich concoctions to treat night blindness. Later, in Greece, Hippocrates, the father of modern medicine, did pretty much the same when he prescribed various preparations of liver to treat the same malady because liver, too, is rich in vitamin A. (Night blindness, or nyctalopia, is a condition in which your eyes lose their ability to adequately adjust to dim light.)

Such antiquated home remedies prospered through the ages but did little to clarify vitamin A's role as a chemical. That type of specific research didn't yield appreciable results until the early 1900s.

Definitive findings on vitamin A came in 1913, when four scientists operating independently in two labs discovered vitamin A by demonstrating that there was an essential substance in fatty foods. Elmer V. McCollum and Marguerite Davis of the University of Wisconsin discovered vitamin A in butter fat and egg yolks, while Thomas B. Osborne and Lafayette B. Mendel of the Connecticut Experiment Station discovered it in cod-liver oil. In those two landmark experiments, the four scientists found that the absence of vitamin A caused eye problems in animals. Two years later, McCollum and Davis fine-tuned their research to directly link vitamin A deficiency with night blindness, thus answering for good the real reason that Hippocrates was such a liver fan.

Following this pioneering work, vitamin A attracted the attention of scientists all over the world within two short decades. In 1920, an English scientist proposed the official "vitamin A" name. It was previously called fat-soluble A. Other scientists discovered

A or B-C?

When it comes to taking supplements, most experts agree that you're better off taking them to round out a healthy, nutritious diet—not to take the place of a healthy, nutritious diet. That is, except when it comes to vitamin A and beta-carotene.

Enormous amounts of vitamin A can be toxic. Too much beta-carotene, while not toxic, can turn your skin orange. The question is, if you want extra A, what do you do?

For starters, talk to your dietitian or physician. After that, consider taking beta-carotene supplements in addition to vitamin A, says Michael Janson, M.D., president of the American Preventive Medicine Association and director of the Center for Preventive Medicine in Barnstable, Massachusetts, and author of *The Vitamin Revolution in Health Care*. That's because beta-carotene is converted into vitamin A by your body at its leisure.

Beta-carotene is nontoxic, so for higher levels of intake, stick to that. But look carefully at labels that say vitamin A *with* beta-carotene. If the label doesn't specify, you can't be sure how much of each you're getting.

similar substances in other foods, like sweet potatoes and corn. These substances would later be called carotene.

Despite these exciting findings, the true defining moment for vitamin A—and a defining moment in the history of vitamins and nutrition in general—came in

1931, when a Swiss researcher isolated the active substance in halibut-liver oil and analyzed it for its chemical content. His work resulted in vitamin A being the first vitamin ever to have its chemical structure decoded. For this, researcher Paul Karrar received the Nobel prize.

A Recipe for Confusion

In comparison with that larval state of research in the early twentieth century, science today has much to say about vitamin A and carotene. Today, for example, the relationship between vitamin A and the carotenes is clear. The problem, however, is that the details are clear to scientists but not necessarily to laymen, says Maye Musk, R.D., an international nutrition consultant, speaker, and author of *Feel Fantastic*.

"Most people aren't really sure about vitamin A and carotene or beta-carotene, and rightly so," Musk says. "More than 600 carotenoids are found in nature, and 50 of them have the potential for vitamin A activity. When you say that—and throw in the fact that beta-carotene can be found in orange fruits and vegetables, like mangoes and carrots, and in green leafy vegetables, like broccoli, and that vitamin A is found in animal products—you have a recipe for confusion."

Here's the scoop: Vitamin A is a misleading name. It's not truly one substance. There are, in fact, several forms of vitamin A, each with varying degrees of potency. The two main types of vitamin A are retinol and dehydroretinol. Then there are the carotenes. These are the precursors to vitamin A, the substances found in fruits and vegetables. Carotenes help us make vitamin A through metabolism.

The four most powerful carotenes vitamin A–wise are called alpha-carotene, beta-carotene, gamma-carotene, and crypto-xanthine, which is a carotene found in corn. Of these four heavy-hitting carotenes, beta-carotene has the highest potential to create vitamin A, alone providing about two-thirds of the vitamin A that your body needs to survive. That's precisely why it gets all the attention when talk turns to vitamin A.

"These carotenes give some of those fruits and vegetables their characteristic colors," Musk says. "But just because you don't see yellow or orange doesn't mean they're not present. In other foods, like broccoli, for example, the carotene is there. It's just masked by chlorophyll, the substance that gives plants their green color."

As for its utility, vitamin A serves the body in several important ways. In addition to its well-known role in maintaining healthy vision and in preventing blindness and night blindness, vitamin A does the following:

♦ Spurs overall growth. In addition to helping growth at the cellular level, vitamin A is indirectly responsible for your sense of taste. Without enough vitamin A, the cells that make up your taste buds dry out, or keratinize, because there isn't enough vitamin A to help those cells properly develop. Because your taste buds are on the fritz, you lose your sense of taste and thus your appetite and ability to grow.

♦ Develops bones and teeth.

♦ Helps specialized cells. Vitamin A helps epithelial cells develop. These are special cells found in your skin and in the lining of mucous membranes, like those in your throat, digestive system, and of course, your eyes.

♦ Helps prevent cancer. Experts aren't exactly sure how, but vitamin A, either in its retinol or carotene form, seems to play a crucial role in warding off cancer, especially cancer of the epithelial cells.

♦ Neutralizes the nasties. Beta-carotene and vitamin A also seem to possess antioxidant properties. Antioxidants hamstring the body's rampaging free radicals, which are unstable molecules that potentially cause everything from cancer to the effects of aging.

Getting the Alpha Vitamin

Here's how to feel A-OK.

Take it easy. Your body excretes some vitamins, like C or B, when you get too much. This isn't necessarily so with vitamin A, which is why doses above 15,000 IU should be taken under medical supervision. In fact, says Musk, getting too much may result in vitamin mortality, rather than vitamin vitality.

"I generally feel that people who take supplements are the people who often need them the least," Musk says. "But with vitamin A, supplements can be even more dangerous.

"I warn people about excess vitamin A intake, which affects the central nervous system and, in extraordinarily large doses, can cause death," Musk says. "Most toxicity occurs through unhealthy and unwise supplementation."

Be careful with beta-carotene. Avoid taking too much beta-carotene, too. Despite its near-mystical appeal, you may look like a walking carrot.

"I've seen this in a few clients of mine," Musk says. "They're drinking too much carrot juice because someone told them to. Too much won't kill them, but it will turn their skin an orange-yellow because all that carotene gets stored in the skin."

Liver and Let Live

We know that this is asking a lot, but next time you're trekking through the Arctic and are tempted to hunt a polar bear, overcome the urge to fry up its liver after the field dressing.

Since 1596, Arctic explorers have known that dining on polar bear liver, or feeding it to their pack dogs, can be lethal. No one ever knew why until polar bear liver was examined in a laboratory. Then scientists discovered that polar bear liver contains up to 18,000 international units of vitamin A per gram. So when a hungry explorer or sled dog eats a modest 500-gram serving, he's consuming a staggering 9,000,000 international units of vitamin A—1,800 times the amount the human body needs in a day, according to the U.S. government, and more than enough to ruin the expedition.

Incidentally, your own liver is where most of your vitamin A is stored. Right now, if you're eating a healthy diet, your liver has enough vitamin A to last you roughly 4 to 12 months. But you can bet that it doesn't have enough to poison a polar bear.

Seek a variety of food sources. Not only will you get healthier amounts of vitamin A and beta-carotene that way but also you'll be on the road to an overall healthy diet that will serve you well. Moreover, eating a varied, healthy diet—especially one rich in produce—will expose you to more of the carotenes than just beta-carotene.

"This is the reason why I recommend eating a variety of produce. Why limit yourself to just one carotene when you can benefit from many?" Musk says.

Look it up. Although vitamin A deficiency isn't something to worry about in the United States, about half of the more than 80,000 children in Third World nations who go blind each year from a lack of vitamin A eventually die. Make sure to get enough in your diet—but not too much—and be thankful that you can.

Don't let your food get fresh air. Although vitamin A and carotenes are relatively hardy, they do lose potency when exposed to the air. Store animal fat products in cold, dark places. And keep fish-liver oils, like cod-liver oil, in dark bottles (also in dark places) to preserve their levels of vitamin A and carotene.

Don't let Baby get too much A. Too much vitamin A supplementation taken in the first three months of pregnancy has been linked with birth defects, even when the amount was 4,000 IU, which is 1,000 IU less than the Daily Value. If you're pregnant, make sure you stick to the prenatal vitamins that your doctor prescribes to make sure you're not getting more vitamin A than you need, warns Musk.

Vitamin B Complex

Think of the B vitamins as the little wooden blocks in the game Jenga, where you attempt to dismantle and then rebuild a tower—piece by piece—without causing a collapse. Without the right piece in the right place, the rest of the tower crumbles or is in danger of crumbling. Only together, in unison, can the separate pieces attain their ultimate goal of working together.

That's a pretty good picture of how the B-complex vitamins work. Yet the B vitamins are so often broken down into their individual pieces that people rarely get to know or appreciate them as a whole. To be sure, those individual pieces are important—vital, even. But in the case of the B vitamins, you have to see the whole to understand the parts, and you have to understand the parts to appreciate the whole. But frankly, it's tough to figure out what the parts even are. Some go by letters (B_6, B_{12}), some by names (riboflavin, thiamin). It can all seem so, well, complex.

"Most energy metabolism pathways use one or more of the B vitamins, so you can understand their importance," says Cindy J. Fuller, R.D., Ph.D., assistant professor of food, nutrition, and food service management at the University of North Carolina at Greensboro. "One reason why the B vitamins as a whole are difficult to understand is because they have so many names. The reason is historical."

Here's the history and the mystery of the B vitamins revealed.

Eight Is Enough

As Dr. Fuller said, the vitamin B family, called the vitamin B complex, can be difficult to understand, in part, because of its many names. So let's start from the beginning.

The vitamin B complex is comprised of eight members. All the B vitamins are water-soluble, meaning that they dissolve in water. Why is that important? Because solubility affects your body's ability to absorb vitamins. Water-soluble vitamins, which include vitamin C and the vitamin B complex, are absorbed directly into the blood. Fat-soluble vitamins aren't.

"In concert, the B vitamins are a fascinating lot in that they're all necessary in fat, carbohydrate, and protein metabolism," says Mara Vitolins, R.D., Dr. P.H., nutrition research coordinator for the Bowman Gray School of Medicine of Wake Forest University in Winston-Salem, North Carolina.

"While you need certain individual B vitamins for specific reasons—niacin, for example, or you run the risk of adverse effects such as fatigue, irritability, or digestive and skin disorders—you also need the B vitamins as a whole," Dr. Vitolins says. In general, the B vitamins are found in green leafy vegetables and whole grains. "However, B_{12} is unusual because you can only get it from animal products, which is why there are sometimes B_{12} deficiencies in pure vegetarians," Dr. Vitolins says.

"The funny thing is that there are millions of dollars spent every year on vitamin B research, and a lot of the time it comes down to this: You need them all, so

Mom was right. Your best approach is to eat a variety of healthy nutritious foods," Dr. Vitolins says.

The role that many of the B vitamins play in the body is what you'd call an official helper-outer. We'll spare you more technical jargon, but suffice it to say that the B vitamins are crucial in providing coenzymes that assist in metabolism. (Coenzymes assist enzymes, protein catalysts that spark vital chemical reactions in the body.) Some B vitamin coenzymes facilitate energy-releasing reactions. Others build new cells to help deliver oxygen and nutrients.

In short, the eight members of the vitamin B complex perform thousands of functions in the body, including the creation of DNA and thus the creation of new cells. Moreover, they act interdependently, meaning, for example, that a lack of riboflavin (one B vitamin) will inhibit the work of vitamin B_6, which needs riboflavin to change into coenzyme form.

"B vitamins, in general, are particularly good for your nervous system, and that's how they'll enhance your functioning," says Richard F. Gerson, Ph.D., a health and fitness consultant in Clearwater, Florida. "But, again, you need the entire B complex. You can't just pick and choose which B vitamins you want to get without doing your body a disservice."

The only problem is that it's hard to tell the B vitamin players without a program. So here it is. On the following pages, we'll detail each of the "Killer Bs" for you.

Folic Acid

Where you get it: Liver, beans, green leafy vegetables.

What it does for you: Helps in DNA synthesis

and cell growth, is a major player for red blood cells, and is crucial in creating amino acids.

What You Need: Daily Value of 400 micrograms.

Cautions: Too little can cause anemia and gastrointestinal problems. It's almost impossible to get too much; however, supplementation in amounts greater than 400 micrograms can mask a vitamin B_{12} deficiency.

Next time you're walking through the woods on a crisp autumn afternoon, take a mind-cleansing breath of fresh air and pause under the cobalt blue sky. Then take a gander at the trees and observe nature's palette of colors. The reds, the yellows, the greens, the browns, and all the in-betweens.

Now think of folic acid.

The connection between leaves and the vitamin called folic acid isn't merely a product of our overactive imaginations. It's a real link, one that scientists made decades ago when they discovered folic acid in 1941. A group of researchers in Texas coined the term *folic acid* after finding a mysterious substance in spinach that spurred growth in bacteria. They suspected, correctly, that the substance was widely available in green leafy plants, so they called it *folic*, from the Latin word *folium*, meaning "foliage or leaf."

Like an autumn leaf, folic acid in its pure form is colorful. It's bright yellow, crystalline, and powdery. It's also unstable, unable to withstand even something as innocuous as light, which destroys it immediately. Yet folic acid is strangely powerful. Without it, you'd be destroyed immediately.

Passing the Folic Acid Test

Folic acid—known as folate when it's found naturally in food—is responsible for more than a half dozen

The Fickleness of Folic Acid

For such a critical vitamin, folic acid suffers from an identity crisis. It goes by more names than an escaped felon.

Here's a list of folic acid's most commonly used aliases.

■ Folic acid: The first name given for folate. It's what people generally mean when they talk folates.

■ Folate: This designates a group of closely related substances. It's the vitamin found naturally in foods and is essential for all animal life.

■ Folacin: *See* Folate.

■ Pteroylglutamic acid: The chemical name for folic acid.

■ Wills' factor: Named after Lucy Wills, an early folic acid researcher in Bombay, India, who, in 1931, discovered that pregnant women with anemia became less anemic after being given yeast.

■ Vitamin M, vitamin B_c, vitamin B_9, vitamin B_{10}, vitamin B_{11}, vitamin U: Labels given to folate by early researchers.

■ SLR factor, factor R, factor U, *Lactobacillus casei* factor, citrovoram factor, and yeast Norit eluate factor: Other early names for folate.

life-sustaining functions in the human body. It's pivotal in creating several types of amino acids, the building blocks of protein and the stuff that we're made of. It's also critical in creating heme, the iron-laden substance in hemoglobin. Hemoglobin is the mainstay of red blood cells, which are crucial to every breath we take.

Folic acid plays an important role in cell division and protein synthesis, two functions that you need to live. Without enough folic acid, your cells wouldn't grow or function. One of the first things to falter is red blood cell production. Another thing to go would be your gut. It follows, then, that the first two symptoms of folate deficiency are generally anemia (where your body produces large but ineffective red blood cells) and stomach problems, including diarrhea, heartburn, and constipation.

Experts are discovering that folic acid might be important to your heart. Researchers in Ottawa, Canada, examined data from more than 5,000 middle-age and older men and women and found that those with the most folic acid were 69 percent less likely to die of heart disease than those with the least folic acid. "Folate may have some promise in treatment and prevention of heart disease, but all the scientific data is not there yet," says Dr. Fuller.

What's more, folic acid may help protect against cancers of the lung, colon, and cervix. Folic acid also protects a woman's fetus from life-threatening birth defects of the brain and spine. Unfortunately, a survey by the March of Dimes found that 90 percent of women of reproductive age are unaware of this fact, and only 15 percent are aware that the federal government has recommended that all women capable of bearing children get 400 micrograms of folic acid every day.

Here are some folate-related things that may be of personal interest.

Have a cup. At dinnertime, turn to the right stuff to get most of the folate you need. Your best bets are green leafy vegetables (especially spinach) and lentils, two of the most folate-packed foods around. A half-cup serving of cooked lentils has nearly all you need for a day, while a cup of cooked spinach packs in almost 50 percent. Other good bean sources are pinto, navy, lima, and kidney beans.

Keep it fresh. Cooking kills between 50 and 95 percent of your food's folate. While you shouldn't lose a tooth filling crunching on uncooked kidney beans, avoid cooking folate-rich food whenever possible—or cook it as little as possible. Lightly steam, instead of boiling, your broccoli or consider a fresh spinach salad instead of boiling it as a side dish.

Don't wait for folate. Folic acid is not a fine wine. It doesn't improve with age. Raw vegetables stored at room temperature for two to three days may lose 50 to 70 percent of their folate.

Don't let your folate go up in smoke. Smoking retards your body's ability to use folic acid, especially in a localized way. It has been shown that smokers' lungs show a localized deficiency compared with the lungs of nonsmokers. (Reason Number 6,770 to quit.) Certain drugs such as aspirin and antacids also can inhibit folic acid. Most healthy adults eating a good diet shouldn't worry about taking an occasional aspirin or antacid, but chronic users, such as people with arthritis or ulcers, should question their doctors.

Vitamin B₆

Where you get it: Rice bran, wheat bran, sunflower seeds, avocados, bananas, lean meat, fish, corn, brown rice, whole grains.

What it does for you: Helps metabolize protein, carbohydrates, and fats. Involved with hemoglobin formation, the absorption of amino acids, and the central nervous system.

What you need: Daily Value of 2 milligrams.

Cautions: Too little can cause irritability, depression, muscle weakness, and greasy scaliness of the skin around the eyes, nose, and mouth. Too much is nearly impossible, but megadoses of 50 milligrams to 2 grams daily can result in an unstable gait, numb feet, sleepiness, and physiologic dependence when taken over the long haul.

As you're probably learning is the case with many vitamins, vitamin B_6 isn't just one substance. It's actually three chemically similar substances—pyridoxine, pyridoxal, and pyridoxamine—collectively called B_6, by virtue of international agreement. Its need was first demonstrated in laboratory rats, and it has since been found necessary to sustain life in pigs, chicks, dogs, and other animal species, including microorganisms and, of course, humans.

The key breakthrough in discovering B_6 came in 1926, when two scientists tried to reproduce pellagra in rats. (Pellagra, from *pelle*, meaning "skin," and *agra*, meaning "rough," is a vitamin B deficiency marked by scaly, flaky dark skin; dementia; and diarrhea.) They succeeded, and eight years later a Hungarian scientist produced a cure from yeast extract. The substance extracted was not one of the recognized B vitamins—niacin, riboflavin, or thiamin—so he named it vitamin B_6. By 1940, five independent laboratories, working alone, isolated vitamin B_6 in crystalline form; it was also called pyridoxine, after its chemical makeup. Two years later, further research revealed two similar substances, which were named pyridoxal and pyridoxamine.

Today, we know that all three white crystalline substances are rightfully called vitamin B_6. We also know that these compounds are easily absorbed in the upper part of the small intestine and are present in almost all body tissue, with a high concentration in the liver. They're secreted into milk during lactation and excreted primarily through urine. Vitamin B_6 is easily dissolved in water, quite resistant to heat and acid, but easily destroyed by oxidation, exposure to alkalis, and ultraviolet light.

Of the three forms, pyridoxine is the most resistant to food processing and storage conditions and is probably the form that you're getting most in your food.

As for what B_6 does, the question is more like what it doesn't do. Vitamin B_6 is involved in a large number of physiologic activities, many of which are crucial to survival. Vitamin B_6 plays a large role in protein metabolism, helps form hemoglobin, and aids in absorbing amino acids from the intestine. It also plays a part in metabolizing fat and carbohydrates. Moreover, scientists have linked vitamin B_6, or the lack thereof, to several clinical maladies, including the following:

♦ Central nervous system breakdowns. Vitamin B_6 helps with energy transformation in the brain and nerve tissue. When it's lacking, the result can be convulsive seizures.

♦ Autism. Although more research is needed, a number of experiments show promise that megadoses of vitamin B_6 under a doctor's supervision may ameliorate autism, a severe disturbance of mental and emotional development in young children.

♦ Kidney stones. Lack of vitamin B_6 has been linked to an increased formation of kidney stones.

Here is more on how you can make the most of vitamin B₆.

Watch for losses. Wheat loses more than 75 percent of its vitamin B_6 when it's milled into white flour. Beef loses 25 to 50 percent of its B_6 stores when it's cooked (more through oven braising than oven roasting). And cooking vegetables and fruits at home results in losses of 50 percent or more. Keep this in mind next time you make a B_6-conscious eating decision—the less processed your food, the better it will be B-wise.

De-emphasize diabetes damage. If you have diabetes, ask your doctor about vitamin B_6 supplements. "People with diabetes experience less of the numbness and tingling of diabetes-related nerve damage if they get supplements of B vitamins, most notably B_6," says John Marion Ellis, M.D., a retired physician in Mount Pleasant, Texas, who spent most of his professional life researching vitamin B_6.

See the light at the end of the carpal tunnel. If your job has you pounding a keyboard for eight hours a day—or doing any other repetitive task for hours on end, like working on an assembly line—you have a vested interest in knowing more about vitamin B_6 because it may be helpful in preventing carpal tunnel syndrome.

"You couldn't say enough about carpal tunnel and vitamin B_6—the evidence is that positive," says Dr. Ellis. He contends that the swelling and inelasticity of the sheath surrounding nerves in the wrist may be caused by a lack of vitamin B_6.

Get to the meat of the matter. About 41 percent of all available vitamin B_6 comes from meat, poultry, and fish. That's not to say that you should overdo it on the meat or that there isn't a world of good from a diet rich in vegetables. But it's something to keep in mind when someone castigates you for enjoying your once-a-month rib eye.

Vitamin B_{12}

Where you get it: Liver and organ meats, muscle meats, shellfish, eggs, cheese, fish.

What it does for you: Aids in red blood cell formation and in the prevention of pernicious anemia (impaired absorption of vitamin B_{12} in the intestine), maintains nerve tissue, and helps metabolize carbohydrates, fats, and proteins.

What you need: Daily Value of 6 micrograms.

Cautions: Too little, sometimes seen in strict vegetarians, can cause sore tongue, weakness, weight loss, back pain, and apathy. There are no known toxic effects from too much—leftovers are excreted through urine.

Like vitamin B_6, vitamin B_{12} isn't just one substance. It's actually several compounds, all of which contain cobalt, giving them the generic name of cobalamins. When not otherwise indicated, the substance assumed to be in question when talk turns to B_{12} is cyanocobalamin, the most active compound. The other compounds are hydroxocobalamin, nitritocobalamin, and thiocyanate cobalamin.

As you'd probably guess from its tongue-twisting names, B_{12} has the distinct honor of having the largest and most complex chemical structure of any vitamin known to man. Just looking at a diagram of its chemical components is dizzying, so you can imagine the enigma that it presented to early researchers.

The first B_{12} research was the result of work by Thomas Addison, a London physician, who first described an illness that was later determined to come from a lack of B_{12}. Dr. Addison described in 1849 a type of anemia that progressed slowly and killed its victims in two to five years. It was so insidious that it was described as pernicious anemia and later became known as Addisonian pernicious anemia in his honor. It took more than 70 years for something to be done about pernicious anemia, starting in 1925 with research by George Hoyt Whipple, M.D., former dean of the University of Rochester School of Medicine and Dentistry in New York. Dr. Whipple showed that liver was beneficial in treating anemia in dogs. A year later, two researchers from Harvard Medical School elaborated on Dr. Whipple's findings, determining that four to eight ounces of raw liver a day overcame pernicious anemia. For their discoveries, they and Dr. Whipple were awarded the Nobel prize in 1934.

It wasn't until 1948, however, that researchers isolated a red, crystalline substance that they called vitamin B_{12} from a liver. Later that same year, researchers at Columbia University in New York City found that B_{12} abated pernicious anemia, and seven years later, a second Nobel prize was awarded for B_{12} research, this time going to Dorothy Hodgkin and co-workers at Oxford University in England, for deciphering the complex chemical structure of B_{12}.

Today, we know many more fascinating things about B_{12}. Unlike any other vitamin, it cannot be synthesized by plants, which is why it's found almost exclusively in meat and meat products. It is the only vitamin that requires specific juices from your gastrointestinal tract to be absorbed. And B_{12} absorption takes a remarkably long time—about three hours, compared with just seconds for other water-soluble vitamins.

Moreover, vitamin B_{12} is remarkably potent and durable. In the cooking process, only 30 percent of a food's B_{12} content may be lost. Its synthetic form has a potency level some 11,000 times that found in the standard liver concentrate once used to treat pernicious anemia. Deficiencies of vitamin B_{12} have been linked to two major areas of health concerns. They are:

♦ Central nervous system problems. A raft of problems have been linked to vitamin B_{12} deficiencies, including memory loss, confusion, delusion, fatigue, loss of balance, decreased reflexes, numbness and tingling in the hands, and ringing in the ears. It has also been linked to multiple sclerosis–like symptoms and dementia. "In a severe deficiency, there is actually a degeneration of the myelin sheath. The stuff begins to literally erode," says John Pinto, Ph.D., associate professor of biochemistry in medicine at Cornell University Medical College and director of the nutrition research laboratory at Memorial Sloan-Kettering Cancer Center, both in New York City. (Myelin is a fatty sheath of tissue that insulates nerve fibers, keeping electrical pulses humming through your body.)

♦ Dangerous chemical imbalance. Research shows that a lack of B_{12} raises the levels of a substance called homocysteine. Homocysteine, in high doses, is toxic to the brain, raising questions about its potential role in Alzheimer's disease; it has also been suggested as a primary cause of heart disease.

Here's how not to be a B_{12} bomber when it comes to getting the nutrition you need.

Be a dairy king. Pure vegans—people who eat only plant foods—may be seriously deficient in vitamin

B_{12}. But if you stopped eating foods that contain B_{12} today, it might take up to 20 years to show signs of deficiency. That's because your body will continue to recycle its B_{12} for as long as it can, reabsorbing it over and over. And even when that stops happening, it will take some 3 years to deplete your body's extreme emergency conservation supplies.

If you opt for a vegetarian lifestyle, consider being a lacto-ovo vegetarian, meaning that you permit yourself eggs and milk. (Just one cup of milk, one egg, or $3\frac{1}{2}$ ounces of cheese a day is all you need to protect against B_{12} deficiency.) Or, says Dr. Vitolins, include meat replacement foods in your diet, like vegetarian burgers, which are textured vegetable-protein products fortified with nutrients often found in real meat.

Don't hit the bottle. As if you'd really need a reason not to drink excessively, here's one vitamin-wise: Excess alcohol, especially when coupled with an unhealthy diet, can rob your body of B vitamins, especially B_{12}, according to international nutrition consultant and speaker Maye Musk, author of *Feel Fantastic*. "The people who have come to see me have not been alcoholics. They may have been heavy drinkers, but they wanted to follow a healthy lifestyle," Musk adds. "They can by making better food choices and drinking less."

Don't let your B_{12} dry up. Milk is a good source of B_{12}, as we mentioned before. But stick to regular, low-fat milk. Pasteurization results in a loss of only 10 percent of B_{12}, whereas evaporated milk loses up to 90 percent of its B_{12}.

Add B_{12} as you age. Because the inner workings of your digestive system change as you grow older, there is serious concern that there might be a grand-scale B_{12} deficiency among the elderly. Even when they do eat meat and drink milk, up to one-third of all people over age 60 can't extract the B_{12} they need from their food because their stomachs no longer produce enough gastric acid. (Remember that B_{12} requires specific gastric juices to be absorbed.) If you're over age 60 or have a loved one who is, ask your doctor about the feasibility of getting a B_{12} shot or using supplementation to curb these effects.

Get it in food. It's easy to put away a health food store–size helping of B_{12} and not get sick—in simply eating your meals. Vitamin B_{12} has no known toxic effects, and because it's easy to get adequate amounts of B_{12} from food alone, there's probably no need to take a B_{12} supplement unless you're told to do so by your doctor.

"B vitamins are widespread in healthy diets. If a B vitamin is lacking, it's probably because your diet is poor," says Musk.

Thiamin (Vitamin B₁)

Where you get it: Enriched cornflakes, sunflower seeds, peanuts, wheat bran, enriched rice, enriched white bread, beef liver, egg yolk, lima beans, refried beans.

What it does for you: Necessary component in energy metabolism, nerve maintenance and functioning, and muscle maintenance and functioning. Maintains healthy appetite and healthy mental attitude.

What you need: Daily Value of 1.5 milligrams.

Cautions: Too little can lead to fatigue, apathy, loss of appetite, depression, and numbness in legs. Extreme deficiency can lead to beriberi, a serious inflammation of the nerves. No known toxic effects.

When it comes to turning the starches and sugars in your breakfast bowl into energy that your body can use, this vitamin is number one. Or to be precise, number B_1. But you can just call it thiamin.

Discovered during the long years of research that led to a cure for beriberi, this vitamin was first dubbed water-soluble B by researcher Elmer V. McCollum of the University of Wisconsin in 1916. Ten years later, two researchers in Holland isolated the exact chemical, which, in 1936, was chemically identified and synthesized by American Robert R. Williams, who named it *thiamine*, because it contained sulfur—from *thio*, meaning "sulfur-containing," and *amine*, the name for organic compounds derived from ammonia. (The final "e" was later dropped.)

Since then, we've learned a lot more about this beriberi-important vitamin, including the following:

♦ Thiamin is a crystalline white powder, with a faint yeastlike odor and a salty, nutty taste.

♦ Thiamin is the least stored vitamin in the body. Your liver, kidneys, heart, brain, and muscles hold the most, but there's still only about 30 milligrams total in the entire body. Moreover, your thiamin reserve can be depleted in just one to two weeks without continual reinforcement.

♦ Thiamin provides one of the most miraculous cures known to modern medicine. A patient ridden with wet beriberi can lie in bed, apparently dying, breathless, and virtually drowning from edema, an internal accumulation of body fluids. But within two hours after being given a thiamin injection, that patient can be back on his feet, almost fully recovered.

♦ Thiamin is necessary for muscle tone and nerve function. It's also responsible for energy production, for without thiamin, there could be no metabolic energy. Likewise, it plays a critical role in maintaining a healthy mental attitude.

"If you dramatically reduce thiamin intake, you reduce the ability of the brain to use glucose and to make neurotransmitters. And if you reduce that, you have impaired mental function," says Gary E. Gibson, Ph.D., professor of neuroscience at Cornell University Medical College's Burke Medical Research Institute in White Plains, New York.

Here are details on getting more thiamin.

Eat extra well if you're active. Active bodies need more energy (and thus more food) than sedentary ones. Make doubly sure that your diet is rich in an array of healthy foods and is especially heavy on the grains, fruits, and vegetables. The healthier food you'll be eating should ensure that you're getting enough thiamin to keep you active.

Pour a bowl of thiamin in the morning. Breakfast cereal is commonly fortified with thiamin and other nutrients, making it a good way to start the day. Ditto for enriched and whole-grain breads, which make a nice complement to healthy cereal. Since the U.S. government began the enrichment plan for flour and bread in 1941, more than 40 percent of every person's daily requirement of thiamin is supplied by these foods.

Convert now. Converted rice—rice that's soaked and parboiled—is a better source of thiamin than rice that was milled from its raw state. Parboiling causes thiamin and other water-soluble nutrients to move from the outer layers to the inner layers of the rice kernel, so fewer of them are removed in the milling process.

Don't add soda to preserve the green. There's an old wives' tale that adding baking soda to the water in which you're boiling green vegetables will preserve their color. Maybe so, but it kills their thiamin. Baking soda is an alkali, and alkalies easily destroy thiamin.

Riboflavin (Vitamin B₂)

Where you get it: Organ meats, enriched corn-flakes, almonds, cheese, eggs, lean meats (beef, pork, lamb), enriched white bread, milk.

What it does for you: Helps the body use oxygen; assists in metabolizing amino acids, fatty acids, and carbohydrates; helps activate vitamin B_6; helps create niacin (vitamin B_3); aids the adrenal gland.

What you need: Daily Value of 1.7 milligrams.

Cautions: Too little isn't much danger but can contribute to other B vitamin deficiencies. Some deficiency symptoms include sore, swollen, chapped lips; painful tongue; oily, scaly skin; and redness and congestion of the cornea. No known toxicity.

Riboflavin's roots lie in milk scum. Maybe that sounds pretty gross, but it's not far from the truth. Pure riboflavin was first isolated in 1933 from milk by a German scientist as part of an ongoing process to identify a yellow-green fluorescent substance in milk whey that had been identified as early as the late 1800s. The substance had previously been identified as some type of pigment—a pigment subsequently found in a variety of other sources, including liver, heart, and egg whites. Called flavin, the pigment remained an enigma to researchers, who couldn't find a biological reason for its existence.

It wasn't until the mid-1930s, thanks largely to German and Swiss researchers, that scientists learned more about this mysterious pigment, which was later named riboflavin because it has ribitol as part of its flavin chemical structure.

Not much has changed since then. Unlike research on the other B vitamins during that era—and research on the antioxidant darlings of today (vitamins A, C, and E)—riboflavin research has remained fairly low-key. "It's not fashionable per se, but you're going to be hearing more about it," says Jack M. Cooperman, Ph.D., clinical professor of community and preventive medicine at New York Medical College in Valhalla. "The key concept to remember here is that riboflavin is one of the essential B vitamins necessary for antioxidant activity inside the body."

We know today that riboflavin is absorbed in the small intestine and that the body has a limited capacity for storing it. What little is stored is stored in the liver and kidneys. Whatever else the body needs must be taken in on a daily basis through diet. Leftovers are primarily excreted through the urine. In pure form, riboflavin looks like fine orange-yellow crystals, bitter-tasting and virtually odorless. In water-based solutions, they impart a strange green-yellow glow. Riboflavin is easily destroyed by light, which is partly why milk isn't stored in clear, glass bottles anymore.

In the body, riboflavin's main role is in energy release, which it accomplishes along with a group of enzymes called flavoproteins. Riboflavin is also thought to be a component in the retinal pigment in the eye, involved in the function of the adrenal gland and in the production of corticosteroids in the adrenal cortex.

Here's how to maximize your riboflavin for ultimate vitamin vitality.

Don't make special attempts. Most people easily meet their recommended amounts and don't need to make a special effort to get more riboflavin in their diets. The average person gets one-half of his riboflavin from milk and milk products, one-fourth from meats, and the rest from green vegetables, whole-grain or enriched bread, and cereal products.

Choose cartons when you can. When you buy your milk, choose cardboard cartons. They won't let riboflavin-robbing light in. Opaque plastic jugs work well, too, but avoid glass bottles and other clear containers. Two hours of light can destroy 50 percent or more of milk's riboflavin.

Niacin

Where you get it: Liver, lean meats, poultry, fish, rabbit, enriched cornflakes, nuts, peanut butter, milk, cheese, eggs, sunflower seeds.

What it does for you: Serves as important coenzyme necessary for cell respiration. Helps release energy from carbohydrates, fats, and proteins. Aids growth, reduces cholesterol, and may protect against heart attack.

What you need: Daily Value of 20 milligrams.

Cautions: Too little can cause pellagra. Too much is usually not seen, except when given medicinally. Large doses, over 100 milligrams, should be taken only under medical supervision because they can cause flushing of the skin, itching, liver damage, elevated blood glucose, and peptic ulcers.

Niacin's discovery came almost single-handedly

from mankind's fight against pellagra, a disease that results in diarrhea, dementia, and a darkening flaking away of the skin. Initially uncommon in Europe, pellagra was first described by Spanish physician Gaspar Casal in 1730, soon after corn was introduced to the European diet. By the nineteenth century, pellagra was widespread in Europe, Africa, and the Americas, particularly in the impoverished, post-Civil War South, where corn was the only sustenance widely available. So widespread and insidious was pellagra that doctors thought it was caused by an infectious agent or a toxic substance found in spoiled corn.

In a strange twist, the cure for pellagra—niacin—was discovered in 1867 by a German chemist, who extracted nicotinic acid (a natural form of niacin) from nicotine in tobacco. However, it would be another 70 years before the connection between niacin and pellagra would be made. By the early 1900s, pellagra had reached epidemic proportions in the southern United States, killing 10,000 people in 1915 and accounting for some 200,000 cases between 1917 and 1918.

In 1914, the U.S. Public Health Service dispatched a team of physicians and researchers to find a cure. By 1925, Joseph Goldberger, M.D., the initiative's leader, found that pellagra resulted from a dietary deficiency, not an infectious agent, and that certain foods—notably yeast, lean meats, and milk—helped prevent it. By 1937, thanks to the initial pioneering, researchers at the University of Wisconsin discovered that two substances, collectively called niacin, were essential when it came to preventing pellagra.

Today, nutritionists know that niacin is actually a collective name for two essential substances, nicotinic acid and nicotinamide, both natural forms of niacin.

Since this discovery, pellagra is rare in the United States. It's also rare in Latin American countries and Mexico, despite the prevalence of corn in their diets. This rarity stems from the ancient Mexican tradition of soaking corn flour in limewater to make it easier to knead. This process releases the corn's niacin, which would otherwise be chemically bound and inaccessible to the body. Africa is the only continent where pellagra remains a public health concern.

Biologically, little niacin is stored in the body. Your body uses what it needs and excretes the rest in urine. What is used goes toward energy metabolism. It also seems helpful in lowering cholesterol, though its boon here is a double-edged sword.

"In the right hands, it's very useful medication. It lowers harmful cholesterol and raises good cholesterol better than any drug we have," says James McKenney, Pharm.D., professor of pharmacy at Virginia Commonwealth University Medical College of Virginia School of Pharmacy in Richmond. "But taken indiscriminately by an uninformed person without a professional monitoring his condition, it can be dangerous."

According to Robert C. Atkins, M.D., founder and director of the Atkins Center for Complementary Medicine in New York City who publishes *Dr. Atkins' Health Revelations* newsletter, a daily dose of 1,500 to 3,000 milligrams can reduce low-density lipoprotein (LDL) cholesterol (the "bad" kind) by 10 to 25 percent, while raising high-density lipoprotein (HDL) cholesterol (the "good" kind) by 15 to 35 percent. However, supplementing at these high doses should be attempted only under strict medical supervision.

Large doses of nicotinic acid have a druglike effect on the nervous system and on the blood. They can dilate blood vessels so much that you feel a tingling sensation, sometimes painful, known as a niacin flush. (The nicotinamide form of niacin doesn't have this effect.) High doses of niacin may also damage the liver and possibly produce diabetes.

Here's what you need to know about niacin.

Take top natural sources. Aim to get most of your required niacin from natural sources. Prized picks include beef liver, tuna (in water), mushrooms, chicken breast, salmon, and asparagus.

Go easy on the water. Because niacin, like all B vitamins, is water-soluble, some 15 to 25 percent of it can disappear quickly if you're cooking with water. That said, it's the most stable of the B vitamins and will otherwise remain resistant to just about every type of food preparation you're bound to do on a given day.

Serve up cereal. Cereal and cereal products are fair sources of niacin because the government in the 1940s mandated that these products be fortified with niacin. Ditto for enriched white flour. (Incidentally, thiamin and riboflavin are added, too.)

Pour a strong cup of niacin. Coffee is a good source of niacin—a cup of dark-roast alone provides some 3 milligrams. In some areas of the world, where diets are low in niacin, a large consumption of coffee is thought to prevent widespread cases of pellagra.

Biotin

Where you get it: Cheese, beef liver, cauliflower, eggs, mushrooms, chicken breast, salmon, spinach.

What it does for you: Metabolizes fats, proteins, and carbohydrates; helps in the transfer of carbon dioxide; and assists in various metabolic chemical conversions.

What you need: Daily Value of 300 micrograms.

Cautions: Too little can lead to dry, scaly skin; loss of appetite; vomiting; nausea; mental depression; tongue inflammation; and high cholesterol. No known toxic effects.

Biotin plays an important role in metabolism by acting as a coenzyme that helps transport carbon dioxide from compound to compound. (Coenzymes assist enzymes in making metabolic reactions come to fruition.) It also helps convert various substances that are chemically important in processes like protein synthesis, the formation of long-chain fatty acids, and in the Krebs cycle, which is the process that releases energy from foods.

The average U.S. biotin intake is estimated to be 100 to 300 micrograms a day, and you're probably getting all you need by eating a healthy, well-rounded diet.

"The people who need to worry about biotin most are bodybuilders who eat raw eggs," says Musk. The reason is because raw eggs contain a biotin-binding substance called avidin. That can keep the body from absorbing the biotin it needs. "It's rare and I've never come across it, but it happens," Musk says. There are no known toxic levels of biotin.

Pantothenic Acid

Where you get it: Liver, wheat bran, rice bran, nuts, mushrooms, soybean flour, salmon, blue cheese, eggs, brown rice, lobster.

What it does for you: Helps create energy by breaking down fats, proteins, and carbohydrates; helps form a substance that is important in transmitting nerve impulses; and helps synthesize cholesterol and steroid hormones formed in the adrenal gland.

What you need: Daily Value of 10 milligrams.

Cautions: Too little leads to irritability, loss of appetite, abdominal pains, nausea, headache, mental depression, fatigue and weakness, muscle cramps, tingling in hands and feet, insomnia, respiratory infections, and a staggering gait. Doses of 10,000 to 20,000 milligrams per day are not toxic but can cause occasional diarrhea and water retention.

Pantothenic acid is involved in more than 100 different steps in the creation of lipids, neurotransmitters, steroid hormones, and hemoglobin. It's also a factor in growth and is essential for human life. Moreover, pantothenic acid is common, found in many foods. (Its name comes from the Greek word *pantothen*, meaning "everywhere.")

Pantothentic acid functions in the body as part of two enzymes, indirectly aiding in the building and breakdown of fatty acids; the creation of antibodies; the metabolism of fats, proteins, and carbohydrates; and energy metabolism. It's also influential on the endocrine glands and the hormones they produce.

Though found in many foods, pantothenic acid has one major drawback: It's easily destroyed in massive amounts by food processing. A study done at Dartmouth Medical School in Hanover, New Hampshire, found that 58 percent is lost from milling wheat into all-purpose flour; up to 79 percent is lost by canning vegetables; and just over 26 percent is lost by canning meat and poultry. Canning seafood destroys almost 20 percent of the pantothenic acid.

Here are a couple of other things to keep in mind about pantothenic acid.

Stick to cereal grains. Pantothenic acid is reasonably stable in natural foods during storage. Some cereal grains may be kept for up to a year without appreciable loss.

Gut it out. Sticking to a healthy diet and lifestyle ensures that your intestinal flora—the bacteria naturally occurring in your digestive system—stay healthy. That's important when it comes to pantothenic acid because it is synthesized by intestinal bacteria. However, scientists aren't sure how much pantothenic acid is produced by the body or how much is used, a strong argument in favor of doing all you can to keep those bacteria—and the rest of you—healthy.

Vitamin C

Where you get it: Green leafy vegetables (broccoli, Brussels sprouts), red cabbage, citrus fruits (oranges, grapefruits, lemons), guavas, parsley, mustard greens.

What it does for you: Helps form and maintain collagen. Is an excellent wound healer. Metabolizes amino acids, fats, and lipids. Helps iron absorption. Promotes strong teeth, bones, and capillary walls. Possibly boosts immunity and prevents colds, infections, and cancer.

What you need: Daily Value of 60 milligrams, 100 milligrams a day if you smoke.

Cautions: Too little causes scurvy, which may lead to massive internal bleeding and heart failure. Too much is hard to do, but side effects, reported at levels more than 33 times the Daily Value, include cramps, nausea, diarrhea, destruction of red blood cells, and kidney and bladder stone formation.

In today's world, James Lind's brand of science wouldn't get past the gate guard at a major university. Yet Lind, a British naval surgeon who lived in the mid-1700s, is responsible for discovering the most compelling thing we know about vitamin C today: Without it, you die a slow, painful, bloody death.

Lind's early experiments with vitamin C hardly met today's scientific criteria. It wasn't what you'd call a randomized, controlled, double-blind clinical trial, the gold standard of modern testing. "In other words, from the scientific community's standpoint, there was no significant compelling evidence," says Michael Janson, M.D., president of the American Preventive Medicine Association and director of the Center for Preventive Medicine in Barnstable, Massachusetts, and author of *The Vitamin Revolution in Health Care*.

Lind tested six pairs of sailors ravaged by scurvy, a vitamin C deficiency that literally destroys the body from the inside out. (Of course, no one knew that at the time.) He treated each pair with doses of either cider, vinegar, sulfuric acid, seawater, oranges and lemons, or a spice mixture. Sailors treated with the citrus fruits recovered within a week. The rest, presumably, wound up resting with Davy Jones on the ocean floor. Despite their promise, Lind's findings weren't published for 6 years. More astonishing, they weren't put to use for another 50 years.

The Old Man and the C

Vitamin C today is perhaps the most widely studied vitamin. It gets its scientific name, ascorbic acid, from "anti-scurvy acid." Of all substances in Nutritionland, it's the reigning media darling, thought to reduce the risk of heart disease, reverse aging, bolster the immune system, strengthen bones, fight cancer, treat asthma, and even cure the common cold, depending, of course, on what you read or to whom you talk.

Yet for something that has attracted so much attention and so many devotees, vitamin C could have used a better public relations firm because it—or, rather, its deficiency—has been known since 1550 B.C. Scurvy symptoms were described then on medical papyrus rolls discovered in Thebes by George Moritz Ebers, a nineteenth-century "Indiana Jones" and novelist. Descriptions of vitamin C deficiency also make appearances in the Bible's Old Testament; the writings of Hippocrates, the father of modern medicine; a chronicle of the Crusades; and the logbooks of Vasco da Gama, the Portuguese sailor who established the first European trading colony. Da Gama reported losing to scurvy 100 of his 160-man crew on one trip alone.

In time—thanks, in part, to Lind—sailors everywhere began to recognize the importance of vegetables and citrus juice in preventing scurvy. In 1795, the British Navy mandated that all their sailors get a one-ounce serving of lime juice daily, earning them the nickname "Limeys." This practice grew and more experiments were conducted, though it wasn't until 1932 that vitamin C itself was discovered. Charles Glen King at the University of Pittsburgh then answered the age-old

Meet Linus of the C-nuts

Early vitamin C pioneer Linus Pauling, Ph.D., is one of history's rare overachievers. He was a respected chemist and a winner of two—count 'em, two—un-shared Nobel prizes: one in 1954 for chemistry, the other in 1962 for peace. He is also the father of the vitamin C movement.

Dr. Pauling wrote his seminal best-seller *Vitamin C and the Common Cold* in 1970 and, with it, started the craze for vitamin C. He further fired the C frenzy by finding that vitamin C–treated terminal patients lived four times longer than patients not receiving the vitamin. Dr. Pauling's study involved 1,100 cancer victims, 100 of whom were given 10,000 milligrams of vitamin C a day. Even one year after he published his results, Dr. Pauling said, "Thirteen of these 'hope-less' patients are still alive, some as long as five years after having been pronounced untreatable, and most of them are in such good apparent health as to sug-gest that they now have normal life expectancy."

Dr. Pauling himself took 12,000 milligrams of vi-tamin C in his orange juice every morning, enjoying enviable health up to the age of 93, when he died just one year after weathering a bout of prostate cancer, something he says that he postponed for decades by taking vitamin C. After all, Dr. Pauling never said that vitamin C makes you immortal—just healthier.

question of what exactly cured scurvy by isolating a crystalline substance from lemon juice.

Thanks to all the down-and-dirty research through the centuries—and lots of lost teeth and bleeding gums—a vitamin, and thus a nutritional sensation, was born.

How It Works

As it turns out, the ravages of vitamin C deficiency aren't a disease at all. Scientists have learned that humans and certain other animals need vitamin C because of a genetic shortcoming.

Man, monkeys, guinea pigs, fruit-eating bats, and certain birds lack a gene responsible for producing oxidase, an enzyme that otherwise would permit us to live fulfilling lives without ingesting vitamin C in our food. This is precisely why your son's garter snake doesn't need fruits and vegetables to say "fangs" for dinner.

Inside your body, vitamin C does a lot of good. It's crucial in creating and maintaining collagen, a fibrous protein that binds cells together much like mortar binds bricks. Consequently, vitamin C is an incomparable ally in healing wounds and burns and in strengthening the walls of capillaries and blood vessels. Vitamin C also helps metabolize the amino acids tyrosine and tryptophan, increase the absorption of iron, promote sound teeth and bones, and quite possibly, stave off infection, common colds, and even cancer.

How does vitamin C do all these wondrous things? Scientists aren't exactly certain, and research continues. But they're reasonably sure that part of it is because of vitamin C's well-established antioxidant properties. Antioxidants are substances that neutralize free radicals—Tasmanian devil–like rogue molecules thought to cause everything from the ravages of aging to cancer.

"Not that all free radicals are bad. White blood cells, for example, use them like bullets in fighting foreign invaders," Dr. Janson says.

"Free radicals are like sparks in your fireplace. They're okay as long as they stay where they're supposed to stay. Once they get on the living-room rug, there's trouble," he adds.

Vitamin C and other antioxidants tame beastly free radicals by offering up one of their electrons to neutralize the blighters. That way, free radicals don't prey on electrons from the body's healthy molecules.

"If the free radicals are like the sparks from the fireplace, vitamin C and other antioxidants are like the asbestos gloves you'd wear to handle them," Dr. Janson says.

Richard F. Gerson, Ph.D., a health and fitness consultant in Clearwater, Florida, has heard the "Pac-Man" analogy applied to vitamin C and other antioxidants. Under this theory, vitamin C and other antioxidants are likened to the star of the computer game of the same name, where a voracious little creature gobbles everything in sight. Antioxidants, as the theory goes, similarly scoff up free radicals as fast as can be. Dr. Gerson prefers a more constructive, empowering perspective.

"I'd rather look at vitamin C and the others as builders. By taking them and keeping a good healthy diet, you're building a defense against things that could go wrong," Dr. Gerson says.

Regardless of how you view antioxidants, it begs the question: Can you get too much of a good thing? With vitamin C, probably not. Dr. Gerson, for example, takes 1,000 to 5,000 milligrams a day.

And Dr. Janson? He takes as much as 13,000 to 14,000 milligrams a day, although he doesn't routinely recommend that dose to others. And why not? "Because based on what I know about vitamins and what I know about myself, it's a reasonable experiment to make," Dr. Janson says.

But doses akin to what early vitamin C pioneer and double Nobel prize–winner Linus Pauling, Ph.D., took or the doses that Dr. Janson takes aren't recommended by everybody.

"While there certainly is a wide range of supplement levels out there, I don't recommend that my clients go above 500 milligrams," says Maye Musk, R.D., an international nutrition consultant, speaker, and author of *Feel Fantastic*.

You need only 10 milligrams to avoid scurvy. If you take 100 times that amount, you might run into adverse reactions such as diarrhea. Taking 2,000 milligrams or more can lead to cramps, nausea, destruction of red blood cells, and even the creation of kidney and bladder stones in people who are prone to them.

Going to the Right Source

Getting the vitamin C that you need is easy. "And if nothing else, taking a reasonable amount of vitamins and minerals might have a placebo effect," Dr. Gerson says, meaning that something good might happen just because you *think* something good might happen.

Here's how C-ing is believing.

Seek food sources first. Getting your vitamin C from food sources is a good idea because you'll be on the path to an all-around healthy diet. The best vitamin C sources—green leafy vegetables and citrus fruits—are healthy for many reasons, including being low in fat and high in fiber.

"By sticking to a healthy diet, you'll be getting vitamin C and doing many other good things for your body that will keep you healthy and maybe even looking and feeling younger than you really are," says Dr. Gerson.

A single serving of broccoli, green peppers, cauliflower, cantaloupe, or strawberries provides more than 50 milligrams of vitamin C for fewer than 60 calories. Other excellent food sources include papaya (more than 180 milligrams), orange juice, and grapefruit juice.

C is for "care." Handle vitamin C with care, since it's water-soluble and easily destroyed by heat, alkalinity, and exposure to air. Here's how to preserve your C.

♦ Buy vegetables in small quantities and eat promptly. Cut your vegetables minimally because more cutting means more vitamin C loss to the air. Keep the skins on.

♦ Use frozen foods immediately. Plunge them directly into boiling water—don't thaw first.

♦ Don't use iron or copper pans. They hasten vitamin C breakdown.

♦ Broil or steam vegetables instead of boiling. If you do boil, do so for as short a time as possible.

Be a spud-lover. Potatoes and other tubers are respectable vitamin C sources because they retain vitamin C longer than green leafy vegetables. A new potato, for example, will have 30 milligrams of vitamin C per 100 grams of weight and lose just 70 percent of that in nine months.

Supplement your nutritional income. Don't ignore the benefits of taking vitamin C supplements. "If you lived in a perfect world in a perfect environment eating a perfect diet and had perfect genes, you *might* still benefit from supplements," Dr. Janson says.

Watch out for withdrawal. Researchers have eyeballed a potential pitfall with taking megadoses of vitamin C: addiction. Not like drug addiction, but more like dependence. Your body grows so accustomed to

More C, Please

The U.S. government may finally vindicate researchers and scientists who have been carrying the torch for vitamin C.

The current Daily Value of 60 milligrams a day is too low, according to a study performed by the National Institutes of Health (NIH) in Bethesda, Maryland. Subjects were given different doses of vitamin C over time, ranging from 30 milligrams to 2,500 milligrams a day.

When researchers observed their immune system cells and blood, they found that they appeared to be optimally saturated with vitamin C at a daily dose of 200 milligrams. Perhaps more interesting, they found that at doses of 400 milligrams and more a day, the subjects retained no more vitamin C in their cells than they did at 200 milligrams.

"It's almost as if we're programmed to have a certain amount of vitamin C and no more," says the study's lead researcher, Mark Levine, M.D., senior investigator at the Cell Biology and Genetics Laboratory at the NIH and director of the Nutrition Program of the National Institute for Diabetes and Digestive and Kidney Diseases of the NIH. "We don't recommend daily doses higher than 500 milligrams a day."

The NIH study and its recommendations carry a lot of weight. As for exactly when the government will increase its vitamin C recommendations, stay tuned.

high C levels that it becomes adept at disposing of the excess.

If you suddenly drop to a more moderate amount, your body's disposal system might not adjust fast enough, resulting in a potential deficiency and even scurvy. This is yet another reason not to take megadoses without the guidance of your physician.

Vitamin D

Where you get it: Fortified milk, fatty fish (herring, kipper, mackerel), liver, egg yolk.

What it does for you: Increases calcium absorption, aids bone growth and integrity, and promotes sound teeth.

What you need: Daily Value of 400 international units (IU).

Cautions: Too much causes elevated calcium levels, which may be characterized by low appetite, increased thirst, nausea, vomiting, and weakness. Because vitamin D can be so toxic, do not take more than 600 IU daily unless your doctor prescribes a higher dosage. Too little can soften and deform bones and cause muscle twitching and convulsions.

Vitamin D is a bit of an oddball in the ranks of vitamins and minerals that your body needs to survive. What's special about vitamin D, and what makes it so autonomous?

Simply put, many scientists don't consider vitamin

D a vitamin at all. The substance we call vitamin D acts and functions more like a hormone than a vitamin, and by hormone we mean a substance produced by the body for the body. Like other hormones (and vitamin A, another oddball), vitamin D affects you at the cellular level. It does this with its ability to penetrate the inner sanctum of a cell, the nucleus, where it dances with DNA or its protein-based wrapping to make its mark on the body's physiology.

Also unlike its brethren B, C, and E, vitamin D stands alone because it's not an essential nutrient. That doesn't mean that it's unnecessary, mind you; it just means that you may not have to add any extra to your diet. As strange as it sounds, no trace of vitamin D need ever cross your lips again—in theory—for you to lead a happy and healthy life. Because the one thing that truly separates vitamin D from its alphabet family is that it's possible for most adults, especially in sunny locales, to get sufficient vitamin D from sunlight exposure.

"If you're working long hours behind a desk, not getting outside and seeing the sunlight, then that's certainly going to be a factor when it comes to vitamin D," says Mara Vitolins, R.D., Dr. P.H., nutrition research coordinator for the Bowman Gray School of Medicine of Wake Forest University in Winston-Salem, North Carolina. "Sunlight is what converts those endogenous stores of vitamin D into something you can use."

Seeing the Light

Just how your body uses sunshine to make vitamin D is about as arcane as how the IRS computes your annual standard deduction. Suffice it to say, though, that the four-step process takes about 36 hours and uses the ultraviolet portion of the sun's rays and your own body heat.

In this process, the body first goes to work on a precursor to vitamin D. Oddly enough, the precursor, the raw material from which vitamin D is made, starts out as cholesterol in the liver. It's a fine and often understated example of the human body's "good" uses for cholesterol.

Going through the motions of converting a vitamin D precursor into the real thing takes work, and the body wouldn't go through these motions unless it were important. Indeed, it is. Vitamin D plays a crucial role in bone formation, especially in children, which is why experts suggest that kids get twice as much vitamin D as grown-ups.

Considering all the work it does in keeping you literally standing tall, you need to make sure that you're getting enough vitamin D.

"Because your body can manufacture vitamin D doesn't mean that you should ignore it," Dr. Vitolins says. "I always recommend dairy products. Milk really does do the body good."

Unfortunately, it takes about a quart of milk to give you what you need in any given day. Still, a couple of glasses a day are a good start. Here are other ways that you can play D like a pro.

Let the sun shine. No, this isn't a *Hair* revival. As we said before, sunlight is critical in helping your body synthesize its own vitamin D. Ten minutes of summer sun on your hands and face provide enough exposure for one day, says H. F. DeLuca, Ph.D., chairman of the department of biochemistry at the University of Wisconsin in Madison. If you're dark-skinned, you'll have to prolong your exposure, because dark-pigment skin takes about 3 hours to reach the same level of vitamin D synthesis that fair skin reaches in 30 minutes.

The State of Vitamin D

Researchers in Boston have determined that the further north you live, the more vitamin D you might need in your diet during certain times of the year. "If you're living in a low-sunlight area during the winter, you could stand outside naked all day and still not make any vitamin D," says Michael F. Holick, M.D., Ph.D., director of the General Clinical Research Center and chief of the Section of Endocrinology, Nutrition, and Diabetes, both at Boston University Medical Center, and director of the Vitamin D, Skin, and Bone Research Laboratory at Boston University School of Medicine.

What do you do if you're Nanook of the North in the winter? Make sure that you get at least 200 international units of vitamin D a day from the food you eat or the supplements you take, if you live in an area of low sunlight, says Dr. Holick.

"It depends on where you are in relation to the equator, but in northern climates during the winter, the sun is at such an angle that the right rays don't penetrate the skin to make vitamin D," Dr. DeLuca says. "You can store up quite a bit of vitamin D in your fat cells, so if your diet is good, it will probably last you through winter."

Note that sunlight through a window doesn't count. Glass filters out the rays that you need most.

Don't lay on the lotion. If you're out in the sun, make sure that you cover up with a sunscreen, since too much exposure prematurely wrinkles your skin and possibly puts you at risk for skin cancer. Because sunscreens with a sun-protection factor (SPF) of 8 or higher stymie vitamin D synthesis, your best bet is to apply sunscreen after enough time has passed for adequate vitamin D production.

Get egg-cited. Egg yolks also are a good source of vitamin D, as are liver, fatty fish, butter, and fortified margarine. That's not to say you have free rein to mainline these foods. They still may present a risk to your heart's health. But realize that, in moderation, they can help boost your vitamin D levels, Dr. Vitolins says.

Vitamin E

Where you get it: Salad and cooking oils (except coconut oil), seeds and nuts, wheat germ, asparagus, avocado, beef and organ meats, seafood, apples, carrots, celery.

What it does for you: Antioxidant powers protect your cells from oxidation. Essential for red blood cells; aids cellular respiration; protects lung tissue from pollution.

What you need: Daily Value of 30 international units (IU).

Cautions: Deficiency is very rare. Also, it's hard to get too much. (Doses above 300 IU sometimes cause nausea and gastrointestinal problems.) If you are considering taking amounts above 600 IU, discuss this with your doctor first.

Vitamin E is among the most popular of vitamins

and perhaps the most sensationalized, threatening to topple even the reigning media darling, vitamin C, in the fight for limelight.

But what do you really know about vitamin E other than it's supposed to be pretty good for you? If it weren't for two university researchers and a roomful of frisky laboratory rats, you and the rest of us might not know anything.

It all started in California. The year was 1922. The school, the University of California. Two scientists were working on a piece of lettuce and wheat germ. That is, they were studying it—it was laboratory time, not lunchtime. The scientists were trying to isolate a nutritional substance from lettuce and wheat germ that helped rats reproduce. Eventually, the intrepid duo struck gold. Or more precisely, they struck upon a gold-colored, fat-soluble chemical, which they promptly named Factor X. Two years later, researchers at the University of Arkansas renamed Factor X vitamin E, presumably because Factor X sounded like a bad science fiction flick.

It wasn't until 12 years later that anyone knew anything more about the substance. In 1936, those wily California researchers said "lettuce experiment more" and got their X in gear. Herbert McLean Evans, along with some new co-workers, isolated a crystalline substance from wheat germ oil. Evans dubbed this new substance *tocopherol*, from the Greek words *tokos*, meaning "offspring," and *pherein*, meaning "to bear." Evans named the substance thus for the role it played in rat procreation, meaning it helped "bring forth offspring" in his whiskered companions.

Thanks to that pioneering groundwork and a lot of modern research, we know today that tocopherol is really a group of substances collectively called vitamin E. In other words, there is no such thing as vitamin E. In reality, vitamin E is a compound of eight chemical cousins, consisting of the tocopherols (the more active substances) and the tocotrienols (the less active substances). The leader of the pack is alpha-tocopherol, the most biologically active substance and the one commonly considered *the* vitamin E when nothing else is specified. Likewise, alpha-tocopherol is the compound most often reproduced as a synthetic supplement.

In its natural form, vitamin E compounds are yellow viscous oils that are insoluble in water. They also stand up pretty well to light, heat, and acids but are destroyed easily by oxygen and ultraviolet light.

In the body, vitamin E requires bile and fat for proper absorption, most of which takes place in the small intestine, where 20 to 30 percent of vitamin E is whisked away into the body's lymph channels. (Lymph, as you'll recall from seventh-grade science, is a body fluid that contains white blood cells and plays an important role in the immune system.)

Vitamin E storage in the body is generally confined to fatty tissue, the liver, and muscles. Vitamin E excretion takes place almost exclusively through defecation.

Hero of the Heart

You'd think that a vitamin so heavily researched would hold little wonder for a researcher who has seen it all.

Not so.

"The thing I find most fascinating about vitamin E is that vitamin E, a fat-soluble vitamin, might actually slow the development of atherosclerosis," says Mara Vitolins, R.D., Dr. P.H., nutrition research coordinator for the Bowman Gray School of Medicine of Wake Forest

Know What You're Taking

When it comes to boosting your vitamin E with supplements, make sure that you know what you're getting. And make sure that you're getting the most—for your money and for your health.

Most supplements will be of alpha-tocopherol, the most biologically active of the eight substances collectively known as vitamin E. If your vitamin jar label has a "d-" before "alpha-tocopherol," it means that the vitamin is from natural sources. It also means that you paid a little more. A "dl-" before the "alpha-tocopherol" means that it's synthesized and thereby a little less potent (and less expensive). "The 'dl-' or 'd-' refers to the chemical structure of alpha-tocopherol," says Cindy J. Fuller, R.D., Ph.D., assistant professor of food, nutrition, and food service management at the University of North Carolina at Greensboro. "In lay terms, there's only one form of the vitamin in d-alpha-tocopherol, and it's the one found in natural sources. The dl type is synthetic, and it comes in eight forms, or isomers, which is where things start to get confusing."

Does your body care if you're popping a d or dl variation of vitamin E? Probably not, Dr. Fuller says. And because you'll have to take a little extra of the synthetic form to equal the potency of the natural form, you'll wind up shelling out about the same amount cash-wise for the same effect health-wise.

"This sounds very confusing, but most vitamin E supplements are sold on an international units (IU) basis, so the bottom line is that 400 IU of d equals 400 IU of dl," Dr. Fuller says. "As long as that's the case, you might as well buy the less expensive version."

University in Winston-Salem, North Carolina. "In other words, it's interesting to me that a vitamin you get from fats and oils—which can cause hardening of the arteries—might actually help prevent heart problems, which have long been associated with these factors."

Two joint studies looking at more than 127,000 people reported that those who took vitamin E supplements for at least two years had a 40 percent lower risk for heart disease than those who didn't. Another study, this one by Japanese researchers, found that 74 volunteers given 100 milligrams of vitamin E daily showed a definite decreased risk for heart disease, compared with a control group of 73 volunteers taking just 3 milligrams a day.

Experts believe that part of vitamin E's power is the role it plays as an antioxidant in the body. Antioxidants are substances that neutralize oxidation, the process that causes intercellular breakdown and, perhaps, everything from cancer to the ravages of aging. An antioxidant like vitamin E works by giving up one of its electrons to stabilize a nasty electron-deficient molecule called a free radical.

Free radicals, in their search to become stable, can rob healthy molecules of their electrons, resulting in damage. Vitamin E, as an antioxidant, inhibits oxidation of polyunsaturated fatty acids, Dr. Vitolins says.

Another fascinating thing about vitamin E is the role it plays in helping other antioxidants. Like a vitamin vigilante, vitamin E protects vitamin C, vitamin A, and carotene (along with a few other things) from being oxidized, allowing them to perform their critical roles unhindered by a free radical ambush.

"This is why most people talk about the 'ACE' vitamins when they're talking about antioxidants. Vitamins A, C, and E tend to work so well together," says

Richard F. Gerson, Ph.D., a health and fitness consultant in Clearwater, Florida.

Other fascinating facts about vitamin E include the following:

♦ Research at the University of Arizona College of Medicine's Health Sciences Center in Tucson has found that vitamin E might reduce age-associated damage in both the immune and central nervous systems. "The results suggest that vitamin E, and possibly other antioxidants, may reduce damage associated with aging," says Marguerite Kay, M.D., professor of microbiology, immunology, and medicine at the university and the study's lead investigator.

♦ Researchers think that vitamin E might prevent lung damage associated with smoking. One study of 83 male smokers and 65 nonsmoking men found that, while both groups had about the same levels of vitamin E in their blood, the smokers' bodies showed an increased need for E, apparently to make up for the damage that smoking was causing their lungs.

♦ One Harvard study tracking 40,000 male health professionals over four years found that those with diets highest in vitamin E developed 36 percent fewer cases of heart disease than those who consumed the least amount of vitamin E. Moreover, those who took supplements of 100 IU a day for at least two years were 37 percent less likely to develop heart disease than those who took no supplements.

Eat Your Fill

Getting the vitamin E you need is pretty easy. It starts with eating a healthy diet in general, but you can supersize your E levels with a little help.

Cut your losses. A lot of your food's natural vitamin E is gone before it ever gets to you. That's because processing and packaging destroy E in many ways. Milling grain to convert whole wheat to white flour, for example, removes 80 percent of the grain's vitamin E. Canning causes losses of 41 to 65 percent in meats and vegetables, and roasting nuts robs them of up to 80 percent of their vitamin E.

You may not have any control over what the processing and manufacturing companies do, but you can cut your own losses by not deep-frying your food. Deep-frying destroys 32 to 75 percent of a food's E.

Chip in for extra E. Believe it or not, potato chips are an excellent source of E—but know that your chips will lose up to 70 percent or more if stored for over a month. (That's still no reason to eat them all at once.)

Clean up smog-E situations. Life in the concrete jungle is hell. You not only have to watch out for errant taxicabs and wayward muggers but you have to watch what you breathe, too. Vitamin E helps do that for you. Studies show that vitamin E protects lung tissue from nasty things in the air, like nitrogen dioxide, which can oxidize cells in your lungs. It's not clear whether E is good against pollution in general, but it shows promise.

Defend against diabetes. Vitamin E might be a friend in warding off adult-onset diabetes. One study from Finland looked at almost 1,000 men ages 42 to 60, none of whom had diabetes.

Four years later, the men were again evaluated, and researchers found that 45 developed diabetes within that time, mostly those with the lowest blood levels of vitamin E. In fact, below-average levels of E indicated a 400 percent increase in risk to develop diabetes.

E-rase scars. Vitamin E's positive effects on cells may help when it comes to healing scars, too.

In one study of people ranging from age 18 to 63, researchers added vitamin E to silicone gel sheets that were used to treat scars. Ninety-five percent of the 40 people who got E showed 50 percent improvement after eight weeks, compared with the same level of improvement in 75 percent of the 40 patients who didn't get vitamin E.

Vitamin K

Where you get it: Green tea, turnip greens, broccoli, lettuce, cabbage, spinach, liver, asparagus, bacon, coffee, cheese.

What it does for you: Controls blood coagulation; essential for synthesizing liver proteins that control clotting.

What you need: Daily Value of 80 micrograms.

Cautions: Too little results in delayed blood clotting and hemorrhagic disease in newborn infants. Natural forms of vitamin K are seemingly nontoxic, but synthetic versions have caused jaundice when given in doses of more than 5 milligrams a day. In rare instances—primarily with infants and pregnant women—toxicity can result when water-soluble substitutes are prescribed. Can result in jaundice or brain damage.

Like many other vitamins, vitamin K is actually one name representing several compounds, all of which are vital to human life. The compounds, known as the quinones, help create blood clotting substances manufactured in the liver.

Vitamin K was discovered in the 1930s by Danish biochemist Carl Peter Hendrick Dam of the University of Copenhagen, who noticed that certain diets in baby chicks caused lethal and uncontrollable hemorrhages. In 1935, Dam named the substance he believed was responsible for controlling clotting the *Koagulation* vitamin, from the Danish word for coagulation. The name later was shortened to vitamin K, and Dam received a Nobel prize in physiology and medicine in 1943 for his discovery.

Natural vitamin K comes in the form of a light yellow oil. Synthetically, it's a yellow crystalline powder. Strangely, clotting seems to be the only use that science has identified for vitamin K. Not that it does the job single-handedly—at least 13 different substances are involved in blood clotting. But vitamin K helps create at least 4 of those substances, including the biggie, prothrombin, which is created in the liver as a precursor to thrombin, the material that actually spins the clot, so to speak.

Here's how to keep K in your life.

Reach for fresh food. Fresh food is the best source for vitamin K. Frozen foods tend to be lacking. Stick to the produce aisle when you're shopping for fresh broccoli, spinach, and asparagus.

Go for home-grown goodness. Vitamin K also comes from naturally occurring bacteria in your intestine. Unfortunately, the amount produced there isn't enough to meet all your needs, so don't neglect a nutritious diet. (Interestingly, newborn babies are born without intestinal flora. They're given a 1-milligram shot of vitamin K at birth.)

Check with your doctor if you're taking anti-coagulants. Sometimes a physician will prescribe an anticoagulant to keep a patient's blood from clotting. There are cases on record where a vitamin K–rich diet was enough to counteract the effect of the medication. Ask your doctor if your vitamin K intake should be a concern if you're ever prescribed an anticoagulant.

But don't cut the K from your diet arbitrarily. And be wary if your doctor suggests that you do cut the K, says John W. Suttie, Ph.D., professor and chairman of nutritional science at the University of Wisconsin in Madison.

The key, says Dr. Suttie, is to keep your levels of vitamin K consistent so that the medication dosage can be prescribed with that consistent K level in mind.

Don't cut all the fat. As far as vitamin K is concerned, a little fat is a good thing. And a little goes a long way. The body absorbs vitamin K only when there's a bit of dietary fat present, so if you're eating K-consciously, make sure that you include a little fat to make it worth your while. A little means a dollop of oil-based dressing on your spinach salad, not drenching it with dressing or scarfing down half a loaf of heavily buttered bread.

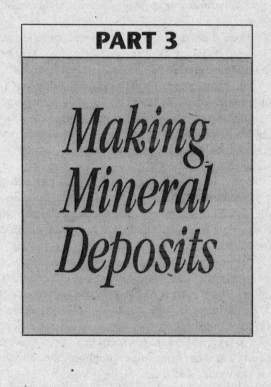

PART 3

Making
Mineral
Deposits

Boron

Where you get it: Wine, prunes, dates, raisins, honey.

What it does for you: Works with calcium, magnesium, and vitamin D to prevent bone loss. May help you stay more alert.

What you need: There is no Daily Value, but 1 to 2 milligrams a day is safe and possibly advantageous.

Cautions: Contrary to popular opinion, boron does not help build muscle. If you see it advertised as a strength-building supplement, the company is misleading you.

Boron is one of the most recent additions to the list of possible essential mineral elements, because researchers have discovered that it enhances the body's ability to use calcium, which may help maintain better bone health.

"We can't say that boron is an essential mineral, because a specific biochemical effect hasn't been discovered yet," says Forrest Nielsen, Ph.D., director of the U.S. Department of Agriculture–Agricultural Research Service Grand Forks Human Nutrition Research Center in North Dakota. "But it does seem that boron makes vitamin D and other bone-improving hormones and minerals more efficient."

Oddly enough, boron's history began as a food preservative in the 1870s, when it was used in the form of borax and boric acid. Although boron was first considered innocuous, countries actually began to outlaw its addition to foods when it was found that dosages of 500 milligrams a day caused appetite disturbances.

Today, researchers understand that boron is beneficial, if not essential, to humans.

Its main benefit seems to be maximizing the body's use of calcium and magnesium. This is good news for those people at risk for osteoporosis.

Just as important, boron seems to play a role in brain function. "When people who normally eat low-boron diets supplement with 3 milligrams a day, they report feeling more mentally alert," says Dr. Nielsen. "Motor function is improved." In fact, the low-boron diets seem to cause electrical changes in the brain that are similar to those found in people with malnutrition. There is evidence that boron may play a role in cognition, he says.

Unfortunately, boron has been misrepresented in the press as a muscle-building mineral, says Dr. Nielsen. "It's hogwash," he adds. "In 1987, I reported that when postmenopausal women were given a boron supplement, there was a slight increase in testosterone, but it was a small increase up to normal levels for women. I've since looked at men in the other studies, and it had no effect on testosterone. In terms of boron being a muscle-builder, it's bunk."

Because boron is an essential nutrient for plants, you can find it in numerous foods, such as fresh fruits and nuts. The western United States has more boron in its water than the eastern states. One glass of wine has slightly less than 1 milligram of boron. Your body absorbs boron easily, and no other mineral seems to counteract the work that it does.

The average American seems to consume 0.5 to 3.1 milligrams a day through food and water. However, since boron has yet to be labeled essential, you won't find it in all multivitamin/mineral supplements. And if you do find it in a multi, the amount will be small, such as the 150 micrograms found in Centrum.

"I recommend a daily intake of 1 to 2 milligrams," says Dr. Nielsen. "I am concerned about that small percentage of the population that gets less than 0.5 milligram a day."

Boron is safe up to 10 milligrams a day, says Dr. Nielsen, but there doesn't seem to be any reason to supplement to those numbers.

Calcium

Where you get it: Cheese, molasses, yogurt, beans, bread.

What it does for you: Builds strong teeth and bones and stimulates nerve impulses (magnesium relaxes them).

What you need: Daily Value of 1,000 milligrams.

Cautions: Taking more than 2,000 milligrams a day may cause constipation and kidney stones and inhibit zinc and iron absorption. Calcium supplements can cause bloating, gas, and confusion, especially in the elderly. When taken together, calcium and tetracycline form an insoluble chemical complex that impairs both mineral and drug absorption.

Sometime after your thirtieth birthday, you start to lose a little backbone with each passing year. That's not a commentary on your psychological state. It's a medical fact.

As you age, you naturally lose bone mass. Your best defense is to make sure that you get enough calcium in your diet. "Aside from calcium, bone consists of high levels of phosphorus and a good quantity of magnesium as well as trace elements of zinc" says Mona Calvo, Ph.D., a member of the clinical research and review staff for the Food and Drug Administration in Washington, D.C. "And vitamin D must be present for the body to efficiently absorb calcium."

In fact, adults usually absorb only 20 to 30 percent of the calcium they consume. But here's what you really need to know: Your body has a complex mechanism to maintain sufficient calcium levels in your blood, which is essential to keep muscles and nerves healthy. To keep this level of calcium constant, the body either takes calcium from the bone and puts it into the blood or absorbs calcium from the blood and puts it into the bone.

If you don't get enough calcium in your diet, your body pulls the mineral from the calcium reserves in your bones, weakening them. As you get older, if you don't eat enough calcium, your body gradually takes more calcium from your bones than it puts in them. Left unchecked, that gradual erosion can lead to osteoporosis, a degenerative disease in which the bones become so fragile that they break in response to even slight trauma. You may have seen elderly people walking around in a stooped position. That's because some of the vertebrae in the spine have collapsed or broken, and this causes the spine to curve.

Whenever you lose height, it usually means that you have experienced a collapsed vertebra as a result of bone loss in the spine. This loss happens over a long period of time. Although women have traditionally been the ones at risk for osteoporosis, as men live longer, they too may feel its ravages.

Research suggests that half of us are getting less than 800 milligrams of calcium a day, well under the 1,000 milligrams recommended. And what a difference a few hundred milligrams can make. Robert Heaney, M.D., professor of medicine at Creighton University in Omaha, Nebraska, and a leading calcium expert, estimates that getting enough calcium could prevent as many as half of all osteoporotic fractures.

Aside from creating strong teeth and bones, calcium is critical for the proper functioning of other organ systems, such as muscle contraction and blood clotting. So a shortage of calcium will prevent you from attaining optimal health in other ways, too.

Even if you do get enough calcium in your diet, caffeine, alcohol, and cigarette smoke can contribute to the body's loss of calcium. On the other hand, weight-bearing exercise, such as walking or running, will help the bones maintain their density over the years.

Your Calcium Plan

Make it your business to consume milk and other foods rich in calcium and vitamin D, and foods fortified with calcium, Dr. Calvo says. "Not only is milk rich in calcium but the vitamin D and protein in milk facilitate absorption," she says. You can also choose cheese and other low-fat dairy foods to get calcium.

Today, manufacturers are adding calcium to a variety of foods. Orange juice, for example, often has it. "It's very hard to keep calcium in a solution. Citrus juice is actually a good medium, but make sure you shake it up and drink it fairly quickly," says Dr. Calvo. Why? So that the calcium doesn't settle to the bottom of the container. The same is true for fortified lactose-free milk drinks, such as Lactaid.

Other products with added calcium include some cereals, corn tortillas, and English muffins. Green vegetables such as kale, broccoli, and Chinese cabbage (bok choy) are also good sources of naturally available calcium.

That doesn't mean, however, that you can stop drinking your milk. "Orange juice doesn't give you vitamin D, and many people in the United States don't get enough D," says Dr. Calvo. "African-Americans and others with darker skin can't always synthesize enough vitamin D (the sunshine vitamin), especially during the winter months when there's little sunshine available." That's why milk is also important to most adults.

Supplementing Your Stores

If you just don't eat any type of dairy product, then you may want to consider taking calcium supplements. And if you head to the store for calcium supplements, you'll find lots to choose from. But you won't find a considerable amount in most multivitamins because calcium is a bulky mineral and is hard to fit in a multivitamin tablet that is small enough to swallow.

Calcium supplements come from a variety of original, natural sources, including oyster shells, ground bone, and limestone. Manufacturers can purify these to varying degrees or combine them with other compounds such as citrate or gluconate. Your body absorbs and uses these various types of calcium supplements differently, so you need to choose wisely. Based on limited research, it seems that most healthy people absorb calcium equally well from calcium supplements that are a combination of amino acids bonded with calcium, calcium phosphate dibasic, or calcium acetate, carbonate, citrate, gluconate, or lactate. People don't absorb calcium as well from oyster shell calcium fortified with inorganic magnesium, from chelated calcium-magnesium combinations, calcium carbonate fortified with vitamins and iron, or a mixture of calcium and magnesium carbonates.

To aid absorption, calcium citrate should be taken on an empty stomach, while another popular form, calcium carbonate, is best taken with food.

"Your calcium tablet may not have the other things required for proper calcium absorption," says Dr. Calvo. Some people take combined calcium and vitamin D products. Other products contain essential trace minerals good for bones, such as magnesium and zinc. Some supplements have side effects, so if your stomach is queasy after taking one, consider drinking a glass or two (eight ounces each) of milk.

Some men are concerned that calcium supplements may cause kidney stones. Kidney stones affect more men than women for reasons that are not entirely clear. We do know that those who are prone to form and pass stones may also hyper-absorb calcium. Most men don't find out they are hyper-absorbers of calcium until they pass a stone. Men with family histories of kidney stones should talk to a doctor about calcium intake; but chances are that he'll advise keeping it to at least the Daily Value of 1,000 milligrams.

Chromium

Where you get it: Blackstrap molasses, apple peels.

What it does for you: Acts cooperatively with other substances to control insulin and certain enzymes.

What you need: Daily Value of 120 micrograms.

Cautions: Do not supplement above 200 micrograms unless you are under your doctor's supervision. Also, if you have diabetes, do not supplement with chromium without doctor supervision, since high intakes can cause your blood sugar levels to drop dangerously low.

Why do those chrome fenders shine so? Because of chromium, a mineral that derives its name from the Greek word *chroma*, meaning "multicolored." And that same mineral can help keep you shining in good health.

Most important is chromium's role as a component of glucose tolerance factor (GTF), a hormonelike agent that also contains niacin and some amino acids. GTF enters the blood when there is an increase of insulin in the bloodstream. It enhances the effect of insulin by making the sugars pass more easily into the cells. If there isn't enough GTF in the system, the sugars may stay in the blood, which can lead to diabetes.

Chromium levels in the body decline with age, and the ability to convert chromium to GTF may also decline with age and could be one of the explanations for adult-onset diabetes. The average diet with plenty of refined flour and sugar also leaves people with lots of sugar to process but very little chromium to help get the job done.

"If you eat a whole grain, you get chromium. But when grain is processed to remove the fiber and the bran, the chromium is also removed," says Cathy Kapica, R.D., Ph.D., associate professor of nutrition and clinical dietetics at Finch University of Health Sciences/Chicago Medical School. "Those processed grains use up the chromium in your body without replacing it, so over the years, you can develop a chromium deficiency that may mimic diabetes."

Although the Daily Value for chromium is 120 micrograms, the U.S. Department of Agriculture estimates that most adults get only about 33 micrograms of chromium every day in their diets. Many multivitamin/mineral supplements include chromium, but some contain less than the Daily Value.

Chromium's reputation as a carbohydrate burner has left many weight lifters with the mistaken belief that chromium burns fat and builds muscle and strength. Chromium picolinate is one of the hottest supplements on the market.

"Studies have shown that we absorb only about 1 percent of the chromium that we consume, and chromium picolinate is one of the best absorbed of the different types of chromium," says Forrest Nielsen, Ph.D., director of the U.S. Department of Agriculture–Agricultural Research Service Grand Forks Human Nutrition Research Center in North Dakota.

But, adds Dr. Nielsen, you only see an increase in chromium's effectiveness if you have a deficiency. "Anything above an adequate intake won't help you. It's a fairly ineffective supplement for bodybuilding." He believes that the amount in a typical multivitamin is more than enough, especially if it's complementing a diet containing whole grains.

"You can take too much chromium; 200 micrograms a day would be the maximum amount," adds Dr. Kapica. "And people who are taking large amounts of supplements aren't helping themselves as much as they would be if they were eating more whole grains and less refined flour and sugar."

Iron

Where to get it: Meat, fortified cereals consumed with orange juice.

What it does for you: Makes your blood nice and red. Aids in the transportation of oxygen throughout the body.

What you need: Daily Value of 18 milligrams.

Cautions: Too much iron has been linked to higher risk of heart disease and cancer in men. Iron supplements are the leading cause of pediatric death from poisoning. So if you have supplements with iron in the house, keep them away from children. A fatal dose of iron for a toddler can be as little as 600 milligrams, which is how much iron you might find in as few as four iron supplement tablets.

There's no doubt that many of us can use more iron than we're getting. Roughly 20 percent of Americans are deficient in this mineral. The group most likely to be coming up short: women in their reproductive years.

"I would say that women need to be a little more thoughtful than men about iron, probably in the same way that women should be a little more cautious about calcium intake because of osteoporosis," says Adria Sherman, Ph.D., professor and chair of the Department of Nutritional Sciences at Rutgers University in New Brunswick, New Jersey.

Iron, which is absorbed in the intestines, comes in two forms: heme and nonheme. Found in meats, the heme form is well-absorbed. Men get about two-thirds of their iron needs met by heme iron; the amount varies for women. Nonheme iron is found in vegetables and isn't absorbed as well.

Most of the iron you consume goes to form hemoglobin, the substance that helps your red blood cells transport oxygen from your lungs to the rest of your body. The rest is stored in the bone marrow, liver, spleen, and other organs.

Because iron also plays a key role in helping prepare your immune system's infection fighters for battle, a deficiency may lead to colds. Low iron levels can also cause fatigue, pallor, and listlessness—hallmarks of anemia, says Dr. Sherman. In children, low iron levels can cause stunted growth and impaired learning. Other symptoms of iron deficiency include split nails, a sore tongue, and cold hands and feet. An annoying condition called restless legs has also been linked to low iron.

Some experts even believe that vague gastrointestinal problems such as gas, belching, constipation, and diarrhea may be rooted in iron deficiency. If you suspect that you may be deficient in iron, ask your family doctor or your gynecologist to test your blood at your yearly exam.

Using Iron Safely

Here's a fact about iron supplements that should encourage healthy respect: Researchers studying 10 years of records at a large Winnipeg, Manitoba, hospital found that an average of five iron supplement poisonings occur each year.

Although accidental iron poisonings occur most often in children who ingest supplements containing iron that are formulated for adults, high levels of iron can also be toxic to adults. Therefore, most experts recommend that you don't take iron supplements unless your doctor confirms the need with a blood test.

A daily intake of 25 milligrams or more for an extended period of time may cause undesirable side effects. Symptoms of acute iron poisoning include pain, vomiting, diarrhea, and shock. Still, doctors normally recommend iron supplementation for pregnant women and for infants.

Among the variety of iron supplements, experts say that those made with ferrous salts are better absorbed. Among them, ferrous sulfate is considered best.

Slow-release and coated iron tablets may cause less diarrhea, nausea, and abdominal pain, but since the site of maximum absorption is the beginning of the small intestine, delaying the time of release decreases the overall amount of iron absorbed by your body. Taking the tablets with a meal could go a long way in helping to reduce stomach upset, but then again, the food may interfere with the iron absorption. Therefore, since it is advantageous for absorption, experts recommend taking iron supplements between meals if you do not experience side effects or if you can tolerate iron taken in this manner.

Men, Take Note

"Few men, if any, need more iron," says David Meyers, M.D., professor of internal medicine and preventive medicine at the University of Kansas School of Medicine in Kansas City. "In fact, almost all men need less iron than they are consuming."

Studies have begun to show that heart disease, the number one killer of men, may somehow be linked to high iron levels in men. "Women only have 30 to 50 percent of the rate of arteriosclerosis as men do, and they get it 10 to 15 years later," says Dr. Meyers. "We have traditionally ascribed that protection to the presence of estrogen, but studies have shown that it isn't just estrogen that seems to protect women, but their periods. Maybe women get less heart disease because they lose iron every month."

This, however, is just a hypothesis, says Janet Hunt, R.D., Ph.D., research nutrition scientist for the U.S. Department of Agriculture–Agricultural Research Service Grand Forks Human Nutrition Research Center in North Dakota. "We haven't seen proof yet. In the studies conducted so far, persons with heart disease and high iron stores may have been different in other important ways that were not even identified. It would be useful to do a long-term study looking at men who are otherwise similar, but with some who are instructed to donate blood and some who aren't, to see if there's a difference in their rates of heart disease."

Magnesium

Where you get it: Meats, green leafy vegetables, brown rice, legumes, nuts, whole grains.

What it does for you: Helps form bones and teeth. Relaxes nerve impulses that cause muscles to flex (calcium stimulates them) and is essential for cellular metabolism and energy production.

What you need: Daily Value of 400 milligrams.

Cautions: Overuse of magnesium supplements, antacids, or laxatives can cause magnesium buildup in those with poor kidney function, which can lead to slowed breathing, coma, and sometimes death. Always check with your doctor before taking supplemental magnesium if you have kidney or heart problems.

Although the Romans used magnesia alba (white magnesium salts from the Magnesia district of Greece) to cure many ailments, the element magnesium wasn't isolated until 1808. Today, it is recognized as an essential mineral that is second only to potassium in terms of concentration within individual cells of the body.

"Magnesium helps the muscle tone of the heart," says Lisa Ruml, M.D., assistant professor of medicine and a researcher in the department of mineral metabolism at the University of Texas Southwestern Medical Center at Dallas. "It's very important for all muscle function, and if you're low in magnesium, it's harder to control blood pressure."

In fact, when a researcher at the University of North Carolina in Chapel Hill reviewed years of magnesium studies, she found ample evidence that stress—both physical and emotional—can increase the body's need for magnesium. The hormones catecholamine and corticosteroid are released during stressful episodes and can cause the heart muscle to lose some of its stored magnesium. In turn, a high magnesium level may help fight the strains of stress.

"Although it's not easy to become chronically deficient in magnesium, I think that magnesium is worth using as a supplement," Dr. Ruml advises. Aside from blood pressure problems, low magnesium levels can, over time, rob your bones of vital minerals, leaving them porous and weakened.

You can find 100 milligrams of magnesium in many multivitamin/mineral supplements. But you also can get a supplement of magnesium alone or with its related bone-building nutrients, such as calcium and zinc. Although the Daily Value is 400 milligrams, most people fall short.

"When magnesium is low, the parathyroid gland doesn't work well, and that's what processes vitamin D to better absorb calcium," Dr. Ruml says. "In other words, you can have trouble conserving your calcium in the presence of low magnesium." In fact, when magnesium intake is extremely low, calcium is sometimes deposited in the soft tissues, leading to calcified lesions.

Supplementation may be particularly important because of the link between magnesium and calcium. Magnesium relaxes nerve impulses and muscle contraction, while calcium stimulates them. The two must be in balance to allow the body to function at optimum levels.

Picking the right magnesium supplement may save you a lot of time in the bathroom. Dose for dose, magnesium gluconate causes one-third the amount of diarrhea of magnesium oxide and one-half the frequency of diarrhea of magnesium chloride, says Herbert C. Mansmann Jr., M.D., professor of pediatrics and associate professor of medicine at Jefferson Medical College of Thomas Jefferson University in Philadelphia.

Molybdenum

Where you get it: Milk, lima beans, spinach, liver, breads, cereals.

What it does for you: As a component of three different enzymes, it's involved in the metabolism of nucleic acids (DNA and RNA), iron, and food into energy. Helps break down toxic buildups of sulfites in the body. May help prevent cavities.

What you need: Daily Value of 75 micrograms.

Cautions: Deficiencies rarely happen unless there is an excess of copper or sulfate in the body. Toxicity is also rare, but high concentrations of molybdenum in the environment can cause symptoms of diarrhea, slow growth, and anemia.

With a name like molybdenum, you've got to be tough. And it is. The adult body has about 9 milligrams of molybdenum (pronounced mo-LIB-duh-num) spread fairly evenly throughout it. Even when intake was lowered to 25 micrograms per day—just one-third of the Daily Value—levels of this hardy mineral in the body remained steady, according to a study conducted by the U.S. Department of Agriculture (USDA).

"No natural deficiency of molybdenum in humans

has ever been described," says Forrest Nielsen, Ph.D., director of the U.S. Department of Agriculture–Agricultural Research Service Grand Forks Human Nutrition Research Center in North Dakota. "And toxicity is also rare in humans, although it is more common in cows that graze on land rich in molybdenum."

Some multivitamin/mineral tablets now contain molybdenum. Up to 250 micrograms of molybdenum a day is estimated by the U.S. National Research Council to be safe and adequate, but there's no reason to take that much. It isn't a mineral that you even need in a supplement, Dr. Nielsen says. The average American diet includes about 93 micrograms a day, well within the recommended limits. However, the body easily rids itself of excess amounts, so don't worry if you see it listed on a supplement label. If you use a multivitamin/mineral that contains molybdenum, make sure that it has no more than 250 micrograms, says Dr. Nielsen.

Amounts higher than 500 micrograms of molybdenum can interfere with your body's metabolism of copper and also can lead to symptoms of gout. On the other hand, too much copper, tungsten, or sulfate can drain the body of molybdenum. This deficiency scenario has only been seen in animals.

"Molybdenum seems to help the body rid itself of the potentially dangerous effects of sulfites and other toxins," Dr. Nielsen says. "We are starting to see evidence that molybdenum may have some antioxidant properties because it fights foreign compounds or drugs that come into the body. If molybdenum isn't there to help your body metabolize them, they can cause cancer, for example. Molybdenum seems to be involved in the detoxification of compounds."

Molybdenum is part of sulfite oxidase, an enzyme

that helps the body detoxify sulfites, compounds found in protein foods and used as chemical preservatives in some foods and drugs. People who can't break down sulfites have toxic buildups of this chemical in their bodies, says Judith Turnlund, R.D., Ph.D., of the USDA Western Human Nutrition Research Center in San Francisco.

Some people are supersensitive to the sulfites used as additives, developing asthma and other life-threatening breathing problems.

Molybdenum also is part of two other enzymes: xanthine oxidase and aldehyde oxidase. Both are involved in the body's production of genetic material and proteins. Xanthine oxidase also helps the body produce uric acid, an important waste product.

Phosphorus

Where you get it: Milk, cereal, meat.

What it does for you: Helps form bones and teeth, builds muscle, and is involved in almost all metabolic actions in the body.

What you need: Daily Value of 1,000 milligrams.

Cautions: There is no known toxicity for phosphorus, but too much can cause a deficiency of calcium in the blood.

Phosphorus is the second most abundant mineral in our bodies, behind calcium. Unlike calcium, phosphorus is naturally found in the majority of foods. It's also available in the beverage section of any grocery store. However, it makes a huge difference whether you get your phosphorus from a can of soda or a glass of milk. And the reason is calcium.

"There is a constant balancing act going on in your blood and bones to keep calcium and phosphorus in balance," says Mona Calvo, Ph.D., a member of the clinical research and review staff for the Food and Drug Administration in Washington, D.C.

The ideal phosphorus-to-calcium ratio (milligrams to milligrams) is 1 to 1, says Dr. Calvo, because the Daily Value for both calcium and phosphorus is the same—1,000 milligrams. You can find a level close to the ideal ratio in a glass of milk.

But drink a can of cola and all you get is phosphorus, and no calcium. Phosphoric acid is used to hold the carbonation in colas and some root beers.

"Phosphorus works with calcium, the most abundant mineral in our bodies, to build bone," Dr. Calvo says. When it isn't busy creating bone, phosphorus is part of many components of the cells like adenosine triphosphate, which is the key compound that stores energy and operates in metabolism. It also functions in almost every other metabolic pathway in the body.

Intake estimates show that while most men consume more than the recommended amount of phosphorus, they sometimes don't get enough calcium.

And according to some studies, when that phosphorus-to-calcium ratio is thrown out of whack, it may lead to decreases in bone mass. More research needs to be done, however, in order to establish this fact in humans.

"Adding to this problem, I believe, is the underreporting of phosphorus levels," Dr. Calvo says. "The more processed foods you eat, the more phosphorus you're getting. It is not required to include phophorus levels in nutrition labels. Because phosphorus food additives are so useful and serve many functions to improve the food supply, it's almost impossible to avoid getting the Daily Value. The same is not true for calcium.

"You need a number of different minerals to help your bones stay strong," Dr. Calvo says. You can find many of these in a glass of milk rather than a pill.

Some food sources with good ratios of calcium to phosphorus include apples, broccoli, carrots, corn, ground beef, roasted turkey, strawberries, and tuna. Dairy products are the best sources overall, Dr. Calvo states.

The phosphorus in meats and dairy foods is more bioavailable than the phosphorus found in cereals, fruits, and vegetables. Unlike calcium, phosphorus is very efficiently absorbed.

Although aluminum hydroxide, which is the main ingredient in a number of antacids, can interfere with absorption, deficiencies of phosphorus are almost unheard of.

"At this point phosphorus seems to be everywhere in the food supply," Dr. Calvo says. "And that's more of a problem than any deficiency issue."

Potassium

Where you get it: Dried fruits, most raw vegetables, citrus fruits, molasses, sunflower seeds.

What it does for you: Helps keep blood pressure down and aids muscle contraction, healthy electrical activity in the heart, and rapid transmission of nerve impulses throughout the body.

What you need: Daily Value of 3,500 milligrams.

Cautions: Don't supplement without a physician's consent if you have kidney problems or diabetes or are taking digitalis, some diuretics, or blood pressure medication. A normal kidney will excrete any excess potassium that the body doesn't need, so it is not necessary to take large amounts of potassium. A normal, balanced diet is more than adequate for most people.

If you're taking in too much sodium every day—and most of us are—potassium helps give it the bum's rush from your body and flushes out excess fluid from your blood. And along with sodium, magnesium, and calcium, potassium helps keep your heart beating nice and strong. If these minerals are not in balance, the blood vessels may become stiff, creating high blood pressure. "One of the first things you may notice, though, if you are low in potassium, is muscle weakness or a loss of stamina overall," says Lisa Ruml, M.D., assistant professor of medicine and a researcher in the department of mineral metabolism at the University of Texas Southwestern Medical Center at Dallas.

So here's the problem: Most of us have thrown that delicate balance way out of whack. While the Daily Value for potassium is 3,500 milligrams, we get an average of about 2,500 milligrams a day. Meanwhile, the Daily Value for sodium is 2,400 milligrams, but we consume anywhere from 2,000 to 6,000 milligrams daily.

"Most people need to cut down on sodium and increase their intake of natural potassium, such as dried fruits or citrus fruits and bananas," says Dr. Ruml. "We used to think that you just needed to watch sodium to control high blood pressure, but now we know that potassium is also important."

This is especially true for African-American men, whose diets tend to be lower in potassium and who also have higher rates of high blood pressure. Researchers gave 43 African-American men potassium supplements (3,120 milligrams a day) and another 43 placebos. The men who took the potassium had an average drop in their blood pressures of 6.9 points. The men who took placebos showed no changes.

It's rare that anyone will suffer from a potassium-deficiency disease, Dr. Ruml says, but when you're sick with the flu or anything that upsets your digestion, you might need more potassium, since vomiting and diarrhea can deplete your potassium reserves. The main symptom of potassium deficiency is weakness.

"When a person goes to the doctor complaining of fatigue, weakness, or a lack of stamina, his doctor will look at the potassium and calcium levels in his blood because these electrolytes control the work that muscles do," Dr. Ruml says.

Electrolytes, which include sodium and potassium, dissolve in water. Potassium, calcium, and magnesium live within cells, while sodium sets up house mainly in the bloodstream. While only sodium and potassium are electrolytes, all four minerals work with muscles. Potassium and magnesium relax muscles, while sodium and calcium contract them.

Go to the Food Bank

If you work out, it's even more important to give potassium its proper respect.

You've probably heard that it's a good idea to eat a banana after a particularly strenuous workout. Why? Because potassium is essential for cell growth and for every pound of muscle you gain, your body needs more potassium.

It's also important because as an electrolyte, potassium is lost through sweat as well as urine. If you perspire, then you also have the potential to lose some potassium.

Increasing your potassium is as simple as peeling a banana or eating a nectarine. Experts agree that your body will respond better to potassium from food than to potassium taken in supplement form.

If you do decide to go with a supplement, check with your doctor first because low potassium levels can signal a variety of serious problems, including adrenal gland dysfunction, renal disorders, and intestinal dysfunction. Also, our bodies tolerate the various versions of potassium very differently. You can choose between potassium bicarbonate, potassium chloride, and potassium gluconate.

"It's often not necessary to go to such lengths as supplementation unless you are on certain medications that make you lose potassium or have a medical problem causing potassium deficiency," Dr. Ruml says. "Citrus fruits are better than pills. Drink a glass of orange juice or add lemons to your water." In fact, a glass of orange juice, grapefruit juice, carrot juice, or tomato juice will give you between 400 and 700 milligrams. And eating the five to nine servings of fruits and vegetables recommended daily in the Food Guide Pyramid should increase your potassium to about 3,500 milligrams daily.

Selenium

Where you get it: Lobster, clams, crabs, whole grains, Brazil nuts, oysters.

What it does for you: Selenium works with vitamin E as an antioxidant and binds with toxins in the body, somehow rendering them harmless.

What you need: Daily Value of 70 micrograms.

Cautions: Severe toxicity and deficiency are rare in the United States.

When a horse grazing in Kansas starts acting woozy and wobbly, his owner knows that he has eaten too much locoweed—a plant rich in selenium.

But while a horse in Kansas might be getting too much selenium, a horse in Florida might not get any at all—and both extremes are dangerous. The same is also true for people: Getting too much or too little selenium can be hazardous to your health.

"Selenium is an essential trace element that enters into an enzyme group that works primarily as an antioxidant defense system of the body," says Vladimir Badmaev, M.D., Ph.D., vice president of scientific and medical affairs for Sabinsa Corporation, a nutraceutical research company in Piscataway, New Jersey. Selenium deficiencies have been shown to compromise the body's ability to fight back against heart disease, cancer, and arthritis—in general, against chronic debilitating disorders.

In general, the soil in states east of the Mississippi River and west of the Rockies is low in selenium.

Dr. Badmaev believes that people, particularly in selenium-poor regions, should supplement at the recommended level of 50 to 200 micrograms of elemental selenium a day.

Other researchers agree with him. "There is evidence to suggest that supplementing up to 200 micrograms a day may prevent certain types of cancer," says Forrest Nielsen, Ph.D., director of the U.S. Department of Agriculture–Agricultural Research Service Grand Forks Human Nutrition Research Center in North Dakota. "However, supplementing in higher amounts could lead to problems." You should consult your doctor before taking more than 100 micrograms of selenium.

When researchers at the University of Arizona in Tucson gave 200-microgram selenium supplements to people with a history of skin cancer, they found that the supplements seemed to ward off lung, colorectal, and prostate cancers. But the supplements did not change the rates of skin cancer. All the people in the study, however, were from the eastern coastal plain of the United States, an area well-known for its lack of selenium-rich soil as well as its high rates of skin cancer.

If you do choose to supplement, Dr. Badmaev suggests combining a selenium supplement with vitamin E, beta-carotene, and vitamin A. Experimental evidence shows that persons with low levels of vitamin E, beta-carotene, and vitamin A—combined with low levels of selenium—are at higher risk of developing cancer. Selenium's antioxidant functions may enable it to terminate cancer cells, Dr. Badmaev says. So combining selenium with other antioxidants can improve the anti-cancer effect.

Sodium

Where you get it: Table salt, anchovies, bacon, bologna, pickles, Parmesan cheese.

What it does for you: Regulates and balances the amount of fluids outside the cells in your body. Aids in muscle contractions and nerve function.

What you need: Daily Value of 2,400 milligrams.

Cautions: Too much dietary salt over a long period of time can cause your body to lose excessive amounts of calcium. A high-salt diet can also lead to high blood pressure. Sometimes this doesn't show up until people reach their forties and fifties, and then to an even greater extent when they reach their sixties and seventies. Normally, sodium needs to be replaced in the body only if you have thrown up, had diarrhea, or were profusely sweating.

For years, sodium has been cast as the villain in the battle against high blood pressure. The reason is that scientists who conducted early studies on high blood pressure found that people who ate a lot of salt—sodium chloride—frequently had slightly higher blood pressure readings. The answer seemed obvious: Cut back on salt and you'd reduce your risk of high blood pressure. It didn't work out that way, though.

Further studies found that using less salt didn't guarantee a drop in blood pressure. In fact, one study in Germany found that a low-salt diet did not appear to lower blood pressure in about 80 percent of those involved. And another study at Albert Einstein College of Medicine and Cornell University Medical College, both in New York City, showed that people with high blood pressure who ate the least salt (about 5,000 milligrams) each day were four times more likely to have a heart attack—precisely the health consequence a low-salt diet was supposed to prevent—than those who ate more than twice as much salt every day.

These days, researchers understand that high blood pressure (also known as hypertension) is more complicated than merely eating too much salt. They are more inclined to believe that low potassium, calcium, or magnesium levels as well as other lifestyle habits, such as exercise, alcohol use, and body weight, contribute more clearly to hypertension than sodium intake.

However, that doesn't change one very important fact: Excessive salt intake is potentially dangerous and, at the very least, seems pointless.

"I don't know what to make of the studies that find that salt isn't as important to hypertension, and I haven't changed my view on the subject," says Louis Tobian, M.D., head of the hypertension department at the University of Minnesota Hospital in Minneapolis.

"We have very clear numbers showing that Western societies that consume a lot of salt have higher blood pressure rates than those of primitive societies with little access to salt—but the case rates don't show up until people are in their forties or fifties," Dr. Tobian says.

However, that doesn't necessarily mean that your blood pressure will drop if you switch to a low-salt diet after years of eating a high-salt diet, Dr. Tobian cautions. Based on studies with rats, he believes that the reason blood pressure doesn't decrease is that the long-term, high-salt intake somehow produces irreversible changes in the brain, which helps regulate blood pressure.

Dr. Tobian believes that the discrepancy in study results may reflect the body's inability to adapt to a drop in sodium intake. In other words, since it takes decades for high blood pressure to show up in the body, it would take just as long for sodium restriction to change hypertension rates. Even those researchers who found that excessive sodium restriction is unwarranted for the high blood pressure population concede that high sodium intake has little, if any, benefit.

So what should a person do? "There's no doubt that we get too much salt in our diets," according to Lisa Ruml, M.D., assistant professor of medicine and a researcher in the department of mineral metabolism at the University of Texas Southwestern Medical Center at Dallas.

"It's one of the first things we measure when we look at minerals in the body. It plays such a big role in calcium imbalances as well as other problems. And everyone should look at the total amount they eat every day to see if they can cut back," Dr. Ruml adds.

That's because aside from its association with high blood pressure, too much dietary sodium can threaten your body's store of calcium. And that can lead to osteoporosis later in life.

Packaged Goods

If you want to know at a glance how much sodium a product contains, here's what the terms on the front of the package mean.

Sodium-free: less than 5 milligrams per serving

Very low sodium: no more than 35 milligrams per serving

Low-sodium: fewer than 140 milligrams per serving

Less sodium: 25 percent less per serving than similar food

Light: 50 percent or less per serving than the regular product

Both potassium and calcium work to lower blood pressure, but when too much sodium is in the blood, it forces the levels of potassium and calcium down.

It Isn't Easy

Sodium is one-half of table salt, that ubiquitous taste enhancer flavoring everything from sushi to American cheese. It is also a mineral within our bodies, an electrolyte to be exact, which means that it dissolves in liquid. Half the sodium in your body is within your blood vessels and in fluids surrounding your cells, another 40 percent is on the surface of your bones, and the remaining 10 percent is in your cells.

Although our taste for excess salt seems to be acquired, human beings appear to crave a certain level of sodium. Most Americans get about 3,000 to 6,000 milligrams each day, well above the Daily Value of 2,400 milligrams. "Ideally, you'd like to keep your intake to the Daily Value, which means about half an inch of salt from a diner-style saltshaker," Dr. Ruml says. This amount includes the salt that's already in the foods you eat. Most people eat about an inch of salt a day.

But the problem isn't caused by the salt you shake on your food; it's the salt stirred in much earlier that causes the problem. Canned chicken noodle soup? Around 1,000 milligrams a serving. Lunchmeat? About 350 milligrams a slice. You get the picture.

"It's difficult to control your salt consumption if you eat out a lot," adds Dr. Ruml. "Sodium is a great preservative. Restaurants and food manufacturers tend to use a lot of it.

"Look at the label and count up how much you're eating in a day," advises Dr. Ruml. "Don't worry about each serving at first. Instead, focus on your total. Aim to keep the amount in the 2- to 3-gram range, rather than having it push up to 5 grams or more."

Zinc

Where you get it: Meats, poultry, eggs, dairy products, oysters, spices.

What it does for you: Essential for normal growth, development, and immunity. Helps maintain skin, hair, and bones. Keeps the reproductive organs functioning and helps in the perception of taste and the ability to see at night.

What you need: Daily Value of 15 milligrams.

Cautions: Ingesting 2 grams or more of zinc can make you sick to your stomach. Long-term, elevated levels of zinc can cause anemia, lower your immunity, and interfere with your body's ability to absorb two other essential minerals—copper and iron.

So, was lunch tasty today? Did you really enjoy the steak you had for dinner last night? Thank zinc. This trace mineral has a lot to do with your ability to taste. In fact, zinc plays a large role in anything that exists on the surface area of the body, such as skin, hair, mucous membranes, and taste buds.

While depletion of zinc is rare, a slight zinc deficiency is common for older men, people on diets, vegetarians, and people who drink a lot of alcohol, who exercise a lot, or who are under a lot of stress. That's because zinc is easily lost through urine and sweat. Symptoms of a zinc shortage include white spots in the fingernails, dull-colored hair, stunted growth, skin changes, delayed wound healing, and small sex glands in young boys.

"Overt zinc deficiency is quite dramatic," says Janet Hunt, R.D., Ph.D., research nutrition scientist for the U.S. Department of Agriculture–Agricultural Research Service Grand Forks Human Nutrition Research Center in North Dakota. "There is a reduction in growth in children, failure to repair tissues, and dermatitis."

Since there are no stores of zinc in the body, getting the right amount from your diet and possibly supplementation is very important. "Zinc helps keep the skin healthy and intact. If you get enough zinc, blood will flow to your skin more easily," says Lisa Ruml, M.D., assistant professor of medicine and a researcher in the department of mineral metabolism at the University of

Put Zinc on Your Nose

Not only does zinc work in your nose and throat but it also works on your skin to prevent sunburn. Zinc oxide, that white stuff you see on the faces of life-guards, won't let the sun's dangerous ultraviolet rays permeate the skin.

"Zinc oxide is insoluble," says Nancy J. Godfrey, Ph.D., of Godfrey Science and Design, a food supplement consulting service based in Huntingdon Valley, Pennsylvania. That means it won't dissolve in water—a helpful characteristic, indeed, when you're at the ocean.

Texas Southwestern Medical Center at Dallas. "People prone to canker sores may benefit from taking zinc, too."

A number of things can inhibit zinc absorption, including too much calcium and copper as well as phytic acid and fiber in food. Phytic acid is a phosphorous compound that can bind to zinc and carry it out of the body. It's found in whole grains but not in meats, which is one reason why animal products are better sources of zinc than plant foods.

"You should still eat whole grains because the zinc in grains can add to the zinc found in meats," Dr. Hunt says. "Vegetarians are at risk because their only source of zinc is grains." Most foods have the correct ratio of zinc and copper, which will prevent the minerals from counteracting one another. But not all supplements include both. This can be a problem, Dr. Hunt warns.

While whole-wheat bread will have some zinc, the

mineral is removed from processed flour and is not replaced in cereal or bread.

Can Zinc Zap the Common Cold?

Maybe vitamin C has a better press agent. When it comes to the common cold, vitamin C gets all the accolades. But there is increasing evidence that zinc gluconate may have true star potential.

"We've known since 1984 that zinc gluconate could soothe sore throats and decrease the severity of colds," says John C. Godfrey, Ph.D., a medicinal chemist and president of Godfrey Science and Design, a food supplement consulting service based in Huntingdon Valley, Pennsylvania. "The problem was that the taste was repulsive."

So Dr. Godfrey and his wife, Nancy J. Godfrey, Ph.D., did what any good scientists or inventors would do. They turned to the recipes of candy makers. But none of the ideas involving sugar or ascorbic acid panned out.

"I had to find a way to fix the flavor and not let the zinc's effectiveness suffer," says Dr. John Godfrey. "There's a small amino acid called glycine that has a very pleasant taste. It's what makes meat, particularly lamb, taste good." Voilà! Dr. Godfrey had his patent, and Cold-Eezer Plus was born.

Make no mistake, Cold-Eezer Plus—which debuted on the market in the winter of 1994–1995 and has since been revised as Cold-Eeze—still has a strong taste. But let it dissolve in your mouth and your throat will feel better. If you swallow the tablets, there is no effect.

"You want to have lots of zinc ions in the mouth and nose," says Sabrina Novick, Ph.D., assistant professor of chemistry at Hofstra University in Hempstead, New York.

Why? Dr. Novick explains it this way: When it comes to your cold's progression, the rhinovirus associated with the common cold contains the key and your cells have the lock. They attract each other. The positively charged zinc ion temporarily blocks the key from entering the lock. But it is only temporary. That's why you need to take another lozenge every two to four hours. "It's not curing the cold; it's stopping the progression," Dr. Novick says.

The bottom line, according to Dr. Godfrey, is that the zinc lozenges—taken correctly—can cut the duration of your cold in half. However, you have to start taking the lozenges as soon as you feel a little tickle in your throat to get the full effect.

Taking one Cold-Eeze every three to four hours, as recommended by the manufacturer, will give you more than the Daily Value for zinc over the course of a day. This is harmless for the few days it takes to treat a cold, says Dr. Godfrey. Safety of the new "second generation" lozenges is increased by the addition of a trace of copper, just sufficient enough to reverse any possible zinc interference if lozenges are used for more than a few days. These lozenges are meant to be taken for only a short period of time, so be sure not to exceed the manufacturer's directions.

The Best
of the Rest
Copper

Where you get it: Black pepper, blackstrap molasses, Brazil nuts, cocoa.

What it does for you: Helps prevent anemia by assisting the body to release and absorb iron. Contributes to the release of energy, the synthesis of red blood cells (hemoglobin) and the proteins collagen and elastin, the neurotransmitter noradrenaline, and the pigment in your hair.

What you need: Daily Value of 2 milligrams.

Cautions: Numerous other minerals, including calcium, iron, lead, and zinc, reduce the utilization of copper. Toxicity occurs when water or other beverages have been stored in copper containers.

When it comes to building a strong body, copper is like pennies from heaven. Too bad most of us act as if the precious mineral were only worth one red cent.

"Copper is an element that doesn't receive as much attention as it deserves because we haven't looked at it in the right way," says Forrest Nielsen, Ph.D., director of the U.S. Department of Agriculture–Agricultural Research Service Grand Forks Human Nutrition Research Center in North Dakota. "There's no good way to indicate if a person is deficient. I believe that many people are consuming less than 1 milligram a day and that low consumption has a detrimental effect on cardiovascular and bone health."

Copper plays a role in the body's formation of strong, flexible connective tissue; in the production of neurochemicals in the brain; and in the functioning of muscles, nerves, and the immune system. Your body stores most of its copper in your bloodstream. However, other minerals—most notably zinc—can interfere with your body's ability to absorb copper.

"The healthy ratio for zinc to copper is in the range of 8 to 12 parts of zinc to 1 part of copper," says Alexander Schauss, Ph.D., director of the life sciences division of the American Institute for Biosocial Research in Tacoma, Washington, and author of *Minerals, Trace Elements, and Human Health*. "Other things can also lead to an imbalance of copper in your body, including smoking cigarettes, having a lot of stress, and drinking tea." Since tea is a diuretic, it drains the body of trace elements, Dr. Schauss says.

Research has shown that too little copper leads to anemia, a disease involving decreased levels of hemoglobin in red blood cells, and also tiny or a reduced number of red blood cells. Early symptoms include fatigue. Dr. Schauss says that excesses of copper, usually as a result of high levels in water, contribute to incidences of hyperactivity in children. In adults, getting too much copper (more than 3 milligrams a day) can cause vomiting.

Fluoride

Where you get it: Fluoridated water and toothpaste, seaweed, marine fish with bones, tea.

What it does for you: Prevents cavities and helps make bone tissue stronger.

What you need: Estimated Safe and Adequate Daily Dietary Intake of 1.5 to 4 milligrams.

Cautions: Excess fluoride causes the enamel of developing teeth to become chalky and mottled-looking. Deficiency of fluoride results in excess dental cavities in people of all ages and possibly more osteoporosis in older folks.

You'd probably be perfectly content to live the rest of your days without ever hearing the sound of a dentist's drill again. If that's the case, don't make the mistake of thinking that fluoride was something you needed only while sprouting your permanent teeth way back when.

"Sometimes people begin to get more cavities around the age of 40," says Israel Kleinberg, D.D.S., Ph.D., professor and chairman of the department of oral biology and pathology at the School of Dental Medicine at the State University of New York at Stony Brook. "It's usually because either stress or a medication they're taking has caused them to have a drier mouth with less saliva."

Your teeth are more susceptible to the acids in food and drink without enough saliva swishing around, so there is a danger of mineral loss. The fluoride in toothpaste and drinking water can help.

"Keep using fluoridated toothpaste, even if you think you're past the years of getting cavities," Dr. Kleinberg says. "Fluoride can always help."

There is an abundance of evidence supporting fluoride's role in warding off cavities. Ideally, between your water supply, fluoride toothpaste, and other tooth products with fluoride, such as mouthwash, adults should get between 1.5 and 4 milligrams of fluoride a day. Kids four years old and up, however, should get no more than 2.5 milligrams a day because more can damage teeth, according to the Estimated Safe and Adequate Daily Dietary Intakes of the National Research Council.

"Fluorosis, a mottling pattern on the teeth, affects tooth enamel during its formation," Dr. Kleinberg says. "Between fluoridated water, juices made with fluoridated water, and toothpaste, children can get too much."

Aside from your teeth, fluoride has been shown to aid in your body's drive to maintain its calcium stores in your bones. While the fluoride in your toothpaste can't help, there will soon be tablets of slow-release sodium fluoride that have proven effective.

One study showed that the slow-release fluoride in conjunction with calcium citrate supplements decreased the rate of spinal fractures in women who were prone to them because of low-density bone levels. The use of slow-release fluoride as a drug to help fight osteoporosis is still being examined.

Iodine

Where you get it: Iodized salt, lobster, shrimp, breads, milk.

What it does for you: Iodine has only one function: to make the hormones secreted by the thyroid gland.

What you need: Daily Value of 150 micrograms.

Cautions: Oddly enough, too much and too little can lead to an enlargement of the thyroid gland, known as goiter.

The thyroid gland uses iodine to produce thyroxine, a key hormone that helps regulate energy production, body temperature, breathing, muscle tone, and the manufacture and breakdown of tissues. Iodine deficiency and excess usually result in goiter, an enlargement of the thyroid gland that is visible as swelling on the front of the neck.

With iodine-fortified salt, most—but not all—of us easily get more than the Daily Value of 150 micrograms.

"There are a few areas in this country that still have cases of goiter," says Dr. Schauss. "Mostly in mountainous regions, such as the Appalachians." Studies have shown that microorganisms can cause goiter, rather than iodine deficiency itself. However, iodine deficiency in the soil and water is the major cause of goiter.

The most interesting thing about iodine, according to Dr. Schauss, is its role in brain function. "We've found that children who are exposed to radiation, or iodine 131 (I_{131}), have more trouble in school," he says. In fact, when the Soviet Union's nuclear power plant at Chernobyl exploded, the Polish government handed out iodine tablets to everyone in Poland within three to four days.

Other governments such as Sweden and Italy urged their citizens to consume kelp or iodine supplements to protect their thyroid from exposure to I_{131}. Kelp contains iodine 192, the stable form of iodine that we find in our salt.

Manganese

Where you get it: Brown rice, spices, nuts, whole grains, beans, blueberries.

What it does for you: Helps form bones and stimulates growth of connective tissue. Assists in the synthesis of fatty acids, cholesterol, and the activation of various enzymes. Thought to have some role in brain function.

What you need: Daily Value of 2 milligrams.

Cautions: The body absorbs only about 45 percent of consumed manganese from the average diet.

Sometimes good things do come in small packages. Take manganese, a mineral found in humans, animals, plants—and even gingerbread men. Eat a few cookies and you will get a good dose of this humble, yet powerful, element.

Manganese—derived from the Greek word for magic—itself isn't an ingredient of gingerbread cookies. But cloves and ginger are, and they feature whopping doses of manganese. Aside from its role in holiday baking, manganese also is used as an alloy in the production of steel to give it toughness.

This is one of those minerals where you're far more likely to get too much than too little. There's only been one documented case of manganese deficiency, but there have been lots of toxicity reports.

That's because miners and other people who work around minerals have been known to inhale the stuff. It can be poisonous in this form. However, toxicity from ingestion is rare but has been caused by contaminated drinking water or from taking high doses of a dietary supplement.

This also is one of those minerals where you probably should get more than the Daily Value, which is just 2 milligrams, says Dr. Schauss. However, if you plan to take more than 10 milligrams a day, consult your doctor first.

Although manganese has not been studied very often, and rarely with humans, it has been shown to play a role in metabolism, glucose tolerance, insulin response, and brain function. Manganese is found in the mitochondria, our energy cells. And without manganese, the energy might remain stuck.

"Animals with high levels of manganese show higher levels of antisocial behavior," says Dr. Schauss. "Unfortunately, we're more than a decade away from understanding the extent of this relationship."

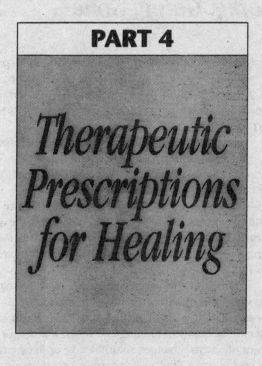

PART 4

Therapeutic Prescriptions for Healing

Age Spots

Going, Going, Gone

O urs is a culture with little appreciation for spots. None of us likes getting a spot on our record, on our reputation, or on our shirt. And we certainly don't like seeing spots when we're looking into a mirror!

But as we age, many of us do begin to see spots, especially on our hands and faces. And whether we call them liver spots, age spots, or sun spots, the reaction is likely the same: We want a spot remover.

Technically known as lentigines, age spots are the result of excess pigment being deposited in the skin during years of sun exposure. So along with treatment, dermatologists also recommend avoiding exposure to the sun.

Note: Though the majority of age spots are harmless blemishes that require no more than a trip to the dermatologist, early stages of skin cancer can masquerade as innocent-looking age spots. If any spot enlarges, thickens, changes color, bleeds, or itches, have it checked by a doctor. For extra protection, also include a skin examination in your annual checkup.

The good news is, if your spots really are just age spots, dermatologists today have an assortment of treatments at their disposal that can fade them, if not remove them completely. These include topical application of tretinoin, a vitamin A acid known as Retin-A.

Fade 'Em Away with Retin-A

Originally developed as an acne medication to unplug clogged pores, Retin-A has found resounding success as an anti-aging ointment. Though not a fountain of youth, Retin-A works to eliminate fine wrinkles, blemishes, and age spots by stimulating cell turnover in a metabolic process that still is not entirely understood, says Retin-A creator Albert Kligman, M.D., Ph.D., professor of dermatology at the University of Pennsylvania School of Medicine and an attending physician at the Hospital of the University of Pennsylvania, both in Philadelphia.

To remove an age spot, dermatologists often recommend applying the strongest dosage of Retin-A that you can tolerate directly on the spot. The area will proceed to peel, and after a few months, the spot should diminish and possibly even disappear.

If you're like the people who were in a research group at the University of Michigan Medical Center in Ann Arbor, you may even see results after just one month. In a 10-month study of 58 people with age spots, researchers found that the majority of people treated with Retin-A experienced lightening of these spots after one month. After 10 months, 83 percent of those treated with Retin-A experienced lightening of their age spots, and 32 percent had at least one spot disappear.

Retin-A can be even more effective when used in combination with other treatments, says John F. Romano, M.D., clinical assistant professor of dermatology at New York Hospital–Cornell Medical Center and St. Vincent's Hospital, both in New York City.

"I often have people apply glycolic acid in the

morning and Retin-A at night. Or I may combine it with a bleaching cream," says Dr. Romano.

Retin-A cream comes in a variety of concentrations, the weakest being 0.025 percent and the strongest being 0.1 percent. It's available only by prescription, so you'll need to work with your dermatologist to find the dosage that's right for you.

And because Retin-A continually sloughs off the outermost, dead layer of skin, it can not only eliminate existing spots but also nip new spots in the bud. The downside of this process is that an area of skin previously sheltered from evaporation and the elements is exposed. That's why a common side effect of Retin-A is dry, sun-sensitive skin that can be irritated and scaly. Though this effect typically diminishes with time, if you're using Retin-A, you'll likely need a moisturizer. Sunscreen is also a must once you start using Retin-A.

Protect Your Skin with Vitamin C

If vitamin D is the sunshine vitamin, then vitamin C is the sunblock vitamin, say some researchers—many of whom also proclaim it the healthy skin vitamin.

"In general, vitamin C is important for keeping the skin younger looking," says Lorraine Meisner, Ph.D., professor of preventive medicine at the University of Wisconsin Medical School in Madison. She recommends a safe daily vitamin C intake of about 300 to 500 milligrams to maintain skin quality.

Medical researchers have also found vitamin C to be of some help when applied topically. It has been shown to significantly reduce the amount of so-called free radical damage that occurs from sun exposure. Free radicals are naturally occurring unstable molecules that steal electrons from your body's healthy molecules to balance themselves. Unchecked, they can cause significant tissue damage. Antioxidants—vitamin C is one—neutralize free radicals by offering their own electrons and so protect the healthy molecules from harm.

"Since vitamin C prevents skin damage from sun exposure, it's reasonable to suspect that it can also prevent the consequences of that damage, including wrinkling and age spots," says Douglas Darr, Ph.D., director of technology development at the North Carolina Biotechnology Center in Research Triangle Park. Dr. Darr advocates using topical vitamin C as an adjunct to sunscreen.

One such topical vitamin C product is Cellex-C, a 10 percent vitamin C lotion. It's available without a prescription from dermatologists, plastic surgeons, and licensed aestheticians (full-service beauty salon operators) and by mail order from Cellex-C Distribution, 2631 Commerce Street, Suite C, Dallas, TX 75226. For optimum sun protection, the lotion should be applied once a day, along with a sunscreen, according to Dr. Meisner, one of the developers of Cellex-C.

Also, though snacking on citrus fruits may help keep your skin healthier, don't count on being able to eat enough oranges to protect you from the sun, says Sheldon Pinnell, M.D., chief of dermatology at Duke University Medical Center in Durham, North Carolina, and another of the developers of Cellex-C. "The cream allows you to get 20 to 40 times the levels that you would achieve by ingesting vitamin C," he says.

Damage Control with Vitamin E

Vitamin E, an antioxidant vitamin added to everything from nail polish remover to shampoo, is also helpful in preventing sun damage.

Researchers have shown that vitamin E oil can prevent inflammation and skin damage if applied within eight hours of sun exposure. Because vitamin E itself produces free radicals when exposed to ultraviolet light, however, researchers recommend that you apply it following, not before, sun exposure.

Vitamin E oil can be bought over the counter in drugstores, as can vitamin E–fortified creams. Research has shown that if the cream or oil contains at least 5 percent vitamin E, it can also be effective in reducing post-sun damage.

You can also reap some of vitamin E's sun-protective properties by taking supplements, adds Karen E. Burke, M.D., Ph.D., a dermatologic surgeon and dermatologist in private practice in New York City. "It's highly effective as an anti-inflammatory agent, and it reduces sun damage to the skin," she says. Dr. Burke recommends that people take 400 international units of vitamin E in the form of d-alpha-tocopherol daily.

Good dietary sources of vitamin E include polyunsaturated vegetable oil, wheat germ, spinach, and sunflower seeds.

Try Some Selenium Sun Protection

You might want to boost your dietary intake of the antioxidant mineral selenium as well, says Dr. Burke.

"Selenium can prevent solar damage, pigmentation, and dark spots, but because the selenium content of soil varies across the country, not everyone is getting enough to be beneficial," says Dr. Burke, citing the Southeast in particular as an area deficient in selenium.

To quench the free radicals caused by sun exposure and to prevent skin damage, Dr. Burke recommends daily supplements of 50 to 200 micrograms of selenium in the form of l-selenomethionine, depending on where you live and your family history of cancer.

To get more selenium in your diet, try tuna; a three-ounce can serves up a full 99 micrograms. Or treat yourself to an ounce of baked tortilla chips for a whopping 284 micrograms.

Medical Alert

Selenium can be toxic in daily doses exceeding 100 micrograms, so if you'd like to try this therapy to protect your skin, you should discuss it with your doctor.

If you're taking anticoagulant drugs, you should not take oral vitamin E supplements.

Aging

A Radical Solution

At age 38, Elizabeth lies on Litchfield Beach in South Carolina, sunscreen carefully smoothed over her wrinkle-free skin, her naturally dark hair tucked under a scarf, and a pair of dense wraparound sunglasses shielding her lovely blue eyes from the morning sun.

Beside her is a cooler containing several bottles of springwater and a fresh fruit salad of watermelon, cantaloupe, and honeydew for lunch. Next to her on the sand is a pair of well-used sneakers for the two-mile walk she takes along the water's edge every day.

Elizabeth knows that she's gorgeous. There are no wrinkles or stretch marks marring her perfect body. And she's determined that there will never be. She'll do whatever it takes to defy aging until the day she dies.

What are the odds that she'll make it? Better than they were a decade ago. Back then scientists had already found the reasons that we deteriorate into wrinkles, bags, age spots, flab, and life-threatening conditions. The reasons were, and still are, genetics, disease, environmental factors such as smoking and diet, and the aging process itself. Today these scientists also know that every single one of these factors may be directly influenced and perhaps even altered by getting enough of the right kinds of vitamins and minerals.

A Chemical Blitzkrieg

Both the diseases that contribute to aging and the physical and mental "damage" that we associate with old age seem to be triggered by a lifelong blitzkrieg of damaging molecules that affect us on many levels.

These molecules, sometimes called free radicals by scientists, are sent zinging through our bodies by cigarette smoke and chronic infection as well as by the normal cell metabolism that converts the carbohydrates and fat we eat into the energy required to power our cells. Yes, just eating your daily breakfast normally produces untold numbers of these harmful molecules. There's no way to avoid them completely.

Unfortunately, free radicals have the nasty habit of stealing electrons from your body's healthy molecules to balance themselves, in the process damaging cells and their DNA, the genetic blueprint that tells a cell how to do its job. And without a perfect copy of that DNA blueprint, a cell doesn't know what it's supposed to do. Yet biochemists estimate that every cell in the body is hit 10,000 times every day by free radicals patrolling the body.

The result?

Depending on how badly they're hit and how quickly they're returned to service by cellular repair squads, the cells may mutate or die, explains researcher Denham Harman, M.D., Ph.D., professor emeritus of medicine at the University of Nebraska College of Medicine in Omaha. And when either of these events happens, it may initiate the underlying biochemical processes that cause many of the diseases that accelerate aging: heart disease, high blood pressure, Parkinson's disease, cancer, cataracts, diabetes, and even Alzheimer's disease.

Some scientists also believe that free radicals affect the aging process even more directly, says Dr. Harman, the man who first raised the possibility. In fact, he adds, "there's a growing consensus that aging itself is due to free radical reactions."

The idea is that there may be an accumulation of damage from the constant cellular bombardment by free radicals. A cell gets hit once, the cellular repair squads come to the rescue and cut out the damage to the cell's DNA blueprint, and the cell bounces back into action. But when the cell gets hit over and over again, there may come a point at which the repair squads can't patch everything back together the way it was. So the cell continues to do its job, but not as well as it had been.

If it's a skin cell, for example, you might end up with wrinkled skin rather than smooth, polished skin.

If it's an eye cell, maybe you just can't see as clearly as you used to.

In any event, scientists have found that 40 to 50 percent of all of the proteins in an older person may be damaged by free radicals. Proteins are involved in a myriad of functions in the body, from guiding chemical reactions to supplying energy to maintaining the body's structures.

And that, plus the fact that laboratory studies indicate that damaged proteins shorten the life span of laboratory animals, has led some scientists to suspect free radicals may directly cause aging.

Natural Antioxidants

Although millions of free radicals bombard your cells on a daily basis, the fact that it takes as long as it does for them to cause damage or disease is a tribute to the natural free radical–fighting systems with which you were born. "These systems are fighting free radicals every moment of every day," says Pamela Starke-Reed, Ph.D., director of the Office of Nutrition at the National Institute on Aging in Bethesda, Maryland.

Each system is ingeniously designed to produce an antioxidant, a naturally occurring chemical that neutralizes the free radical (or the oxidant, as it is sometimes called) by offering its own electrons. In doing so, the antioxidant helps preserve your body's healthy molecules.

Each antioxidant is designed to work in a different way in a different part of the cell, says Dr. Starke-Reed. Its marching orders come from the genetic instructions on your chromosomes, and its power comes from a ready supply of specific nutrients in your diet. One natural antioxidant is dependent upon the availability of copper, zinc, and manganese. Another is dependent on iron, and a third is dependent on selenium.

How much do you need? "You want to keep everything in balance," says Dr. Starke-Reed. But since scientists are just beginning to understand what it takes to keep that balance, "the best that we can do right now is to tell people that they should be taking in at least the Daily Values of all essential vitamins and minerals," she states.

Supplementing the Body's Natural Antioxidants

Although the body produces natural antioxidants to neutralize free radical damage, it doesn't produce enough to handle the free radical bombardment generated by the modern world. Your body's natural antioxidant systems were simply not designed to handle rooms full of cigarette smoke, a diet loaded with fat, and constant exposure to new and more virulent viruses.

This may change once scientists learn how to alter our genes so that we produce more natural antioxidants. But in the meantime, we do have another option: enhancing our natural antioxidants with man-made antioxidants—in a word, supplements.

Laboratory studies indicate that antioxidant supplements, predominantly vitamins C and E plus beta-carotene and selenium, seem to be able to neutralize free radicals that sneak past the natural antioxidants produced in your cells, says Dr. Harman.

"Nobody really knows what the optimum levels are," he adds. "But I recommend daily doses of 200 to 400 international units (IU) of vitamin E and 1,500 to 2,000 milligrams of vitamin C, along with 25,000 IU of beta-carotene every other day. I also suggest that people take one 50-microgram tablet of selenium in the morning and one at night." Some people may experience diarrhea when taking high daily doses of vitamin C.

Will this actually slow the aging process? "Nobody knows," replies Dr. Harman. It does in laboratory animals. But it will be decades before the people who load up on antioxidants live long enough to answer that question for humans, he says.

Yet while we're waiting to find out, one thing seems absolutely clear: Those folks who take supplemental antioxidants or who enrich their diets with antioxidant-rich fruits and vegetables certainly seem to be preventing development of the diseases that can accelerate the aging process.

More than 50 studies conducted during the past decade demonstrated that high intake of foods rich in beta-carotene reduces the risk of cancer. More than 40 studies indicated that vitamin C does the same. And a review of studies that measured the amounts of antioxidants people eat revealed that the one-fourth of the American population consuming the most fruits and vegetables, the primary dietary sources of beta-carotene, vitamin C, and selenium, had half of the rate of cancers of the lung, mouth, esophagus, stomach, pancreas, cervix, and bladder compared with those who didn't consume as much.

What's more, people who got less of the antioxidant vitamins C and E and carotenoids such as beta-carotene were more likely to develop cataracts and macular degeneration, a vision-destroying disease that affects mainly older people. People who got plentiful supplies of these antioxidants were 37 percent less likely to have heart attacks.

So not only do antioxidants seem to prevent the diseases that accelerate us into old age, they also seem to be helping us maintain quality of life.

Getting people to eat more as they age is important, says Jeffrey Blumberg, Ph.D., associate director and chief of the antioxidants research laboratory at the Jean Mayer U.S. Department of Agriculture Human Nutrition Research Center on Aging at Tufts University in Boston. But what you eat is also important, he adds.

"In essence, eating a super high quality diet is crucial if you want to do all that you can to stay young longer," says Dr. Blumberg. "It's especially important to key in on good food sources of vitamins C and E and beta-carotene." Good sources include orange and yellow vegetables, fruits, and whole grains.

"In addition, I'd go so far as to advise people who want to take steps to slow down the aging process to take a daily multivitamin/mineral supplement," he says.

Medical Alert

Doses of vitamin C as high as 1,500 to 2,000 milligrams may cause diarrhea in some people.

If you are taking anticoagulant drugs, you should not take vitamin E supplements.

Allergies

Taming the Savage Sneeze

Faster than a speeding bullet. More powerful than a locomotive. Able to make its victims itch, wheeze, sneeze, weep, cough, and ache in a single attack. Is it the flu? Is it food poisoning? No, it's your pesky allergies bringing you to your knees again.

Allergies can lay waste a mere mortal the way kryptonite fells Superman. The list of potential allergens—substances that people can be allergic to—is quite long: from pollen, cat dander, and dust mites to such seemingly harmless substances as strawberries, shaving cream, and fabrics. The symptoms are just as versatile, affecting the nose, eyes, throat, lungs, stomach, skin, or nervous system, or even causing fatigue or depression—all of which can hit you in varying strengths.

You might not think of yourself as oversensitive, but sometimes the immune system is. Allergy symptoms occur when your body's immune system overreacts to substances you're exposed to. Histamine and leukotrienes, powerful defensive chemicals that your immune system releases, can cause many of the common allergy symptoms, including runny nose and nasal congestion. Mast cells—found in tissues such as skin, lungs, throat, stomach, and intestines—release histamine. And cells called basophils, which hang out in your blood vessels, release leukotrienes when they are exposed to an allergen.

Of course, the best way to put an end to your allergy troubles is to avoid the allergens that affect you in the first place and to take any allergy medicine that your doctor prescribes. But some nutrients may be able to prevent some of your misery, too, provided they are taken before an allergy attack. Here's what the experts say about the most promising ones.

Vitamin C: The Bodyguard

Vitamin C's effect on allergic reactions has been heavily studied. High levels of vitamin C help reduce histamine release from mast cells and also make histamine break down faster once it is released. And when you're low on vitamin C, researchers discovered, your blood levels of histamine rise. But investigators are now seeing a broader picture of just how vitamin C may affect the allergic-reaction process, and there's evidence that it doesn't work alone.

Enter bioflavonoids. Plant foods contain more than 4,000 of these unique natural chemicals, and researchers have been investigating their role in allergy prevention for decades. "Vitamin C works as an antioxidant that protects the bioflavonoids, which look to be what's really reducing the allergy symptoms," says Jeremy E. Kaslow, M.D., assistant clinical professor of medicine at the University of California, Irvine, and an allergy specialist in Garden Grove, California.

It's too early for scientists to make specific recommendations about the kinds or exact amount of bioflavonoids that people with allergies should be taking, says Elliott Middleton Jr., M.D., professor emeritus of medicine at the State University of New York at Buffalo School of Medicine and Biomedical Sciences and founder of the Chebeague Island Institute of Natural Product Research in Maine. But it's still a good idea to regularly consume foods that contain bioflavonoids. They aren't hard to come by if you are eating right to begin with, says Dr. Middleton.

"Foods with vitamin C have bioflavonoids by default, so diet can be a means of getting enough of both nutrients," Dr. Kaslow says. Getting the recommended five to nine servings of fruits and vegetables should make it easy to reach the Daily Value for vitamin C (60 milligrams) and provide a healthy dose of bioflavonoids at the same time. Some doctors suggest that getting 1,000 to 2,000 milligrams of vitamin C a day is beneficial to ward off some allergy symptoms.

Dr. Kaslow recommends that if you are taking a supplement with vitamin C for allergy relief, make sure that the product label also says that it contains bioflavonoids.

Mighty Magnesium

Magnesium helps relieve bronchospasm, or constricted airways, in the lungs. It has been used intravenously to help relieve the symptoms of life-threatening, drug-resistant asthma attacks. Now it seems that this mineral may be valuable in keeping histamines in check.

"The flow of calcium into and out of a cell helps regulate some cell function. Magnesium deficiency may change the permeability of mast cell membranes, allowing calcium to enter cells more easily," says Kay Franz, Ph.D., associate professor of nutrition at Brigham Young University in Provo, Utah, and one of the study's authors. "When that happens, histamine is released."

Regardless of whether you have allergies, experts recommend that you get your Daily Value of 400 milligrams of magnesium. That's because magnesium is an important player in many of the body's functions. Foods like nuts, beans, whole grains, bananas, and green vegetables will help. Don't go overboard with magnesium, though. It is, after all, what gives milk of magnesia its laxative powers.

If you have kidney problems and are considering taking a magnesium supplement, check with your doctor first. Most people with kidney disease have a decreased ability to clear waste products from the blood. Excess magnesium in the diet or from supplements would not be easily excreted and could build up in the blood and tissues to potentially toxic levels.

Remember the Membrane

Now here's a sticky subject. The mucous lining is the body's internal skin. It is a layer of cells containing infection-fighting biochemicals that secrete mucus. Mucus has an important function: It shields cells from direct contact with pollen and other allergens.

"Having an unhealthy mucous lining will promote allergies," says Dr. Kaslow. So make sure that you're effectively countering those attacking allergens by consuming adequate amounts of vitamin A (or its precursor, beta-carotene), selenium, iodine, and zinc. "Those are the ones that we focus on when there is a problem with mucus, but you still need to have good supplies of all nutrients to have a consistently healthy mucous lining," explains Dr. Kaslow.

Antioxidants: Can They Help?

An allergic reaction causes the generation of unstable molecules called free radicals, which injure your body's healthy molecules by stealing electrons to balance themselves. In the process, free radicals injure mast cells and may make them even more twitchy and prone to histamine release, says Dr. Middleton. Vitamins C and E, beta-carotene, selenium, and other antioxidants all help neutralize free radicals by offering their own electrons, thus protecting healthy molecules from harm.

It is still unknown how much of which antioxidants is needed to have an effect on allergic reactions, so Dr. Middleton suggests that people make sure that they are eating lots of fresh fruits and vegetables that are rich in antioxidants. "There may be undiscovered nutrients at work alone or in tandem with known antioxidants in whole foods," he explains.

Medical Alert

If you have heart disease or kidney problems, check with your doctor before taking magnesium supplements.

Taking more than 1,500 to 2,000 milligrams of vitamin C a day can cause diarrhea in some people.

Alzheimer's Disease

Fighting the Memory Thief

Few health problems are as feared as Alzheimer's disease. The fourth leading cause of death in adults (after heart disease, cancer, and stroke), Alzheimer's affects approximately four million Americans. And this figure is expected to more than triple by the middle of the next century.

Alzheimer's is a disease that sneaks up slowly, ever so quietly stealing away an elderly person's memory and personality, eventually eroding his ability to take care of himself. Elderly people with Alzheimer's are then forced to rely on family or health care professionals for survival. Is there no hope?

Actually, yes, there is. A cure is probably decades away. But even in the high-tech world of brain research, some of the most promising treatments on the horizon actually include the use of a few simple vitamins.

Investigating an Elusive Enemy

A look at what's going on in the brain of someone with Alzheimer's disease makes the memory loss and other personality problems at least understandable. Once-healthy brain cells get tangled into knots and die off.

Far less clear is just what's killing those cells. For

years, research focused on microscopic plaques, made of a substance called amyloid, that slowly build up in the area of the brain responsible for memory and mental functioning. Once the plaques start hardening, the havoc begins.

As it turns out, amyloid probably has quite a few partners in crime—and at least one could be hiding in your family tree. Some forms of a blood protein called ApoE that normally ferry cholesterol through the blood also appear to cause more amyloid to be deposited in the brain and may help it harden, says Leonard Berg, M.D., chairman of the medical and scientific advisory board for the Alzheimer's Association and director of the Alzheimer's Disease Research Center at Washington University in St. Louis. And the evidence implicating one form, ApoE-4, as a risk factor for this disease is convincing. Folks with two ApoE-4 genes are eight times as likely to develop Alzheimer's as those who inherit only ApoE-2 or ApoE-3. In one study of 46 adults with Alzheimer's, 21.4 percent had the requisite two ApoE-4 genes compared with 2.9 percent who had no ApoE-4 genes.

Other researchers think that zinc can potentially increase the amount of toxic amyloid deposited in the brain. In laboratory experiments, investigators at Massachusetts General Hospital in Boston found that a slight increase in zinc caused amyloid "to curdle into gluelike clumps" within just two minutes. More information is needed on the role of dietary zinc in Alzheimer's, according to the study's lead researcher, Rudolph Tanzi, M.D., director of the genetics and aging unit at Massachusetts General Hospital and Harvard Medical School. But now there is enough evidence to warn against megadoses of elemental zinc. Because increased dietary zinc has been shown to markedly decrease mental functioning in people with Alzheimer's, Dr. Tanzi suggests that they get no more than the Daily Value of 15 milligrams.

During studies in the 1960s, animals injected with aluminum developed tangles similar to those found in people with Alzheimer's. Since then, studies using advanced measuring devices have found increased concentrations of aluminum in brain tissue obtained from people who had died from Alzheimer's, says Daniel Perl, M.D., director of the neuropathology division at Mount Sinai School of Medicine in New York City. "We still don't know where the aluminum is from or what it's doing there, but we're trying to determine whether it has an active role," he says.

Brain Rust Sets In

No matter what the cause of Alzheimer's may ultimately be, some researchers are convinced that the oxidative damage that your brain suffers over a lifetime also plays a role in the development of this disease. When the body burns oxygen to produce energy, the process also spawns chemically unstable molecules that are known as free radicals. These molecules steal electrons from your body's healthy molecules to balance themselves, damaging all kinds of cells, including brain cells, in the process.

A number of things contribute to the production of free radicals: pollution, cigarette smoke, alcohol—in other words, living in the modern world. "What makes me think that oxidative damage is important is that one of the main risk factors for Alzheimer's is getting old," says Dr. Berg. "Oxidative damage accumulates during aging just from normal metabolism of brain cells."

In fact, 10 percent of people ages 65 and older have Alzheimer's, while 20 percent of those over age 75 have the disease. A whopping 40 percent of those over age 85 have it.

One theory suggests that the oxidation process might make amyloid even more damaging—and might kill some brain cells on its own.

Further complicating the search for an Alzheimer's cure: ApoE-4, zinc, aluminum, oxidation, and even inflammation may each play some small role in causing the disease in all people who have it. "There probably won't be a single solution," says Dr. Berg. "The same symptoms and the same plaques and tangles come about from multiple different causes."

Vitamin E Might Provide Some Protection

While researchers explore different approaches for conquering Alzheimer's, at least one research team has turned to a vitamin breakthrough in stroke treatment for answers.

During a stroke, damaged brain cells release a neurotransmitter called glutamic acid. This chemical causes a chain reaction that destroys more brain cells, releasing even more dangerous glutamic acid.

Exposing brain cells to vitamin E in the laboratory seems to shield them from the effects of a stroke, says David Schubert, Ph.D., professor of neurobiology at the Salk Institute for Biological Studies in San Diego. "Vitamin E actually has a protective effect on brain cells, limiting the number killed by the glutamic acid," he explains.

In another study, Dr. Schubert's laboratory showed

that bathing brain cells in vitamin E protects them from a toxic protein found in amyloid plaques.

How? Just as soaking a peeled apple in lemon juice prevents oxidation from turning it brown, antioxidants such as vitamin E protect brain cells by neutralizing free radicals.

There's a hitch, however, in using vitamin E to prevent and treat Alzheimer's. Vitamin E doesn't cross what's called the blood-brain barrier very well. A natural protective mechanism, this barrier literally shields the brain from most substances. "It's a problem. Vitamin E is not the ideal compound to use in any type of therapy in this respect," says Dr. Schubert.

In the quest for a cure, however, researchers are attempting to fuse vitamin E with something like a steroid so that it can cross your blood-brain barrier more effectively, says Dr. Schubert.

It's too early to tell whether vitamin E supplements alone can help ward off Alzheimer's disease. But Dr. Schubert says there's enough potential to warrant taking supplements. "Vitamin E is pretty hard to get in your diet, because it's primarily in vegetable oils," he says. "And if you don't eat enough, the vitamin E in your blood and brain actually decreases as you get older. That can be elevated somewhat by vitamin E supplements."

Although you should see your doctor first, about 400 international units (IU) of vitamin E a day should be enough for most people, he says. The Daily Value for vitamin E is 30 IU.

The Thiamin Connection

While vitamin E researchers try to protect the brain against the ravages of amyloid plaques, those studying thiamin have taken a different approach: improving the memory of people with Alzheimer's.

In one study, 11 people with Alzheimer's symptoms were directed to take either 1,000 milligrams of thiamin or placebos (look-alike dummy pills) three times a day for three months. (This is a lot of thiamin, as the Daily Value is just 1.5 milligrams.) Tests before and after the study showed that memory improved slightly for those taking thiamin.

That might not seem like a particularly impressive finding. But people in the later stages of Alzheimer's disease generally experience a significant drop in mental functioning every six months. "We found some not very noticeable but clinically measurable positive results," says John Blass, M.D., director of the dementia research service at the Burke Medical Research Institute in White Plains, New York.

In another study inspired by Dr. Blass's work, researchers at the Medical College of Georgia in Augusta treated 18 Alzheimer's patients for five months with megadoses of thiamin ranging from 3,000 to 8,000 milligrams a day, with the dose changing from month to month.

At the end of each month, the participants were given a brief bedside exam that included questions about the date, the name of the hospital, and the city, county, and state, says Kimford Meador, M.D., head of the Section of Behavioral Neurology at the college. When the results were analyzed, Dr. Meador says, the research team discovered that some participants improved slightly the month they took 5,000 milligrams of thiamin a day.

"Overall, even in those whose scores dropped,

they didn't drop as fast as they 'should have,'" says Dr. Meador. In other words, he would have expected people in the later stages of the disease to perform poorly, but while taking the vitamin, they were doing better than expected.

"In particular, on the bedside exam you can expect a three-point drop almost every four to six months. We didn't see that in these people," he explains. "Our people either maintained where they were or dropped a point or two—not as far as they should have. At this stage of the research, this is pretty much the best you can hope for."

Why might something like thiamin help protect memory? It's possible that thiamin helps make an important neurotransmitter called acetylcholine, which helps the nerve impulses that carry thought leap across the gaps between brain cells, more available in the brain, explains Dr. Meador. And acetylcholine is lower in people with Alzheimer's. Interestingly, research shows that thiamin deficiency in older folks may run as high as 37 percent, he says.

Does this mean that people with Alzheimer's could benefit from taking large doses of thiamin? Much more research needs to be done before answering that question for sure, says Dr. Meador. "The effect of the treatment is not tremendous in and of itself, but it looks like it's an innocuous treatment and of mild benefit," he says. "I'd like to stress that it's not a final answer and that we studied small numbers. But until something better comes along, why not?" Taking 5,000 milligrams of thiamin a day caused only mild nausea in some people, says Dr. Meador. If you or a family member would like to try this therapy, make sure you discuss it with your doctor.

Medical Alert

Anyone with Alzheimer's disease should be under a doctor's care.

A dose of 5,000 milligrams of thiamin is thousands of times beyond the Daily Value and caused nausea in some people when it was tested. Make sure you get your physician's approval before trying this therapy.

If you are taking anticoagulants, you should not take vitamin E supplements.

Anemia

Getting Back in the Pink

The old doctors' joke—that the first order of business is to find the pale patient against the white sheet—makes one good point about anemia: It tends to drain the color out of you, as surely as it pulls the plug on your energy supply.

Anemia is a blood disorder that results from a shortage of hemoglobin in the red blood cells, the disk-shape cells that carry oxygen to all parts of the body. No matter what kind of anemia you have—and there are several varieties—the symptoms tend to be the same. Along with being pale and fatigued, you can feel weak and short of breath, your heart rate may climb, and you may find it hard to concentrate.

These symptoms occur because without sufficient hemoglobin in the red blood cells, all parts of the body, including the brain, are starved for oxygen. And the heart tries to compensate by pumping more blood more often, explains Paul Stander, M.D., a doctor of quality management and director of medical education at Good Samaritan Medical Center in Phoenix.

Doctors can usually diagnose anemia by examining red blood cells under a microscope to determine their shape, size, and number and by tests that measure levels of different blood components.

"Even after we've determined the type of anemia, it's important to figure out what's causing it," Dr. Stander says. Everything from excessive bongo playing (the constant impact on the hands damages blood cells) to arctic temperatures and toxic drugs can cause the disease.

"Nutritional deficiencies are a fairly common cause of anemia, too," Dr. Stander says. In addition to iron deficiency, a shortage of folate (the naturally occurring form of folic acid) or vitamin B_{12} can be a culprit. Rarely, the problem turns out to be an inadequate supply of copper, riboflavin, or vitamin A, B_6, C, or E.

Here's what studies show.

Iron Out an Oxygen Shortage

We've all heard about iron-poor blood, and for good reason. Iron deficiency is by far the most common cause of anemia. Up to 58 percent of healthy young women may be short on iron, although not always to the point of anemia.

The problem is that many women don't consume enough iron each day to make up for the 2.5 milligrams or so they lose each month during menstruation. Pregnant women need even more iron. Teens and women nearing menopause also often come up short.

Studies show that women ages 18 to 24 get about 10.7 milligrams a day, which is nowhere near the Daily Value of 18 milligrams.

An iron shortage leads to a reduction in hemoglobin, the iron-based protein in red blood cells that lets these cells pick up oxygen in the lungs and release it in tissues where oxygen is low. "It's simple enough," Dr. Stander says. "These cells simply can't transport the oxygen you need." The cells even look pale under a microscope.

If you do have iron-deficiency anemia, your doctor will initially prescribe large amounts of iron—often 200 to 240 milligrams a day, usually in a form called ferrous sulfate. (Experts caution against taking this much iron without medical supervision.) Avoid using over-the-counter preparations such as enteric-coated iron tablets or capsules containing slow-release granules, experts say. Both can interfere with the body's ability to absorb the iron. And make sure your doctor continues your treatment for a sufficient amount of time. Although your anemia will be corrected in 3 to 4 months, it takes an additional 6 to 12 months of therapy for your body's iron stores to be replenished.

The large amount of iron used to correct anemia is not available through food, says Sally Seubert, R.D., assistant professor of nutrition at the University of Texas Southwestern Medical Center at Dallas. "We still encourage women to eat more iron-containing foods, however," she says. Even liver, a food often avoided since *cholesterol* became a bad word, is recommended occasionally to anemic women, she says. "It's an unbeatable source of easily digested iron," she notes.

Getting Enough Copper

While you're stocking up on iron, you'll also want to make sure that you're getting 2 milligrams of copper, the Daily Value.

Your body needs copper as well as iron to make hemoglobin. Although it's uncommon, copper deficiency can cause a kind of anemia similar to iron deficiency, Seubert says. Most people get less than 1.6 milligrams a day, the amount considered necessary to maintain proper copper balance in the body. Good food sources include shellfish, nuts, fruits, cooked oysters, and dried beans.

And if you're taking zinc supplements, you'll want to pay special attention to your copper intake. That's because zinc actually interferes with copper absorption. For each 10 milligrams of zinc you take, you should make sure that you're getting 1 milligram of copper. (It's also worth noting that people who take more than 30 milligrams of zinc a day are at increased risk of developing anemia. So don't take more than this amount without medical supervision.)

The B$_{12}$ Anemia

There's no doubt that a little bit of vitamin B$_{12}$ can go a long, long way. The Daily Value is only 6 micrograms, the lowest requirement for any of the vitamins. But a dietary deficit of this nutrient causes major problems.

The anemia associated with vitamin B$_{12}$ deficiency is called pernicious anemia. Until 1934, this form of anemia was invariably fatal. People survived for months or even years while growing ever weaker, but they eventually succumbed. Then in 1934, two Boston doctors won the Nobel prize in medicine for demonstrating that a diet rich in lightly cooked liver, which contains a lot of B_{12}, could ward off the deadly deficiency.

Vitamin B_{12} is needed throughout the body to make DNA, a cell's genetic material. So a shortage leads to impaired cell production. Without adequate amounts of B_{12}, red blood cells suffer what is called maturation arrest, Dr. Stander explains. "They grow big, but they never mature into properly working red blood cells," he says. "Often they never make it out of the bone marrow, where they're made."

Fatigue is only one of several possible symptoms of pernicious anemia. Others include a burning tongue, tingling and numbness in the hands and feet, loss of appetite, irritability, mild depression, memory loss, and vague stomach pains.

Today, doctors know that usually it is not a shortage of this nutrient in the diet but an inability of the body to absorb vitamin B_{12} that causes deficiency problems.

As people get older, they may have reduced production in their stomachs of an enzyme called intrinsic factor. Intrinsic factor escorts any vitamin B_{12} that you've eaten across your intestinal lining into your bloodstream. As levels of intrinsic factor drop, less B_{12} gets absorbed, and what's stored in the body gets used up.

"Those who've had stomach surgery or who have Crohn's disease or other stomach or intestinal problems may also lose the ability to absorb vitamin B_{12}," Dr. Stander says.

Most people with vitamin B_{12} deficiencies need injections of B_{12} to bring levels back to normal. "And most will need injections for the rest of their lives," says Dr.

Stander. Only the small percentage of people whose B_{12} deficiencies are caused by dietary shortages, such as strict vegetarians, will benefit from oral supplements or from getting more B_{12} from food to help meet the Daily Value of 6 micrograms.

Folate Shortage Can Cause Problems

They're called tea-and-toasters. And that's a fairly accurate description of the diets of some people who end up with anemia caused by a shortage of folate. Folate is a B vitamin found in brewer's yeast and in spinach and other dark green leafy vegetables—the foliage foods from which this nutrient gets its name.

The body needs folate to make DNA. As with vitamin B_{12}, when folate is in short supply, blood cells never reach maturity. Instead, they become large, egg-shaped cells that just can't do their jobs right, Dr. Stander says.

Unlike vitamin B_{12}, folate is not stored in large amounts in the liver. The liver's supply is used up within two to four months, so symptoms of folate-related anemia can occur much more quickly than symptoms of vitamin B_{12} deficiency.

Blood tests can determine which vitamin is in short supply. "It's important to make this distinction, since supplementing with folic acid when it's actually vitamin B_{12} that's needed can mask symptoms and lead to B_{12}-related nerve damage," Dr. Stander says. So check with your doctor before taking folic acid as a supplement.

People found deficient are given 1,000 micrograms of supplemental folic acid a day to replenish their tissues' supplies. Pregnant women may need as much as

2,000 to 3,000 micrograms, Dr. Stander says. Those amounts are much more than you can get from even the best food sources.

Some research indicates that older people, especially those in not-so-great health, are better able to maintain normal blood levels of folate if they get 400 micrograms a day. That's an amount found in many multivitamin/mineral supplements.

Good food sources of folate include spinach, kidney beans, wheat germ, and asparagus. If you're relying on greens to boost your supply of this nutrient, stick to salads and lightly steamed vegetables. Folate is destroyed by lengthy cooking.

Medical Alert

Talk to your doctor before taking more than 400 micrograms of folic acid daily, as high doses of this vitamin can mask symptoms of pernicious anemia, a vitamin B_{12}-deficiency disease.

Most experts recommend that you consult your doctor before taking more than the Daily Value of iron (18 milligrams). Your doctor can prescribe the amount of iron that's appropriate for you based on a blood test. A daily intake of 25 milligrams or more for an extended period of time may cause undesirable side effects.

In people with vitamin B_{12} deficiencies caused by malabsorption probems, doctors give the vitamin by injection to bypass the faulty digestive system.

Angina

Easing the Squeeze

A ngina is actually a symptom, not a disease. This squeezing or dull, pressurelike pain—a kind of charley horse in the chest—is telling you that your heart muscle isn't getting enough oxygen to meet its needs. The pain is most likely to occur with exercise, stress, or cold weather—or after a big meal.

Just like the pain of a heart attack, angina can radiate to the left shoulder and down the inside of the left arm, straight through to the back, and into the throat, the jaw, and even the right arm. The pain typically lasts for only 1 to 20 minutes. If it lasts longer or gets worse, get to a hospital—fast! You could be having a heart attack.

People who get angina usually have coronary heart disease. The spaghetti-size arteries that deliver blood to the heart muscle have been narrowed or clogged by plaque, which forms from cholesterol and scar tissue. Plaque reduces blood flow to the heart muscle and makes arteries more likely to go into spasm, which reduces the blood flow even more. And if a fatty deposit ruptures or develops a crevice or fissure where blood can enter, it invites clot-forming platelets to congregate at the scene. The end result of this whole mess can be a full-blown blood clot that obstructs blood flow and causes a heart attack.

"Drugs such as nitroglycerin, beta-blockers, and calcium channel blockers offer predictable help," says

Robert DiBianco, M.D., associate clinical professor of medicine at Georgetown University School of Medicine in Washington, D.C. "These drugs dilate blood vessels and reduce the heart's oxygen needs. Nitroglycerin and beta-blockers may also help protect the heart from the damage associated with oxygen deprivation in the early hours of a heart attack." Sometimes cholesterol-lowering drugs are prescribed.

Standard treatment also includes a diet that cuts total fat to less than 30 percent of calories and saturated (animal) fat to under 10 percent of calories—the same fat-trimming diet used to cut your risk of further artery clogging, Dr. DiBianco says.

Some medical experts take these low-fat guidelines to extremes. They recommend that no more than 10 percent of calories come from fat—a diet that in some cases makes cholesterol deposits shrink and that often reduces muscle spasms and clotting. They also call for nutrients that may help prevent atherosclerosis, such as vitamin E. And they add other nutrients, such as magnesium, which is thought to help the heart function better under less than ideal circumstances.

Here's what research shows may help.

Vitamin E: All-Around Heart Help

Vitamin E appears to play a role when it comes to beating heart disease. A study by Harvard University researchers found that men who took at least 100 international units (IU) of vitamin E daily for at least two years reduced their chances of developing heart disease by about 40 percent.

Since angina is a symptom of heart disease, there's good reason to believe that vitamin E can help relieve angina pain. And in fact, British researchers found that people who had the lowest levels of vitamin E in their blood were 2½ times more likely to have angina than those who had the highest levels.

Vitamin E may work directly in helping to prevent the buildup of fatty plaque that restricts blood flow to the heart muscle, says Balz Frei, Ph.D., associate professor of medicine and biochemistry at Boston University School of Medicine. "It helps prevent the oxidation of LDL cholesterol (the 'bad' kind) in the artery wall, which is one of the first steps in the development of heart disease," he says.

Vitamin E also helps prevent blood-blocking clots in arteries by its action on platelets, disk-shape components of blood that regulate coagulation, explains Dr. Frei. "Adequate amounts of vitamin E inhibit the tendency for platelets to stick to each other and to the inside walls of blood vessels," he explains.

The best amount of vitamin E to relieve angina? Doctors who recommend this nutrient suggest 100 to 400 IU a day. These large amounts require supplementation, since most people don't get much more than 15 IU a day from vegetable oils, nuts, and seeds, the usual food sources for this vitamin.

Add On Some Selenium

There's also some evidence that selenium, a mineral that teams up with vitamin E, can offer protection from angina.

One study, by researchers in Poland, found that people with a particularly dangerous kind of angina called unstable angina were more likely than normal to have low levels of both vitamin E and selenium.

Another study found that people with heart disease who took 200 IU of vitamin E and 1,000 micrograms of selenium a day (a very high dose that requires medical supervision) had significant reductions in angina pain compared with patients taking placebos (blank pills).

Doctors who recommend selenium supplements to their heart patients generally stick to 50 to 200 micrograms a day. Supplements in excess of 100 micrograms should be taken only under medical supervision, however. To up your intake from foods, munch on whole-grain cereals, seafood, garlic, and eggs.

Magnesium May Smooth Things Out

Magnesium is well-known for its ability to relax the smooth (involuntarily controlled) muscles. These include the muscles that wrap around blood vessels, bronchial tubes, and the gastrointestinal tract. That's why magnesium seems to be helpful for disorders that may include muscle constriction, such as high blood pressure, Raynaud's disease, migraines, and at least some kinds of angina.

In several studies, magnesium given intravenously was effective in stopping variant angina, spasms in the coronary arteries not related to a permanent blockage.

"Oral magnesium also seems to be helpful, at least for some kinds of angina," says Burton M. Altura, Ph.D., a leading magnesium researcher and professor of physiology and medicine at the State University of New York Health Science Center at Brooklyn.

Unfortunately, magnesium deficiency seems to be all too common in people with heart disease. Studies show that up to 65 percent of all people in intensive care units and 20 to 35 percent of people with heart failure come up short on magnesium.

Magnesium deficiency can be induced by drugs meant to help heart problems, Dr. Altura says. Some types of diuretics (water pills) cause the body to excrete both magnesium and potassium, as does digitalis, a commonly prescribed heart drug. Signs of magnesium deficiency include nausea, muscle weakness, irritability, and electrical changes in the heart muscle.

If you have angina, talk to your doctor to see if your diet is adequate in magnesium. Your doctor might suggest making changes in your diet to increase the magnesium content. If you're still low on magnesium, he may recommend magnesium supplementation, Dr. Altura says. How much magnesium you need to take depends on the results of a so-called magnesium loading test, Dr. Altura explains. For this test, you take a large dose of magnesium, and the doctor checks the amount of magnesium in your urine to see how much your body retains. "Not everyone needs to take the same amount," Dr. Altura says.

Although magnesium is considered to be a fairly safe mineral, even in high doses, don't take supplemental magnesium without medical supervision if you have kidney or heart problems. You could have a dangerous buildup of magnesium in your blood, or your heart could slow down too much.

The Daily Value for magnesium is 400 milligrams. Based on his research, Dr. Altura has calculated that 70 percent of men get only 185 to 260 milligrams daily, while 70 percent of women get 172 to 235 milligrams daily.

Diets rich in vegetables and whole grains are much higher in magnesium than diets that include lots of meats, dairy products, and refined foods.

Medical Alert

If you have angina, you should be under a doctor's care.

People who have heart or kidney problems should not take magnesium supplements without medical supervision.

Selenium in doses exceeding 100 micrograms daily should be taken only under medical supervision.

If you are taking anticoagulants, you should not take vitamin E supplements.

Bladder Infections

Flushing Out Trouble

For some women, the symptoms are all too familiar: burning and stinging during urination and the persistent urge to go, go, go, even when they have just gone. Their urine may be cloudy, smelly, and sometimes tinged with blood. The usual problem: a urinary tract infection, caused by bacteria that have worked their way up the urethra into the bladder and settled in for the duration.

Urinary tract infections are second only to colds

when it comes to infections in women, whose anatomy sets the stage for trouble. (In men, urinary tract infections are much less common but potentially more serious, because they're often tied to prostate problems.)

Women who get bladder infections, particularly women who don't seem to be able to shake them, may have a problem with the cells lining the bladder, says Robert Moldwin, M.D., assistant professor of urology at Albert Einstein College of Medicine in New York City and an attending physician at Long Island Jewish Medical Center in New Hyde Park, New York. Somehow these cells have undergone a change that makes it easier for bacteria to stick to the bladder wall as well as to the vaginal wall. Once the bacteria are on the vaginal wall, it's easy for them to migrate to the bladder.

"Normally, any bacteria that get into the bladder are flushed right back out, but in this case, they're not," Dr. Moldwin says.

Doctors recommend a number of moves to minimize the risk of infection for women who develop recurrent infections. Urinate before and soon after sex, for example. And think twice about using a diaphragm. Women who rely on this birth control method are two to three times more prone to recurrent infections than nonusers, since the diaphragm causes irritation of the vaginal surface, which allows bacteria to adhere, according to Dr. Moldwin.

Spermicidal jellies can also contribute to bladder infections, upsetting the normal balance of "friendly" bacteria in the vagina and the surrounding area. Also, jellies may irritate the vagina, set up inflammation, and let bacteria adhere to the vagina, from where they migrate to the bladder, adds Dr. Moldwin.

Most doctors treat urinary tract infections with antibiotics, which usually work just fine. "And we often tell patients with recurrent problems to take one antibiotic pill each time they have sex," Dr. Moldwin adds.

In addition to these measures, some doctors suggest the following nutritional therapy.

Acidify with Vitamin C

Some doctors believe that pushing the urine's pH (acid-alkaline) balance a bit toward the acid side helps treat a bladder infection by slowing the growth of bacteria in the bladder. "Some doctors recommend vitamin C supplements for this," Dr. Moldwin says. It is unclear how this has an effect, and there are no studies to prove it, but it seems to help some women, he adds.

"Vitamin C also is likely to be prescribed when a woman is taking a urinary antiseptic drug such as methenamine mandelate (Uroqid-Acid) or methenamine hippurate (Hiprex), which work best when urine is acidified," Dr. Moldwin says. These drugs are most likely to be prescribed as long-term therapy to prevent recurrent or antibiotic-resistant infections.

Doctors who recommend vitamin C to prevent or treat bladder infections usually suggest a daily dose of 1,000 milligrams. You would have to eat about 14 oranges a day to get that much. In fact, oranges and orange juice aren't your best sources of vitamin C in this case, and not only because you would OD on OJ.

"Because of the way your body metabolizes it, orange juice does not acidify your urine as efficiently as supplements," says Kristene Whitmore, M.D., chief of the department of urology at Graduate Hospital in Philadelphia and co-author of *Overcoming Bladder Disorders*.

You can check the acidity of your urine with chemically treated nitrazine strips, a sort of litmus paper that's available in many pharmacies. Follow the directions on the package.

Cancer

Prevention Starts on Your Plate

Let's face it: It's really hard to see a light side of cancer. Even jokes about this deadly disease can't help but remind us of our mortality.

But one of the brightest sides of cancer these days is that so much of it seems to be preventable. Many experts believe that at least 50 percent of cancer cases could be averted with changes in diet. But because changing their diets is not an easy thing for people to do, some experts believe that supplements may be needed to make up for existing nutritional deficiencies.

"There's no one magic bullet to prevent cancer, but there are dietary changes you can make that, when combined, will certainly reduce your risk of cancer," says Patrick Quillin, R.D., Ph.D., certified nutrition specialist, nutritional director for the Cancer Treatment Centers of America, headquartered in Arlington Heights, Illinois, and author of *Beating Cancer with Nutrition*.

The sooner you make those dietary changes, the better your chances of never having to battle this deadly foe, Dr. Quillin says. "Cancer usually develops slowly, over many years, and goes through a number of stages," he adds.

Nutrition is most likely to have an impact on the early precancerous stages known as initiation and progression. These stages include potentially stoppable, even reversible, changes in a cell's genetic material, which are often the result of damage caused by chemical reactions in the body. Once the genetic changes are complete, however, and the now cancerous cell begins to multiply, nutrition is no longer a sole therapy option.

Researchers are still figuring out the exact details of a cancer-preventing diet, and they probably will be for a long time to come. Sometimes contradictory findings remind us that much remains to be learned about nutrition and cancer. Nevertheless, certain nutrients stand out as valiant warriors in the war against cancer. Here's what research shows.

Vitamin C Shields Cells

Sure they're tasty, but there's another reason that you might want to down a glass of freshly squeezed orange juice, slice a red pepper over your green salad, and nibble a handful of fragrant strawberries. You'll be getting lots of vitamin C, potentially potent protection against cancer.

"Approximately 90 population studies have examined the role of vitamin C–rich foods in cancer prevention, and the vast majority have found statistically significant protective effects," reports researcher Gladys Block, Ph.D., of the University of California, Berkeley.

"Evidence is strong for cancers of the esophagus, oral cavity, stomach, and pancreas. There is also substantial evidence of a protective effect against cancers of the cervix, rectum, and breast."

One review that looked at the results of several population studies found that women with the lowest risk of breast cancer were getting about 300 milligrams of vitamin C a day, the equivalent of about 4½ oranges or about three cups of orange juice. Their risk was reduced by about 30 percent.

In a study from Latin America, an area with one of the highest rates of cervical cancer in the world, women who got more than 314 milligrams of vitamin C a day had 31 percent less risk of developing cervical cancer than women whose intakes were under 153 milligrams a day.

And in a study from New Orleans, people getting at least 140 milligrams of vitamin C in their diets (about two oranges' worth) every day were only half as likely to develop lung cancer as those getting less than 90 milligrams a day.

"Vitamin C is a potent antioxidant," explains Balz Frei, Ph.D., associate professor of medicine and biochemistry at Boston University School of Medicine.

What's an antioxidant?

"Vitamin C," explains Dr. Frei, "along with certain other nutrients, has the ability to neutralize free radicals, harmful molecules in the body that can be produced during chemical reactions that involve oxygen."

Free radicals steal electrons from your body's healthy molecules to balance themselves, and in the process, they can harm a cell's membrane and genetic material. Antioxidant nutrients such as vitamin C offer free radicals their own electrons and so save cells from oxidative damage. "Free radical damage can occur as the result of normal body processes as we age and can also be the result of exposure to cancer-promoting chemicals," Dr. Frei explains.

Vitamin C helps prevent mouth, throat, stomach, and intestinal cancers by neutralizing cancer-promoting nitrosamines. Nitrosamines are produced during the digestion of nitrites and nitrates. Nitrites are preservatives found in especially high concentrations in meats such as hot dogs and ham, while nitrates are naturally present in vegetables.

Vitamin C helps maintain a healthy immune system, an additional cancer-fighting talent. Plus it may help build up vitamin E, another anti-cancer nutrient, to proper fighting form.

Most experts believe that the average daily intake of vitamin C, 109 milligrams for men and 77 milligrams for women, isn't enough to provide optimum cancer protection. Although vitamin C supplements can easily boost your intake, eating vitamin C–rich foods such as citrus fruits and other tropical fruits, broccoli, and Brussels sprouts provides additional cancer protection with nutrients such as folate (the naturally occurring form of folic acid), beta-carotene, bioflavonoids, and fiber. In fact, evidence of anti-cancer activity is considerably stronger for vitamin C–rich fruits and vegetables than for vitamin C itself.

The amounts of vitamin C supplementation that doctors recommend to optimize the potential for cancer protection vary widely, from 50 to 5,000 milligrams or more a day. Most, however, stay within 250 to 1,000 milligrams a day, taken in two or three divided doses.

Vitamin E for Extra Protection

Wheat germ, almonds, and sunflower seeds: Sure, they're crunchy and delicious, great on yogurt or hot cereal, but they also provide healthy amounts of yet another nutrient that may help protect against cancer—vitamin E.

Studies using experimental animals have consistently shown that vitamin E can help protect cells from damage that can lead to cancer. "Population studies have had mixed findings, however, probably because most people don't get enough vitamin E from foods to get much cancer protection," Dr. Quillin says. More recently, population studies that have also looked at long-term intake from vitamin E supplements have found protective effects.

In the Iowa Women's Health Study, for instance, researchers found that women who developed colon cancer consumed the smallest amounts of vitamin E, averaging less than 36 international units (IU) a day. Women who got almost twice that much of the vitamin—about 66 IU from supplements—had only one-third of the risk of developing this cancer compared with those with low intakes.

Another study, by researchers at the National Cancer Institute in Rockville, Maryland, found that people who said they regularly used vitamin E supplements had half of the normal risk of oral cancer of people who did not take vitamin E supplements.

Studies that have looked at blood levels of vitamin E have also found evidence of protective effects. British researchers, for example, found that women who had the highest blood levels of vitamin E had only one-fifth of the risk of breast cancer compared with women who had the lowest blood levels of vitamin E.

"Like vitamin C, vitamin E has the ability to protect biological molecules from the kind of chemically induced damage that can lead to cancer," Dr. Frei says. "Because it is fat-soluble itself, vitamin E is particularly good at protecting fatty cell membranes from oxidative damage."

"Strong cell membranes may be particularly important in the colon, because the bacteria there produce a lot of free radicals, the unstable molecules believed to harm DNA and promote tumor growth," adds Roberd Bostick, M.D., assistant professor of epidemiology at Bowman Gray School of Medicine of Wake Forest University in Winston-Salem, North Carolina, and co-investigator of the Iowa Women's Health Study.

Vitamin E may also stimulate and enhance the immune system so that it attacks budding cancer cells and inhibits the production of nitrosamines, Dr. Bostick says.

Based on its possible protective effects against some types of cancer, a growing number of researchers believe that vitamin E may prove to be a key player in any cancer prevention plan. Many recommend 400 to 600 IU a day. Such large amounts are impossible to get through dietary sources alone. Even a diet that contains good sources, such as wheat germ and safflower oil, provides only about 30 to 40 IU of vitamin E a day. "Only supplements can provide these large amounts," Dr. Quillin notes.

Selenium: Vitamin E's Partner in Protection

Lots of evidence points to the fact that when selenium intake goes down, cancer rates go up. It seems that getting enough of this essential mineral cuts your risk of most kinds of cancer—lung, skin, breast, prostate, and other types.

Researchers at the University of Limburg in the Netherlands measured the selenium content of people's toenails. (Strange as it may seem, toenail levels of selenium are considered a good indicator of long-term selenium intake.) They found that the people whose toenails had the highest levels of selenium had half of the rate of lung cancer compared with those whose toenails were low in selenium.

Selenium's protective effect was most apparent in people who weren't eating much in the way of beta-carotene and vitamin C.

In another study, people with the lowest blood levels of selenium were more than four times as likely to develop skin cancer as people with the highest levels.

"Selenium acts as an antioxidant, which means that it helps protect cells from harmful free radical reactions that occur when skin is exposed to sunlight or when lungs are exposed to cigarette smoke and pollutants," reports Karen E. Burke, M.D., Ph.D., a dermatologic surgeon and dermatologist in private practice in New York City. Selenium acts together with vitamin E, with selenium protecting within the cells and vitamin E protecting the outer cell membranes, she adds.

The Daily Value for selenium is 70 micrograms. The average daily intake from food is slightly more than 100 micrograms.

For cancer prevention, nutrition-oriented doctors, including Dr. Burke, recommend 50 to 200 micrograms of selenium a day (depending on what part of the country you live in and your personal and family history of cancer), taken in the form of l-selenomethionine. This is the organic form of selenium, which means it is more easily absorbed, with less possibility of adverse side effects.

To treat cancer, doctors at the Cancer Treatment Centers of America use up to 800 micrograms of selenium daily. In very large amounts, selenium can be toxic. Experts recommend that selenium supplements in excess of 100 micrograms be taken only under medical supervision.

Good food sources of selenium include wholegrain cereals, seafood, Brazil nuts, garlic, and eggs. "Foods that are processed lose their selenium," Dr. Burke says. Brown rice, for example, has 15 times the selenium content of white rice, and whole-wheat bread contains twice as much selenium as white bread.

The Beta-Carotene Connection

The real heroes in the war against cancer are fruits and vegetables, hands down. "Studies consistently show that people who eat plenty of fruits and vegetables are less likely to develop cancer than those who avoid fruits and vegetables," Dr. Block reports.

And when fruits and vegetables are broken into their individual nutrients, several components seem to stand out as particularly protective against cancer. One of them, beta-carotene, is the yellow pigment found in a variety of fruits and vegetables.

One study, for instance, found that during the year prior to being diagnosed with cancer, men who got less than 1.7 milligrams (about 2,800 IU) of beta-carotene a day—the amount in about one inch of carrot—were twice as likely to develop the disease as men who got more than 2.7 milligrams (about 4,400 IU) per day.

In another study, breast cancer risk almost doubled in postmenopausal women who ate the fewest carotene-rich foods compared with women who ate more of those foods. The risk appeared to drop off sharply once women reached a beta-carotene intake of more than 5,824 IU per day. That's the amount in a little less than one-third of a carrot or three six-ounce glasses of vegetable juice cocktail.

And in yet another study, researchers at the University of Arizona in Tucson found that more than 70 percent of people with a precancerous condition called oral leukoplakia who took 30 milligrams (about 50,000 IU) of beta-carotene a day for six months reduced the size of their oral lesions. The lesions of 18 of the 25 people in the study decreased in size by 50 percent or more, and there were four complete remissions.

"Laboratory studies support beta-carotene's anti-cancer role," says Norman Krinsky, Ph.D., professor of biochemistry in the department of biochemistry at Tufts University School of Medicine in Boston. "Animals who are given large doses of beta-carotene prior to being exposed to a cancer-causing chemical are less likely to develop cancerous tumors."

In other cases, beta-carotene has slowed the progression of precancerous lesions and has even helped reverse precancerous cell changes, possibly by promoting the cell's repair of genetic material.

Beta-carotene is just one of the disease-fighting compounds known as carotenoids. Plentiful in fruits and vegetables, carotenoids are potent antioxidants. They help thwart the harmful ways of those pesky free radicals just as vitamins C and E do.

In the body, some of the beta-carotene we eat is converted to vitamin A, an important regulator of cell growth and differentiation, Dr. Krinsky adds. "That means vitamin A helps cells mature into their final forms, which helps prevent cells from developing into cancer," he explains.

Unfortunately, a study from Finland found that longtime heavy smokers who took beta-carotene supplements of 20 milligrams (about 33,000 IU) a day were more, not less, likely to die from lung cancer. Although some doctors believe that finding is purely chance, others think it warrants careful consideration.

"This was such a well-designed study, with so much statistical power, that we can't ignore it," says Jerry McLarty, Ph.D., chairman of the department of epidemiology and biomathematics at the University of Texas Health Center at Tyler and lead researcher in an ongoing study of beta-carotene and lung cancer. "Certainly, more research needs to be done to get to bottom of this."

Some researchers say that the study was too little, too late, that the men given the supplements may have already had early lung cancer, still undetectable on x-rays. "Certainly, the finding of this study supports the argument that vitamin supplements alone cannot undo the damage wrought by years of bad habits or act as a substitute for eating well," Dr. McLarty says.

An increasing number of nutritionally oriented doctors are recommending supplements of beta-carotene to help prevent cancer, usually 10,000 to 25,000 IU daily. One 7½-inch carrot contains about 20,000 IU of beta-carotene.

"We recommend these supplements not because they have been proven to prevent cancer but because we believe some beta-carotene is better than none," says David Edelberg, M.D., facilitator of the American

Holistic Center/Chicago, one of the country's largest alternative medicine practices. "Unfortunately, the reality is that many people don't eat enough vegetables each day to get even this relatively small amount of beta-carotene."

Even doctors who recommend beta-carotene supplements, however, urge you to load up on orange, yellow, and dark green leafy vegetables such as carrots, spinach, kale, sweet potatoes, winter squash, and cantaloupe. Having even a single serving of any of these foods every day puts you ahead of the national average when it comes to beta-carotene.

"These foods also contain other, less-studied compounds that may prove to be at least as protective as beta-carotene against breast cancer and other forms of cancer," Dr. Krinsky explains.

For people who've had lung cancer, some doctors may recommend up to 500,000 IU of beta-carotene, says Dr. Quillin. These amounts are considered nontoxic, but you should discuss taking this much with your doctor or health care provider, he adds.

Folic Acid's Cancer-Stopping Power

Kale, spinach, romaine lettuce: These leafy greens are packed with a number of cancer-crushing nutrients. One in particular, folate, appears to help protect cells from cancer-inducing genetic damage caused by certain chemicals.

"Folate deficiency can induce damage to the genetic material in a cell, which can in itself lead to cancer and which also makes the cell more vulnerable to cancer-causing chemicals," explains Tiepu Liu, M.D., Dr. P.H., research assistant professor at the University of Alabama School of Medicine in Birmingham. Folate deficiency also makes it harder for a cell to repair its genetic material, which also sets the stage for cancer, Dr. Liu says.

In one study, researchers at the University of Alabama found that smokers treated with 10 milligrams (10,000 micrograms) of folic acid and 500 micrograms of vitamin B_{12} each day had significantly fewer precancerous cells than an untreated group. (Vitamin B_{12} was added because smokers tend to be deficient in B_{12} and because folic acid needs B_{12} to be active.)

And in a more recent study, Japanese doctors also found that folic acid and vitamin B_{12} provide impressive protection. Smokers who took 10 to 20 milligrams (10,000 to 20,000 micrograms) of folic acid and 750 micrograms of B_{12} daily had significant reductions in the number of potentially precancerous cells found in abnormal spots in the passageways of their lungs. The spots were checked with a lung-scanning scope several times over the course of one year. Seventy percent of initially abnormal spots were reclassified as normal by the end of the year, and not one lesion had gotten worse. In contrast, a control group that took no supplements fared this way: 77 percent of their spots remained the same, 5 percent got worse, and 18 percent got better.

And Harvard Medical School researchers found that men getting 847 micrograms and women getting 711 micrograms of folic acid daily had one-third less risk of precancerous colon polyps compared with men getting 241 micrograms and women getting 166 micrograms a day.

Researchers at the University of Alabama also found that among women who were exposed to a potentially cancer-causing virus, those whose blood levels of folate were low were five times as likely to develop disturbing cervical cell changes (cervical dysplasia) as women with higher folate levels.

"We speculate that adequate amounts of folate may help protect a cell's genetic material from invading viruses," Dr. Liu says. Unfortunately, studies so far show that in women who already have cervical dysplasia, supplemental folic acid is unable to reverse the condition, Dr. Liu adds.

The amount of folic acid given in the University of Alabama study of smokers, 10,000 micrograms, is far above the Daily Value for folic acid, which is 400 micrograms. Some doctors believe that people should be getting at least 400 to 800 micrograms of folic acid a day to prevent cancer. To get that amount, you'd have to fill up on the very best food sources: dark green leafy vegetables, oranges, beans, rice, and brewer's yeast.

Doctors who treat cancer with nutrition recommend about 400 micrograms of folic acid, along with 1,000 micrograms of vitamin B_{12}, every day, Dr. Quillin says. Vitamin B_{12} is available from food sources such as seafood and green leafy vegetables. Supplements may also be helpful.

Finding a doctor who uses folic acid to treat rather than prevent cancer can be difficult. Because methotrexate, an early anti-cancer drug, worked by interfering with folate metabolism, there has been concern among cancer specialists that folic acid could fuel cancer growth. Not so, says Dr. Quillin. In animal studies, folic acid did not increase cancer growth. And according to him, a folate deficiency increases the likelihood that a cancer will spread to other parts of the body. Doctors at the Cancer Treatment Centers of America include 400 micrograms of folic acid in their treatment regimens.

Be aware that high doses of folic acid can mask symptoms of pernicious anemia, caused by vitamin B_{12} deficiency. It's best to work with a doctor if you plan to take much more than the Daily Value of folic acid.

Medical Alert

Talk to your doctor before taking more than 400 micrograms of folic acid daily, as high doses of this vitamin can mask symptoms of pernicious anemia, a vitamin B_{12}-deficiency disease.

Selenium supplements in excess of 100 micrograms should be taken only under medical supervision.

Start with a low dose of vitamin C and work up to the higher amounts. Large doses can cause diarrhea in some people.

If you are taking anticoagulant drugs, you should not take vitamin E supplements.

Cardiomyopathy

Heart-Protecting Nutrients

Cardiomyopathy is a special form of heart disease. It's a breakdown of the muscle tissue in the heart. This muscle tissue, known as the myocardium, becomes inflamed, then scarred and fibrous. As a result, the walls of the heart may become thick and hard or thin and weak. The heart sometimes enlarges and beats faster, trying to play catch-up because it isn't pumping blood efficiently.

People with cardiomyopathy may become breathless when they're active and sometimes even when they're doing nothing at all. They may tire easily, develop ankle swelling, and have chest pains.

Compared with coronary heart disease, which is the most common form of heart disease, cardiomyopathy is rare. But it's one of the main reasons people become candidates for heart transplants. That's because traditionally, there hasn't been a whole lot available for cardiomyopathy. Most doctors use drugs to provide some relief by reducing demands on the heart.

"These drugs are indispensable and have been shown to be remarkably effective in some people," explains Robert DiBianco, M.D., associate clinical professor of medicine at Georgetown University School of Medicine in Washington, D.C.

Unlike coronary heart disease, cardiomyopathy isn't always caused by fat-clogged arteries, although it can be, Dr. DiBianco says. It may be caused by a virus or another type of infection, such as Lyme disease or AIDS; an inherited metabolic disorder; exposure to toxic chemicals such as cobalt, lead, or carbon monoxide; sensitivity to commonly used drugs; toxins such as alcohol or cocaine; or heart damage caused by a disease such as diabetes.

Poor nutrition also seems to play a role in the development of some forms of cardiomyopathy or in worsening its symptoms.

Several of the "classic" deficiency diseases—pellagra (niacin deficiency), beriberi (thiamin deficiency), and kwashiorkor (protein deficiency)—can cause cardiomyopathy. So can imbalances of calcium and magnesium, which play important roles in proper heart function.

And shortages of other nutrients, particularly selenium and vitamin E, make the heart more vulnerable to damage.

Here's what research shows can help this potentially life-threatening problem.

Selenium Shields Hearts

Until 1979, researchers didn't know for sure that the mineral selenium is essential for human nutrition. That year, evidence came from Chinese scientists who reported an association between low selenium intake and a condition called Keshan disease, a form of cardiomyopathy that affects primarily children and women of childbearing age.

People in certain parts of China were getting little selenium in their diets because the soil in their region contains almost none. Since plants don't require selenium, they can grow in selenium-poor soil. But they offer no selenium to the people and animals who eat them, so there is simply no good food source, plant or animal, in the region. In fact, some animals suffered from the same heart condition, and it was Chinese veterinarians who first made the connection between human cardiomyopathy and selenium.

"Chinese doctors soon found that selenium supplements could prevent this potentially fatal problem," says Orville Levander, Ph.D., a research leader at the U.S. Department of Agriculture Beltsville Human Nutrition Research Center in Maryland.

Selenium deficiency alone doesn't seem to cause cardiomyopathy, however, Dr. Levander says. "Researchers now think this condition develops only in selenium-deficient people who have been exposed to certain viruses that zero in on the heart muscle."

Dr. Levander and his colleague, Melinda Beck, Ph.D., professor at the University of North Carolina at Chapel Hill, found that a particular kind of virus called Coxsackie remained its mild-mannered self in laboratory animals that were getting enough selenium. But in selenium-deficient lab animals, it caused extensive heart damage.

"Selenium seems to help protect the heart muscle from viral damage," Dr. Levander says. "We don't know exactly how, but it seems to be related to its antioxidant properties." Viral invasions cause the generation of free radicals, unstable molecules that steal electrons from healthy molecules in your body's cells to balance themselves, thus damaging the cells. Antioxidants disarm free radicals by offering up their own electrons, saving cells from harm.

Most researchers in the United States don't think Americans are deficient enough in this mineral to develop cardiomyopathy, Dr. Levander says. Chinese researchers found that it takes only a small amount, about 20 micrograms a day, to prevent cardiomyopathy. Most Americans get well above that amount, averaging 108 micrograms a day.

But some research shows that so-called adequate amounts of selenium may not be high enough to provide optimum antioxidant or immunity-stimulating protection. That's why some doctors recommend selenium supplements of 50 to 200 micrograms a day.

If you're concerned about deficiency, ask your doctor to check your blood level of selenium, Dr. Levander says. If your blood level is low, you may need to take supplements. Supplements of more than 100 micrograms a day should be taken only under medical supervision, however, since selenium can be toxic in large amounts. Stop taking selenium if you develop a persistent garlic odor on your breath and skin, loss of hair, fragile or black fingernails, a metallic taste in your mouth, or dizziness or nausea with no apparent cause. These symptoms mean that you're getting too much.

Generally, fruits and vegetables don't contain much selenium. On the other hand, seafood and, to a lesser extent, meats are rich in easily absorbed selenium. Grains and seeds, garlic, and mushrooms also offer some selenium, depending on where they are grown.

Vitamin E Adds Antioxidant Protection

If you're concerned about giving your heart all of the protection you can, you'll want to add vitamin E to your arsenal.

"In animal studies, cardiomyopathy problems are more likely to be worse in the animals with simultaneous deficiencies of selenium and vitamin E. These deficiencies can be prevented or cured by supplementation with either nutrient alone," Dr. Levander says. (In animals, vitamin E can also protect the heart against cardiomyopathy caused by magnesium deficiency.)

Like selenium, vitamin E has antiviral and antioxidant properties, so it may help protect the heart against infection and toxins. It may also help prevent the development of atherosclerosis, or clogged arteries, which could make a failing heart even weaker, says Peter Langsjoen, M.D., a cardiologist in private practice in Tyler, Texas, with a special interest in nutrition. He recommends 400 international units daily. That high amount is available only from supplements.

Magnesium May Aid Weakened Hearts

In animals, the evidence is clear. When put on a low-magnesium diet, young animals develop heart muscle damage that leads to heart failure.

"In humans, the picture isn't so clear," says William Weglicki, M.D., professor of medicine and physiology at George Washington University Medical Center in Washington, D.C. "For people, there's no good proof that magnesium deficiency causes cardiomyopathy."

Magnesium is so intimately involved in heart function, however, that getting enough may help a compromised heart work better for a number of reasons, says Carla Sueta, M.D., Ph.D., assistant professor of medicine and cardiology at the University of North Carolina at Chapel Hill School of Medicine.

"Magnesium affects heart muscle contraction, and magnesium deficiency can cause abnormal heart rhythms and/or irregular beats," Dr. Sueta says. "Adequate amounts can help prevent constriction of isolated blood vessels, which can affect the blood supply to the heart muscle."

Apparently, magnesium also offers protection during a heart attack. "Magnesium-deficient animals have greater tissue damage after heart attacks than animals getting enough magnesium," Dr. Weglicki says.

If you are a heart patient concerned about magnesium, have your doctor monitor levels in your red blood cells, Dr. Sueta suggests. "If your levels are low, you know for sure that you're low in magnesium. And if your levels are borderline, you still are probably low in magnesium," she says. You can have normal levels of magnesium, however, and still be low enough to have magnesium deficiency–related heart problems, Dr. Sueta adds.

If you have kidney problems or heart disease, it's important to take magnesium supplements only under medical supervision.

If you're simply concerned about heart health, experts suggest that you make sure to get the Daily Value of 400 milligrams. Nuts, beans, and whole grains are your best food sources, and green vegetables also provide a fair amount. Studies show that most people fall short of the Daily Value.

Medical Alert

If you have cardiomyopathy, you should be under a doctor's care.

If you have a kidney problem or heart disease, it's important to take magnesium supplements only under medical supervision.

Selenium supplements of more than 100 micrograms a day should be taken only under medical supervision. In large amounts, selenium is toxic.

If you are taking anticoagulant drugs, you should not take vitamin E supplements.

Cataracts

Chasing Away the Clouds

Crack open an egg and drop it into a hot frying pan. You'll see the egg white turn cloudy, then white, as normally clear proteins in the egg are irreversibly altered by the heat.

Well, something similar to that happens when you get cataracts. Proteins in the lens of the eye lose their crystal-clear properties, becoming yellowish, cloudy, and about as easy to see through as a fried egg. Of course, cataracts take not seconds but many years to form. And it's not heat but cigarette smoking, a buildup of sugar in the lens (usually associated with diabetes), and especially years of exposure to sunlight that eventually pull the shades on vision for many people.

Many doctors now think that the main cause of cataracts is oxidative damage to cells in the eye's lens. Oxidative damage is the same chemical process that rusts iron and makes cooking oil turn rancid. In the lens, the oxidative process can occur as part of normal metabolism as well as in the presence of light, which creates harmful unstable molecules called free radicals. These free radicals grab electrons from your body's healthy molecules to balance themselves, causing an ever-escalating molecular free-for-all that ends up hurting perfectly innocent cells.

Nutrients Shield the Lens

The lens can partially protect itself from this free radical damage, and it relies on certain nutrients to keep its defense system strong. Vitamins C and E, beta-carotene (a precursor of vitamin A), and minerals such as selenium, zinc and copper—all components of antioxidant enzymes found in the lens—may all play roles in protection. Even B vitamins such as riboflavin and B_{12} as well as an amino acid called cysteine may be involved, but evidence for these nutrients is very slim, says Randall Olson, M.D., professor and chairman of the department of ophthalmology at the University of Utah School of Medicine and director of the John A. Moran Eye Center, both in Salt Lake City.

"Not all of the facts are in, but the evidence to date is mostly positive that nutrients such as vitamins C and E and beta-carotene are helpful," Dr. Olson says. "And the evidence seems to indicate that these nutrients are synergistic, that they work best together."

In fact, several small studies suggest that people who take multivitamin/mineral supplements are less likely to develop cataracts than those who do not. A Harvard University study, for instance, found that doctors who regularly took multivitamin/mineral supplements cut by about one-fourth their risk of developing cataracts compared with those not taking supplements. And a study by Canadian researchers found that supplements reduced cataract formation by about 40 percent.

A 10-year nationwide study now in progress called the Age-Related Eye Disease Study is evaluating whether a mix of vitamins, including E, C, and beta-carotene, really does help keep eyes crystal-clear. "Until the results of that study are in, we can't say for sure whether these nutrients are really helpful," says Emily Chew, M.D., medical officer in the Division of Biometry and Epidemiology at the National Eye Institute in Bethesda, Maryland.

In the meantime, here's what research shows may help slow the development of cataracts.

Take C and See

Researchers have known for some time that the lens of the eye can concentrate vitamin C. Concentrations of vitamin C in the lens and in the aqueous humor, the watery fluid surrounding the lens, are about 10 to 30 times the concentrations in other parts of the body.

"We're very interested in a possible protective effect, especially since vitamin C is a water-soluble antioxidant and the lens is composed mostly of water and proteins," says Allen Taylor, Ph.D., director of the Laboratory for Nutrition and Vision Research at the Jean Mayer USDA Human Nutrition Research Center on Aging at Tufts University in Boston.

In studies using laboratory animals, vitamin C seems to help protect the lens from oxidative damage from light, sugar, and certain drugs, Dr. Taylor says.

And what about people? "It's possible that people are not getting enough vitamin C in their diets to make a difference when it comes to preventing cataracts," says Susan E. Hankinson, Sc.D., associate epidemiologist in the Channing Laboratory at Brigham and Women's Hospital in Boston. And there are a couple of studies that suggest vitamin C supplements can help protect against cataracts.

When Dr. Hankinson and researchers at the Harvard School of Public Health crunched numbers on nutrient intakes for 50,828 nurses, they found that women who had taken vitamin C supplements for 10 years or more (average intake: 250 to 500 milligrams daily) fared better. Compared with women who never took supplements, the supplement takers had 45 percent less chance of developing cataracts bad enough to require surgery.

In another study, people taking 300 to 600 milligrams of supplemental vitamin C a day experienced a 70 percent decrease in risk compared with people who were not taking that much vitamin C.

"Our finding makes sense, because cataracts generally form over a long period of time," Dr. Hankinson explains. "It's reasonable to think that long-term use of preventive agents such as vitamin C would result in lowered risk."

Doctors who recommend vitamin C to people at risk for cataracts suggest from 500 to 3,000 milligrams a day. (Some people may experience diarrhea when taking more than 1,500 milligrams of vitamin C daily.) "Research has yet to determine an optimum amount of vitamin C to take to prevent cataracts, but studies do show that the concentration of vitamin C in the lens continues to increase as people move into the 500-milligram range," says Dr. Taylor.

It's true that many doctors believe vitamin C is harmless even in high amounts. But when it comes to the eyes, one researcher contends that it's best to stay below 3,000 milligrams.

"I've found that intakes of 3,000 milligrams or more of vitamin C are associated with retinal macular puckering and sometimes with increased risk of retinal detachment," says Ben C. Lane, O.D., director of the Nutritional Optometry Institute in Lake Hiawatha, New Jersey. High doses of vitamin C seem to make the gelatinous material inside the eyeball watery, which reduces pressure against the retina, allowing it to more easily pull away from the back of the eyeball, Dr. Lane says. (The retina is a light-sensitive area at the back of the eyeball that receives images.)

It may be wise to get at least some of your daily vitamin C from citrus fruits. That's because chemical compounds called bioflavonoids, which are closely related to vitamin C and are found in the white membranes of oranges and grapefruit, also seem to offer antioxidant protection and, Dr. Lane adds, may even be more important.

14-Carrot Eye Protection

We know. It's an old, old line, but the point is well-taken: The reason (well, maybe one reason) why you've never seen a rabbit with glasses may indeed stem from this long-eared critter's penchant for carrots and perhaps spinach.

When it comes to cataracts, beta-carotene and plain old vitamin A may offer protection. At least that's what Harvard School of Public Health researchers found when, once again, they picked apart the diets of their much-studied nurses. They found that women with the highest beta-carotene and vitamin A intakes had a 39 percent lower risk of cataracts severe enough to require surgery than women getting the least beta-carotene and vitamin A.

It is possible that both beta-carotene and vitamin A may help prevent oxidative damage to the lens. Vitamin A itself is not an antioxidant. But, explains Dr. Hankinson, "it's possible that people who get enough preformed vitamin A in their diets have more beta-carotene and other carotenoids available to act as antioxidants, since these compounds may be converted to vitamin A only as the body needs them." In other words, if you're taking in enough vitamin A, your body won't need to use up beta-carotene to make the vitamin for you. Doctors who recommend vitamins suggest about 25,000 IU of beta-carotene daily.

Many doctors, including Dr. Hankinson, warn that it's too early in the research game to place your bets on any one supplement, such as beta-carotene, to prevent cataracts. Vitamin-rich foods seem to be important, too. "Even though we found that carrots offer protection, we found a stronger protective effect from spinach, which doesn't contain as much beta-carotene but has antioxidant compounds such as lutein and zeaxanthin," says Dr. Hankinson.

Best advice to date: Keep packing in those leafy greens as well as orange and yellow fruits and vegetables.

E Is for Eyes

What do wheat germ and sunflower oil have to do with healthy eyes? Both are good sources of vitamin E, an antioxidant nutrient that works its way into cell membranes and disarms free radicals before they have a chance to attack cells.

"Research in animals and test-tube studies indicate that vitamin E may help protect the lens from oxidative damage from light, sugar, and cigarette smoke," Dr. Olson explains.

In humans, the story seems to be the same. In one study, people taking 400 IU of vitamin E a day had half of the risk of developing cataracts compared with people who did not take vitamin E. In another, people whose blood levels of vitamin E were high had about half of the risk of developing cataracts compared with people with low blood levels.

"Vitamin E is a powerful antioxidant," Dr. Olson explains. "There's reason to believe that combined with other nutrients, it may help slow the progress of lens clouding."

You'd have to plow your way through bowls and bowls of wheat germ to get 400 IU of vitamin E, the amount found in some capsules. So supplementation is in order. "I recommend 400 IU a day," Dr. Olson says. The Daily Value for vitamin E is 30 IU; but most people get only about 10 IU a day from their diets.

The Case for Zinc

Doctors sometimes add a bit of zinc, an essential mineral, to their anti-cataract formulas. There's evidence that zinc is important for the function of the retina and that it may help prevent deterioration of the retina as we age. Plus the body needs zinc to make several antioxidant enzymes found in the eye, including superoxide dismutase and catalase.

Doctors who recommend zinc to prevent or slow cataracts call for a wide range, from 15 milligrams a day (the Daily Value) to 50 milligrams a day, the amount Dr. Olson recommends.

Dr. Lane bases his initial dosage on an individual's zinc status, determined by testing. "It may be necessary to start a person at a fairly high amount, then cut back as his status returns to normal," he says.

One thing is for sure with zinc: More is not necessarily better, and doses exceeding 15 milligrams should be taken only under medical supervision. Too much zinc can deplete your body of copper, an essential trace mineral. You should get about 1 milligram of copper for every 10 milligrams of zinc. Even in fairly small amounts, copper can be toxic. Don't use long-term copper supplementation above the Daily Value of 2 milligrams without medical supervision, Dr. Lane cautions.

Selenium Adds Antioxidant Power

Doctors sometimes round out their antioxidant prescriptions with selenium, a mineral involved in the body's production of glutathione peroxidase, another protective enzyme found in the eye and other parts of the body.

Dr. Lane recommends selenium supplements only to people who have been found to be deficient in glutathione peroxidase activity or in red blood cell selenium or who have been subject to mercury poisoning. Dr. Olson does not recommend individual selenium supplements but does sometimes recommend multivitamin/mineral products that contain selenium, such as Icaps and Ocuvite (available in health food stores).

Doctors who recommend selenium supplements suggest 50 to 200 micrograms a day, no more. In even small amounts, selenium can be toxic, so don't take more than 100 micrograms daily without medical supervision.

If you're a fan of garlic, then you'll be getting a healthy amount of selenium with each bite. Other selenium-rich foods include onions, mushrooms, cabbage, grains, and fish.

Medical Alert

If you have cataracts, you should be under a doctor's supervision.

Don't take more than 100 micrograms of selenium daily without medical supervision.

Some people may experience diarrhea when taking more than 1,500 milligrams of vitamin C daily.

If you are taking anticoagulant drugs, you should not take vitamin E supplements.

Don't take more than 15 milligrams of zinc daily without medical supervision.

Chronic Fatigue Syndrome

Building Energy with Nutrients

Everyone gets tired. But not everyone gets chronic fatigue syndrome (CFS).

People with this disease aren't just tired. They're constantly exhausted, not just for a few days but day in and day out for six months or longer.

And the fatigue is only the beginning. Many people with CFS also have flulike symptoms, such as sore throat, painful lymph nodes, and aching muscles. Others have problems concentrating and bouts of confusion and forgetfulness. And many people with CFS have no tolerance for exercise: Imagine a woman who used to run several miles a day being so exhausted by a walk around the block that she stays in bed for the next couple of days. That's CFS.

While children and older people aren't immune, CFS is most common in younger adults. "About 90 percent of my CFS patients are between ages 25 and 50," says Paul Cheney, M.D., a CFS specialist and director of the Cheney Clinic in Charlotte, North Carolina.

Once it hits, CFS is hard to get rid of. Doctors don't know what causes CFS or how to cure it. And while many people recover on their own within a year or two, some never fully recover.

The Illness behind the Headlines

While CFS has probably been around for a long time, it wasn't until the mid-1980s that a mysterious flulike illness that hit mostly young professional women made headlines. Nicknamed the yuppie flu, it was often written off as burnout or depression. Many people who had CFS looked so healthy that they were told that their symptoms were "all in their heads."

Today most doctors are familiar with CFS, but they still have a hard time diagnosing it. Symptoms vary widely from person to person and often resemble the flu, mononucleosis, or depression. And because no one knows what causes CFS, medical science has not yet developed a definitive test that can prove whether a person has it. In the 1980s, some researchers believed that CFS, like mononucleosis, was caused by the Epstein-Barr virus; while that theory has been rejected, some experts still suspect that a virus may play a role.

These days, most experts consider CFS an immune activation (autoimmune) disorder similar in some respects to lupus and rheumatoid arthritis. In immune activation disorders, the immune system is so cranked up to defend the body against invaders that it actually attacks the body's own tissues. Doctors also see a high incidence of allergies among people with CFS, another sign that their immune systems tend to overreact.

CFS resembles other immune activation disorders in another way: A disproportionate share of people with CFS—probably around 75 percent—are women, says Dr. Cheney. "It could be that women's immune systems are just stronger than men's," he says. "This is an advantage early in life, when girl infants die less often of infections than boys do. But that strong immune system makes a woman more likely to experience immune activation disorders in adulthood."

Like most aspects of this mysterious disease, the reasons that women are more susceptible are subject to much debate. But one thing doctors do agree on is that CFS isn't all in the patient's head. Today CFS is widely regarded as a physical illness, not a mental one.

Getting the Big Picture

No one knows for sure how many people have CFS. The Centers for Disease Control and Prevention (CDC) in Atlanta estimates that 100,000 to 250,000 Americans have seen their doctors for it. But since the CDC uses a very strict definition of the disease in gathering these statistics—unless an individual has the right number and combination of symptoms, the case isn't reported as CFS—many researchers believe that the disease is far more common than the figures indicate.

A study of 3,400 nurses from around the country found that while only 11 met the CDC criteria, 23 believed they had CFS. "We chose nurses because presumably they would be more familiar with CFS than the general population and better able to judge whether they have it," says Leonard Jason, Ph.D., professor of psychology at DePaul University in Chicago, who conducted the study.

In another study of the general population, 0.2 percent were found to have CFS. Based on these results, Dr. Jason estimates that about 387,000 American adults have CFS.

While no one has found a cure for CFS, dietary changes and nutritional supplements can help strengthen the immune system, improve energy levels, and ease some of the symptoms of CFS, says Allan Magaziner, D.O., director of the Magaziner Medical Center in Cherry Hill, New Jersey. Dr. Magaziner has been treating people with CFS for more than ten years.

"Of course, taking a supplement isn't going to cure CFS," he cautions. "People need to understand that they also have to eat right, exercise appropriately, and work with a physician who's knowledgeable about CFS."

Muscling Up with Magnesium

Some people with CFS have benefited from taking supplements of magnesium, a mineral that is involved in the cells' energy production.

One British study found that people with CFS had below-normal blood levels of magnesium. After receiving injections of magnesium, 80 percent reported improvement in their symptoms.

But even if their blood tests don't show magnesium deficiencies, people can still benefit from extra doses of the mineral, according to Dr. Cheney. "Their blood levels of magnesium may be normal, but that doesn't tell the whole story," he says. "Magnesium, like potassium, is pumped into the cell, so normally there's a higher concentration inside the cell than there is in the blood. And that pump mechanism may not work very well in people with CFS, so their magnesium levels can be normal in the blood and low in the cell."

Dr. Magaziner also finds that most people with CFS notice improvement in their symptoms after starting magnesium supplements. "It doesn't work for everyone," he says. "But many of my patients find that it eases their muscle aches and makes them feel less fatigued."

This is probably because people with CFS have enzyme deficiencies that hamper the cells' ability to convert food into energy, according to Dr. Cheney. And extra magnesium improves enzyme function, which results in greater energy production on the cellular level.

If you're interested in trying magnesium, Dr. Magaziner recommends starting with 500 milligrams a day. "This level is perfectly safe, although occasionally a person will develop loose bowels or diarrhea," he says. "If that happens, I would simply reduce the dose to the point where the diarrhea goes away." If you have heart or kidney problems, however, you should check with your doctor before taking magnesium supplements.

Dr. Cheney recommends a chelated form of magnesium called magnesium glycinate. "It's rapidly absorbed in the gastrointestinal tract, so it doesn't cause digestive problems," he explains. "And it tends to be drawn into the cell, where it's needed."

And because taking more magnesium increases the body's need for calcium, Dr. Magaziner suggests taking calcium supplements as well. "I usually recommend taking them in a two-to-one ratio—1,000 milligrams of calcium if you're taking 500 milligrams of magnesium," he advises.

A Boost from B Complex

The B-complex vitamins help support the adrenal glands, which are among the major organs in the body connected with stress, says Dr. Magaziner. "B vitamins also support the central nervous system, to help us cope with stress in general," he explains. "We lose a lot of B vitamins when we're stressed, so we need to replenish them." These nutrients are also involved in energy production, which makes them essential for people with CFS.

Dr. Magaziner recommends a supplement containing the entire B complex. Thiamin, pantothenic acid, and vitamins B_6 and B_{12} are especially important for people with CFS, he says.

You can get the B-complex vitamins in most multivitamin/mineral supplements, says Dr. Cheney. Check the label to make sure the supplement contains at least 50 milligrams each of thiamin, pantothenic acid, and vitamin B_6 and 50 micrograms of vitamin B_{12}. He also recommends taking a separate B-complex supplement whenever you're under stress.

Higher doses of vitamin B_{12}, given through injection by a physician, can also be helpful in cases of enzyme deficiency, says Dr. Cheney. Injected B_{12} doses may be 1,000 times higher than the normal daily dose.

Arm Yourself with Antioxidants

Also helpful in treating CFS are the so-called antioxidant nutrients, which include vitamin C, vitamin E, beta-carotene, and the mineral selenium.

These nutrients form a veritable SWAT team that helps defend your cells against free radicals, unstable molecules that occur naturally in the body and that are also produced by bad habits such as smoking, sunbathing, and drinking alcohol. Free radicals steal electrons from your body's healthy molecules to balance themselves, damaging cells in the process. Antioxidants neutralize free radicals by offering their own electrons, protecting healthy molecules from harm.

"Antioxidants protect the body from deterioration, degeneration, and environmental stresses," says Dr. Magaziner. "And since many people with CFS are unusually sensitive to environmental factors such as household chemicals, food additives, and artificial fragrances, taking antioxidants makes sense."

Damage from free radicals is such an important factor in CFS that some researchers consider CFS a free radical–generated disease, says Dr. Cheney. "I don't think it's caused by free radical damage, but that seems to be one of the factors that maintains it," he says.

To help bolster the immune system and improve stamina, both doctors recommend an antioxidant-complex supplement, available in most drugstores and health food stores. Because dosage varies widely from brand to brand, read the label to make sure that you're getting at least 500 milligrams of vitamin C, 25,000 international units (IU) of beta-carotene, 400 IU of vitamin E, and 50 micrograms of selenium.

People with CFS may also want to try a vitamin C supplement in the form of ester-C, says Dr. Cheney. "Ester-C is much more bioavailable than regular vitamin C," he explains. "Your body absorbs twice as much. People with CFS can take 2,000 milligrams of ester-C twice a day; it's very safe." Taking more than 1,500 milligrams of vitamin C can cause diarrhea in some people, however, so it's a good idea to check with your doctor before exceeding that amount. Ester-C is available in health food stores.

Medical Alert

If you have been diagnosed with chronic fatigue syndrome, you should be under a doctor's care.

If you are taking anticoagulants, you should not take vitamin E supplements.

If you have heart or kidney problems, you should always check with your doctor before taking magnesium supplements.

Doses of vitamin C in excess of 1,500 milligrams a day can cause diarrhea in some people, so it's a good idea to check with your doctor before taking more than that amount.

Colds

Common Nutrients for a Common Condition

A phlegm-filled cough. Nose blowing that rivals any air horn blast. Sneezes so severe that even good china in the next room isn't safe.

All of these, of course, are cold symptoms. But experts think that they're also cold senders, launching tiny droplets of mucus into the air with every wheeze, hack, and honk.

Inside these specks of mucus are soccer ball-shaped organisms called rhinoviruses, so tiny that 15,000 lined up side by side would barely span the space between two words on this page. Whether carried on a finger as you scratch your nose or inhaled through your nose or mouth, some of these malevolent microbes may eventually get the break they're looking for: the chance to get inside your body.

It's all downhill from there, literally. The wavelike downward motion of the tiny hairlike projections that line your throat pushes the virus as well as your normal throat mucus toward your esophagus. If you're fortunate, powerful digestive acids destroy the virus before it can do any harm.

When you do become infected, however, the virus's cold-producing plan begins to unfold. Finding a warm spot in your throat where your own mucus layer is thin and offers little protection, a single virus attaches itself to a cell and commandeers the cell's own replicating capability. Office copiers should work so well: Within a few hours, over 100,000 viruses are created. "That's the reason therapy is so difficult," says Elliot Dick, Ph.D., professor of preventive medicine and chief of the respiratory virus research laboratory at the University of Wisconsin–Madison and one of the country's leading cold researchers. "Viruses essentially become part of us, part of our cells."

And all of that awful sneezing, snorting, and coughing? That's called the host response, your body's way of fighting this unwanted guest from within. Before long, white blood cells, the avenging angels of your immune system, are rushed to the scene of the infection to kill the cells containing the virus. That influx of blood causes swelling in the sinuses. Stepped-up mucus production designed to trap the virus makes for a running nose and eventually a hacking cough.

Chances are, though, that the battle will not be won for another seven days, the average length of the dreaded common cold. Is there anything that you can do to put a stop to all of this mayhem? You could take vitamin C.

What Research Says about Vitamin C

Taking vitamin C to treat a cold is about as common as, well, the common cold.

And yet the controversy over its effectiveness continues, with the general public serving as its strongest advocate.

Ever since Linus Pauling, Ph.D., shocked the medical community with his book *Vitamin C and the Common Cold*, doctors have debated the merits of his recommendations. Among them: taking 500 to 1,000 milligrams of vitamin C every hour for several hours to reduce the length and severity of a cold. Dr. Pauling certainly walked his talk: For six years prior to his death at age 93, the two-time winner of the Nobel prize reportedly took 12,000 milligrams of vitamin C a day.

Dozens of studies of varying professionalism and reliability followed Dr. Pauling's pronouncements, with mixed results. At last count, roughly half supported his megadose claim. The others, testing much lower doses, showed that vitamin C is of little help in ending a cold in progress.

And that is precisely what vitamin C advocates have claimed all along: If you're going to take vitamin C for a cold, you have to take a lot. In fact, a review conducted by a British researcher found that all of the studies done since 1970 in which people were taking 1,000 milligrams or more of vitamin C a day to reduce the symptoms of their colds showed positive results, including a 72 percent reduction in the duration of cold symptoms.

Vitamin C Primes Your Defenses

One study, conducted by Dr. Dick and his colleagues at the University of Wisconsin–Madison, even showed that taking vitamin C before you get a cold can be helpful.

His research team found a way to study the spread of the common cold up close. They gathered a roomful of male volunteers, placed tiny amounts of cold virus directly in the nostrils of 8 and then watched the contagion spread to the other 12 as the men sneezed, coughed, and blew their noses. Along with poker chips and playing cards, they passed cold viruses to each other. Within a week, almost without fail, Dr. Dick says, every man in the virus-filled, windowless room had a cold.

In three separate studies, Dr. Dick didn't just try to get the men sick. He also experimented with vitamin C to see if it offered any protection.

In each study, half of the men were given 500-milligram doses of vitamin C at breakfast, lunch, and dinner and before bed each day, for a total of 2,000 milligrams of vitamin C a day. The rest got placebos (look-alike dummy pills). "Unlike other studies, we didn't have to trust whether they were going to take the vitamin C," says Dr. Dick. "We actually gave it to them. Either they came up to the lab or we went around to where they were housed and gave it to them with a little glass of water."

The pretreatment continued for 3½ weeks; then the poker games began. All of the men caught colds even though they maintained their 2,000-milligram-a-day vitamin C intakes. The study results, however, showed that vitamin C was helpful in reducing their colds' effects.

"We found during those experiments that the vitamin C greatly reduced symptoms of a cold," says Dr. Dick. "The length was a little shorter, but that wasn't the main thing. The main thing was that those who took vitamin C just weren't very ill, while some of the others got real humdingers of a cold."

In fact, only 1 person in the entire vitamin C–taking group came down with a full-fledged cold, while 16 in the placebo group had moderate or severe colds, Dr. Dick says.

So what is it about vitamin C that seems to make it useful for fighting colds?

Your immune system contains a number of natural defenders that spring into action at the first sign of an invading microorganism such as a cold virus. Among them are white blood cells. When your vitamin C levels are high, your white blood cells are apparently reinvigorated, giving them more of the energy that they need to neutralize the virus, explains Dr. Dick. "The best experimentation that I've seen suggests that vitamin C is in some way or another stimulating the white blood cells to function better," he says. "They attack the infected cell, gather around it, destroy it, and then clean up."

And what about the skeptics? "Our results are nice and positive, and a lot of other people's results aren't nice and positive," says Dr. Dick. "But nobody has looked at it in the fashion that we have."

Once a skeptic himself, Dr. Dick now takes 2,000 milligrams of vitamin C an hour for three hours at the first sign of cold symptoms. "Usually the cold is gone by then, but if not, I'll take 1,000 milligrams an hour until it is," says Dr. Dick. "I thought it was a bunch of foolishness, too. Not anymore."

The Daily Value for vitamin C is only 60 milligrams. Doses larger than 1,500 milligrams a day can cause diarrhea in some people.

Zinc: Another Cold Controversy

Long appreciated for its immune-boosting power, zinc attracted considerable attention in the 1980s as a cold remedy, and in a remarkable way.

George Eby of Austin, Texas, observed a three-year-old girl who suffered repeated severe colds. He reported giving her a 50-milligram zinc gluconate tablet at the start of one of her colds in a bid to boost her immune system.

But she refused to swallow the tablet, instead dissolving it in her mouth. Her symptoms were gone within a few hours, far faster than usual. After observing zinc's cold-stopping effect several more times, Eby wondered whether sucking, not swallowing, zinc might actually be the long-sought cure for the common cold.

Eby conducted a scientific study to see if he was on to something. Published in a medical journal, the results of the study were promising. Those who took plain, awful-tasting zinc gluconate tablets reported that their symptoms were gone after an average of 4 days, while those taking better-tasting placebos said that their colds lasted an average of 11 days.

"The results seemed very significant. But the problem was that the zinc gluconate tasted so bad, there was some concern that people had reported their colds were over just because they didn't want to take this awful-tasting stuff anymore," says John C. Godfrey, Ph.D., a medicinal chemist and president of Godfrey Science and Design, a food supplement consulting service based in Huntingdon Valley, Pennsylvania.

In their haste to develop a tastier zinc gluconate cold lozenge, some researchers mixed in additives that apparently rendered the cold-stopping merits of zinc gluconate inactive. "You can take zinc gluconate and add citric acid to it, which is what one pharmaceutical company did, to make something that tastes acceptable. It really does wipe out the nauseating flavor of zinc, but it also inactivates the zinc," says Dr. Godfrey.

Tinkering in his own kitchen with ingredients that he had purchased in a local health food store, Dr. Godfrey combined zinc gluconate and glycine into a lozenge that tasted pretty good to his family—and also seemed to knock out their colds.

"I noticed, and my family reported to me, that when they had colds, as soon as they put one of these lozenges in their mouths, their symptoms disappeared," he says. "It was very dramatic. You would be all stuffed up and sneezing, with a sore throat, and you would put one of these in your mouth, and then you'd actually be getting relief. You could actually hear little crackling noises in your sinuses as they opened up. The postnasal drip is rapidly reduced. Sneezing is not totally wiped out, but it goes way down."

Watching your family get better hardly constitutes a scientific study. Dr. Godfrey followed up his observations, however, with a study conducted at the Dartmouth College Health Service in Lebanon, New Hampshire. Researchers divided 73 college students into two groups: those who were given zinc gluconate and glycine lozenges and those who took similar-tasting placebos. The students were told to suck on the lozenges at two-hour intervals and to take up to eight lozenges a day. Each lozenge contained roughly 24 milligrams of zinc. (The Daily Value for zinc is 15 milligrams.)

Researchers discovered that those students who started taking the zinc gluconate lozenges 1 day after they first felt ill suffered from their colds for only 4.3 days. Those who took placebos suffered for 9.2 days. "Cough, nasal drainage, and congestion were the symptoms most improved," says Dr. Godfrey. "That was an indication that the earlier and more vigorously you treat a cold, the better the result will be. That's where our research since then has been focused."

And what is it about zinc gluconate that causes the improvement? There are at least two theories. The unique shape of the rhinovirus that helps it hook into your cells also fits the active ingredient in zinc perfectly, almost like a bag over a bowling ball. "The geometry fits very neatly," says Dr. Godfrey.

Another possibility: Zinc gluconate concentrations in your mouth may literally short-circuit the nerve in your nose that's responsible for sneezes and other symptoms, says Dr. Godfrey.

Will Dr. Godfrey's results end the great zinc debate? Maybe not. Plain zinc gluconate tastes awful, and just swallowing it isn't enough to treat a cold. You have to suck on zinc gluconate to get its symptom-banishing effects. Stomach discomfort is an occasional side effect that can usually be avoided by eating something first; even a cracker will do, says Dr. Godfrey.

If you're looking for zinc lozenges in a pharmacy

or health food store, here's what you need to know: Steer clear of zinc lozenges that are combined with citrate, tartrate, orotate, or mannitol/sorbitol. They may taste good, but the cold-stopping capabilities of the zinc are completely inactivated, according to Dr. Godfrey. In addition to its bad taste, plain zinc gluconate can cause mouth soreness, but it will do the job. The pleasant-tasting, clinically proven zinc gluconate with glycine is available through the Quigley Corporation, P.O. Box, 1349, Doylestown, PA 18901. No matter which form you choose, a general treatment regimen is one 24-milligram lozenge dissolved in your mouth every two hours (up to eight lozenges a day) to help relieve cold symptoms.

Are zinc lozenges worth taking? "I guess it depends on how you look at a cold," says John H. Turco, Ph.D., director of the Dartmouth College Health Service. "Some people feel like a cold isn't a tremendous setback. But obviously, if you can get rid of some of the symptoms, it's probably worth it."

Medical Alert

Doses of vitamin C larger than 1,500 milligrams a day can cause diarrhea in some people.

Supplemental zinc in doses such as 24 milligrams should only be taken for cold symptoms for a period of 7 to 10 days.

Depression

Dispelling the Darkness

Of course you've been depressed. Hasn't everybody?

The answer is, in a word, no.

The word *depression* is thrown around so much in casual conversation that many people don't realize how serious it can be, says Harold Bloomfield, M.D., a psychiatrist in Del Mar, California, and co-author of *How to Heal Depression*.

"Depression isn't the same as being sad or discouraged," says Dr. Bloomfield. "Those feelings are just part of being alive. Depression is an illness, one that can be controlled with proper treatment or that can ruin your life if you don't get the help you need."

Are You at Risk?

Depression may look and sound like the blues, but it lasts longer and has a more profound impact on a person's life. If you're clinically depressed, you live in a state of sadness and hopelessness so severe that it makes normal activities seem impossible. You may lose interest in friends or hobbies, have suicidal thoughts, or feel overwhelming guilt because you can't "snap out of it." Depression can kill your appetite or make you want to eat all the time. Sleeping more or less than usual and problems concentrating can also be warning signs.

Depression can happen to anyone. It is estimated

that about 15 percent of us will have at least one bout of depression in our lifetimes that's severe enough to require medical attention. Sometimes it's triggered by an emotional blow such as a divorce or the death of a loved one, but it can also appear out of nowhere.

A family history of depression can also put you at risk. "We see depression running in families just as diabetes and high blood pressure run in families," says Dr. Bloomfield. "That doesn't mean that there aren't other causes, but a family history of depression makes a person more prone to it."

Depression often surfaces during times of transition, such as the teenage years, midlife, and retirement. The elderly are particularly vulnerable: Dr. Bloomfield estimates that people over age 60 are four times as likely to be depressed as younger people.

Hormones can also play a role. Some women who take birth control pills or hormone replacement therapy may experience depression as an effect of their pills and should see their doctors for guidance. Premenstrual and postpartum depression are also common.

Feed Your Head

Nutritional deficiencies are common in depressed people, according to Dr. Bloomfield, though which comes first—deficiency or depression—isn't entirely clear. "If people haven't been eating right their whole lives, it can start to catch up with them in their forties or fifties. And if they have a tendency toward depression, it often shows up around the same time."

While poor nutrition probably doesn't cause depression, correcting a deficiency can be beneficial if you're battling it, says Dr. Bloomfield. But nutritional supplements are no substitute for professional evaluation. "If you think you're depressed," he advises, "it's crucial that you see a physician or psychiatrist for help."

A Boost from the B Vitamins

A healthy intake of the B-complex vitamins is important for anyone who wants to keep depression at bay, says Dr. Bloomfield. While the whole B complex apparently plays a role in keeping you emotionally and physically healthy, a few members of the family seem to have particularly strong effects on depression.

"There has been lots of evidence that if you're deficient in thiamin or riboflavin, over time it's going to lead to a depression of the whole functioning of the body, both physically and emotionally," says Dr. Bloomfield.

Symptoms of thiamin deficiency include fear, uneasiness, confusion, and mood changes, which can be signs of depression. A study at the University of California, Davis, found that thiamin supplements improved sleep, appetite, and mood in older women who were only slightly deficient in the nutrient.

Another B vitamin that has been linked to depression is folate (the naturally occurring form of folic acid). Researchers know that people who have low levels of folate are more likely to be depressed than those who have normal levels. And in a study at the University of Toronto, depressed people with higher levels of folate in their systems got over their depression faster than those with lower levels.

Experts advise that it's also important to make sure you're getting enough vitamin B_6. People with depression often don't, according to a study of 101 depressed men and women evaluated by the New York State Psychiatric Institute in New York City. Your body needs B_6 in order to manufacture the hormone serotonin, which seems to play a role in regulating your mood.

Many drugs, including those containing estrogen, can interfere with the absorption of vitamin B_6. This may be why some women experience depression after starting oral contraceptives or hormone replacement therapy. Vitamin B_6 may be particularly helpful for women on the Pill or for those who grapple with premenstrual depression, says Dr. Bloomfield.

Some researchers suggest that the B vitamins are even more effective when taken as a group. One study found that elderly people with depression who took supplements of thiamin, riboflavin, and vitamin B_6 along with antidepressant medication showed more improvement than those taking medication alone.

The safest, most convenient way to get all of your Bs is to invest in a B-complex supplement, says Dr. Bloomfield. Look for a supplement that contains at least 10 milligrams each of thiamin, riboflavin, and vitamin B_6 and 100 micrograms of folic acid, he suggests, and take it twice a day.

Staying Up with Vitamin C

If your diet fails to supply all of the vitamin C you need, doctors know that your mental as well as physical health may be at stake. Depression is a well-documented symptom of scurvy, a disease that results from severe deficiency of vitamin C. And while scurvy is relatively rare in developed countries, there's reason to believe that even a minor deficiency of vitamin C can affect your mental health.

Vitamin C is important for strengthening the immune system, which isn't in top form in depressed people. "We know that depressed people are more vulnerable to illness, so anything that strengthens the immune system is beneficial," says Dr. Bloomfield. He recommends vitamin C supplements in generous doses, up to 4,000 milligrams a day. This amount is many times the Daily Value, but since excess vitamin C is excreted in the urine, Dr. Bloomfield says that this large dose is safe.

Some people may experience diarrhea from this much vitamin C, however, so experts say it's a good idea to check with your doctor before taking more than 1,500 milligrams a day. Also, since vitamin C can interfere with the absorption of tricyclic antidepressants, you should discuss vitamin C supplementation with your doctor if you are taking this type of medication.

Dr. Bloomfield recommends that vitamin C supplements be taken early, first thing in the morning or at lunch, because some people might have difficulty falling asleep if they take these supplements later in the day.

Mind Your Minerals

Evidence is sketchy, but at least one study suggests that the mineral selenium may play a role in depression. Researchers at the University College of Swansea in Wales found that people who took supplements of 100 micrograms of selenium daily felt less fatigue, anxiety, and depression than those who didn't.

Since it's too soon to tell whether selenium is of any benefit in the fight against depression, the best advice is to shoot for getting the Daily Value of this mineral, which is 70 micrograms. Eat a balanced diet and check to see that your multivitamin/mineral supplement contains selenium; that way you can be sure that you're covering all the bases, says Dr. Bloomfield.

Medical Alert

If you have symptoms of depression, you should see your doctor for proper diagnosis and treatment.

Doses of vitamin C exceeding 1,500 milligrams a day can cause diarrhea in some people, so it's a good idea to check with your doctor before taking more than that amount. Also, since vitamin C can interfere with the absorption of tricyclic antidepressants, you should discuss vitamin C supplementation with your doctor if you are taking this type of medication.

Dermatitis

Ending the Irritation

When a husband or wife overreacts at home, the pot roast can end up in the petunias. When your immune system overreacts to an irritant, you get dermatitis.

Dermatitis is simply your immune system flashing its message—"I'm irritated"—on your skin in the form of an itchy red rash. And it doesn't take much to irritate some folks' skin. Culprits include things such as nickel and latex and even certain foods. And such outbursts occur fairly often: 10 percent of all children suffer from dermatitis at one time or another.

Doctors are now aware, however, that immune

system irritation and allergy are not the only causes of dermatitis. In rare cases, vitamin and mineral deficiencies can also help launch dermatological tirades. Deplete your body of vitamin A, biotin, or any of the other B vitamins, vitamin E, or zinc, and it won't be long before a skin rash appears.

"We have known for years that minor deficiencies of certain vitamins and minerals could produce skin, hair, and nail problems in both children and adults," says Wilma Bergfeld, M.D., dermatologist and director of the Section of Dermatopathology (the study of the causes and effects of skin diseases and abnormalities) and Dermatological Research at the Cleveland Clinic. "What's far less clear is just how they cause them."

Zero In on Zinc

Perhaps the best-understood deficiency-dermatitis connection is the link to zinc. Imagine your roof without shingles to protect against the elements, and you get a picture of your skin without zinc.

Take in less than the Daily Value of 15 milligrams of zinc for a few weeks, and the shingles of your skin—your top layer of skin cells—begin to dissolve, says Dr. Bergfeld. Without this protective layer, your skin becomes rough and crusted, opening up opportunities for bacteria, yeast, and other infections to take hold, she explains.

"In a zinc deficiency, your skin simply does not perform the normal barrier function that it otherwise would," says Thomas Helm, M.D., assistant clinical professor of dermatology at the State University of New York at Buffalo School of Medicine and Biomedical Sciences and director of the Buffalo Medical Group. "Zinc is important in regulating the production of proteins, fatty acids, and DNA. Zinc deficiency causes skin rash, loss of appetite, loss of taste, and impaired immunity."

As a result, zinc deficiency can cause dermatitis around the mouths and rectums of young children. Such deficiencies aren't exactly common, but they occur more frequently than other nutrient-related skin problems, says Jon Hanifin, M.D., professor of dermatology at Oregon Health Sciences University in Portland.

Other people who are most susceptible to this kind of dermatitis include those with irritable bowel syndrome (a distressing digestive disorder), those undergoing chemotherapy, alcohol-dependent people, and some moms-to-be. "In all of these cases, their zinc levels may actually go below the normal range even if they are eating enough zinc," says Dr. Helm. "It's just not being absorbed properly."

Fortunately, alleviating problems caused by a zinc deficiency is as simple as adding more zinc to your diet; you should aim for the Daily Value of 15 milligrams. Even when there is a problem with zinc absorption, zinc deficiency can usually be overcome by increasing dietary zinc, Dr. Helm says.

"When zinc replacement is given, most of these rashes clear right up," agrees Dr. Bergfeld.

Give Vitamin E a Go

You probably won't find a scientific study to confirm it, but clinical reports seem to show vitamin E's effectiveness against some kinds of dermatitis.

One such case, published in the British medical journal *Lancet*, described an otherwise healthy 38-year-old man who had dermatitis on his hands for four years. Under the supervision of his doctor, he tried all kinds of approaches to get rid of it, including changing soaps, watchbands, and the wrap on his steering wheel, as well as wearing gloves to the gym and taking a multivitamin/mineral supplement. Then he began taking 400 international units (IU) of vitamin E a day.

Nine days after he started the supplement, the man's dermatitis cleared, says Commander Patrick Olson, M.D., an epidemiologist and preventive medicine specialist at the Naval Medical Center in San Diego. Dr. Olson is the one who treated the man. Since writing about the case, Dr. Olson says, he has received no fewer than 10 letters from people as far away as Britain reporting the same kind of success with vitamin E.

Although all of the letters sound credible, Dr. Olson says that he was most intrigued by one from an infectious disease specialist in Florida who read the article and urged his sister to give it a try. "She started taking 400 IU of vitamin E a day in soft gel form, and it resolved her condition completely for the first time in the six or eight years that it had been diagnosed," says Dr. Olson. "It was very gratifying to hear that."

Dr. Olson theorizes that the antioxidant action of vitamin E prevents damage from free radicals; in this case, the damage is manifested as dermatitis. Free radicals, normal by-products of cell life, are unstable molecules that steal electrons from your body's healthy molecules to balance themselves, damaging cells in the process. Antioxidants neutralize free radicals by offering their own electrons and so protect healthy molecules from harm.

"It's just a theory, but since vitamin E seems completely benign at these doses, there's no reason why this area shouldn't be explored further," says Dr. Olson.

While the Daily Value for vitamin E is only 30 IU, doses of up to 400 IU daily are considered safe. To get that amount from food, you'd have to eat a pound of sunflower seeds, five pounds of wheat germ, or two quarts of corn oil.

Vitamin C Might Help

It's no secret that a vitamin C deficiency can damage gums and skin. And at least one study showed that taking supplements helps people with severe eczema, according to Melvyn Werbach, M.D., author of *Healing through Nutrition*. (Eczema is a type of dermatitis characterized by weeping breaks in the skin that eventually form scales.) Dr. Werbach recommends taking 3,500 to 5,000 milligrams of vitamin C each day for three months. This is a lot of vitamin C, as some people experience diarrhea from only 1,500 milligrams. If you'd like to try this treatment, you should discuss it with your physician.

Most dermatologists don't suggest vitamin C for dermatitis, but there are reasons that it might work, says Dr. Helm. For one thing, doctors are just learning that vitamin C seems to protect the skin from sun damage. Vitamin C speeds wound healing and prevents ultraviolet-induced free radical damage to the skin. Studies show decreased photoaging and susceptibility to sunburn in animals given vitamin C supplementation, Dr. Helm reports. "It's not unreasonable to suspect that vitamin C can help the skin stay healthy when exposed to harmful stresses other than ultraviolet light," he says.

Medical Alert

Some people may experience diarrhea when taking doses of vitamin C exceeding 1,500 milligrams daily.

If you are taking anticoagulant drugs, you should not take vitamin E supplements.

Diabetes

Helping the Body Handle Sugar

When she finally went to the doctor, three months after she first noticed her symptoms, Allene Harris of Valley Mills, Texas, was surprised to learn that she has diabetes. It doesn't run in her family.

"I just didn't feel right," she recalls. "I was very tired, and I thought it was because of the stress I'd gone through when my mother died. But I was happy to hear that it could be controlled by diet. My doctor said that as long as I was willing to make some changes, I probably wouldn't need to take insulin."

Her diet—a careful balance of carbohydrates, protein, and fat that's heavy on fiber and light on saturated fat and sugar, with just enough calories to maintain her weight—perked her up as fast as it dropped her blood sugar. She was feeling better in a matter of days.

"I knew this was something that wouldn't get better on its own, so I found out as much as I could about taking care of it and started doing it," she says. Much of her nutrition information comes from a diabetes support group that includes a nutritionist.

This sort of take-charge approach can make the difference between living a long, healthy life despite diabetes and suffering the potential consequences: heart disease, blindness, nerve and kidney damage, and poor circulation in the hands and feet.

"There's absolutely no doubt that diet is the cornerstone of diabetes care," says Mary Dan Eades, M.D., medical director of the Arkansas Center for Health and Weight Control in Little Rock. "The change in a person's condition as a result of proper nutritional guidance can be dramatic."

Double Trouble with Sugar

Most of us know that people with diabetes have problems with too much sugar in their bodies. But there's a bit more to be aware of in understanding this complex disease. For one thing, diabetes comes in two different forms.

Type I diabetes, formerly called juvenile diabetes, results from a lack of insulin, the hormone that allows cells to take up glucose circulating in the bloodstream. Glucose is the simple sugar that the body uses for fuel. Type I diabetes is also called insulin-dependent diabetes mellitus. (*Mellitus* means "honeyed" in Latin.) The lack of insulin comes about because of damage to insulin-secreting cells in the pancreas. The damage may be caused by a virus or by an autoimmune reaction, in which the body's immune system attacks cells in the body.

Type II diabetes, or non-insulin-dependent diabetes mellitus (formerly called adult-onset diabetes), results because sugar can't get inside cells, a condition called insulin resistance. Most people with Type II diabetes have plenty of insulin, at least in the beginning stages of the condition. But receptor sites, or portals, on the membranes of the cells don't work properly to allow sugar inside. Exactly why that happens nobody knows, but research indicates that the defect in the receptors probably occurs from damage brought about by chronic exposure to high levels of insulin.

In both types, the end result is too much sugar in the blood. "Excess sugar causes tremendous oxidative stress in the body, which leads to all sorts of problems," explains Joe Vinson, Ph.D., professor of chemistry and nutrition at the University of Scranton in Pennsylvania. That simply means sugar molecules react with oxygen to form unstable molecules called free radicals, which cause havoc by stealing electrons from your body's healthy molecules to balance themselves.

This electron pilfering damages cells and sets the stage for heart disease as well as for kidney, eye, and nerve damage. "Oxidative damage is thought to be associated with all of the complications of diabetes," Dr. Vinson says.

Excess sugar also sticks to proteins, causing their structural and functional properties to be significantly changed. "This is another major cause of diabetes complications," Dr. Vinson explains. "It's one reason people with diabetes often have a hard time healing from wounds or surgery. They have trouble making quality collagen, the connective tissue that is the major structural protein in the body."

Nutritional therapy for diabetes covers all the bases. It helps lower blood sugar and blood fats, restores nutrients in people whose diabetes is not well-controlled, and protects against oxidative damage.

Changes in eating habits are considered standard treatment for diabetes, especially for Type II. And individual nutrients appear to play important roles. Here's what research shows may be helpful.

Vitamin C Saves Cells

Diabetes itself doesn't kill people. But those nasty complications, such as heart disease and blindness, can make things rough. And that's where vitamin C comes in.

Studies show that vitamin C helps prevent the sugar inside cells from converting to sorbitol, a sugar alcohol that cells can neither burn for energy nor move out. Vitamin C may also be effective in diminishing the damage to proteins caused by free radicals.

"Sorbitol buildup has been implicated in diabetes-related eye, nerve, and kidney damage," says John J. Cunningham, Ph.D., professor of nutrition at the University of Massachusetts at Amherst. "It accumulates in cells and disrupts a large spectrum of biochemical reactions." In other words, it really gunks up the works.

In a study by researchers at the University of Massachusetts at Amherst, the red blood cell levels of sorbitol in people with Type I diabetes dropped from double the normal amount to normal after they took 100 or 600 milligrams of vitamin C a day for 58 days.

"That's important, because it could mean that over time, people with diabetes who get plenty of vitamin C will have fewer complications," Dr. Cunningham explains. "Given its ability to permeate all tissues in the body and its low toxicity, we believe that vitamin C is a superior choice over drugs that do the same thing."

Sorbitol, by the way, is used as a sweetener in some dietetic foods. But that doesn't pose a danger for people with diabetes, says Dr. Cunningham. "Dietary sorbitol is poorly absorbed, for one thing," he says. "And it's not transported inside cells, the only place it does any harm."

Doctors who recommend vitamin C for diabetes suggest anywhere from 100 to 8,000 milligrams a day. In his study, Dr. Cunningham found that 100 milligrams of supplemental vitamin C a day works just as well as 600 milligrams a day in people already getting at least the Daily Value (60 milligrams) from foods. Dr. Cunningham suggests that you work with your health care team, including a nutritionist, to determine the right amount for you. For some people, doses exceeding 1,500 milligrams a day can cause diarrhea.

Citrus fruits are tops for vitamin C delivery. Or thrill your taste buds by blending orange juice with a cup of cubed guava or papaya. That tasty concoction packs close to 200 milligrams of vitamin C.

Vitamin E Saves Hearts

Vitamin E gets lots of good press for its role in helping to prevent heart disease. That's important for people with diabetes, whose risk of heart disease is two to four times normal.

That high risk results mostly from free radical damage to fats found in the bloodstream, explains Sushil Jain, Ph.D., professor of pediatrics, physiology, and biochemistry in the department of pediatrics at Louisiana State University Medical Center in Shreveport.

The damage, called lipid peroxidation, leads to clogging in the miles of tiny capillaries found in the body, to the reduced life span of red blood cells, and to something called platelet aggregation, in which blood cells tend to stick to each other and to blood vessel walls, causing serious traffic jams.

"People with diabetes may need more antioxidant protection than is available in a normal diet," Dr. Jain says. In his studies, people with diabetes who took supplements of 100 international units (IU) of vitamin E a day had 25 to 30 percent lower blood levels of harmful triglycerides, which are blood fats made of sugar. Vitamin E also reduced the tendency for sugar to stick to proteins in the blood, Dr. Jain says.

Doctors who prescribe vitamin E for their patients with diabetes recommend from 100 to 800 IU a day. "I begin with 100 IU and may go as high as 800 IU," Dr. Eades says. It's important to work with your doctor as you increase levels, she adds. "If you're taking insulin, your doctor may need to drop your insulin dose with each increase in vitamin E. And you should monitor your blood pressure, as there is speculation that vitamin E might increase blood pressure in some people."

The large amounts of vitamin E used for diabetes are not available from even the best food sources: wheat germ and nut and seed oils. Only supplements can provide these large amounts. Doses exceeding 600 IU a day should be taken only under medical supervision.

Magnesium: For Eyes and More

It may be the world's most underappreciated mineral. Magnesium is not a trace mineral but a nutrient necessary for every major biological function in your body. And it offers a long list of potential benefits for diabetes. Low levels have been linked to degeneration of the eye's retina, high blood sugar, high blood pressure, and clotting problems that can lead to heart disease.

Although studies have yet to be done that look at whether supplemental magnesium can prevent diabetic complications such as retinal damage, some research indicates that it could be helpful.

In Italy, for instance, doctors found that people

with Type II diabetes who took 450 milligrams of supplemental magnesium a day produced more insulin and cleared sugar from their bloodstreams better than before they started taking magnesium supplements.

People with diabetes, especially those taking insulin or whose blood sugar is not well-controlled, tend to come up short on magnesium, studies show. One in four may have the kind of marginal deficiency that often goes undetected, even when they're eating enough. "People with diabetes tend to lose magnesium through their urine," Dr. Eades explains.

"I have people take 1,000 milligrams of magnesium twice a day for four weeks to assess their responses," Dr. Eades says. (She also has people take 1,500 milligrams of calcium a day during this period.) But she cautions against taking these amounts unless you discuss it with your doctor first. This is especially important if you have heart or kidney problems. During this therapy, most people experience some improvement in blood sugar and blood pressure and have less fatigue. After four weeks, she reduces the dose to 500 milligrams a day (100 milligrams more than the Daily Value), taken along with 1,000 milligrams of calcium.

Foods rich in magnesium include whole grains, almonds, cashews, spinach, beans, and halibut.

Chromium Helps Insulin Work Better

Chromium is a trace mineral. The very same mineral used to put a shine on car bumpers, it is a key player in the body's use of sugar. It hooks up with insulin to help escort sugar through the cell membrane and into the cell. Deficiencies of chromium make cells resistant to insulin and lead to high blood sugar levels. Of 15 studies that have looked at the effects of chromium supplementation on the body's ability to use sugar, 12 show positive results.

In one study, people with diabetes who took 200 micrograms of chromium or 9 grams of high-chromium brewer's yeast a day had lower blood levels of sugar, insulin, triglycerides, and total cholesterol and higher levels of heart-healthy HDL cholesterol than before they started taking chromium.

"Deficiency of chromium not only worsens sugar metabolism but also may contribute to development of the numbness, pain, and tingling in your feet, legs, and hands that diabetes causes," Dr. Eades says. She recommends daily doses of 200 micrograms of either niacin-bound chromium or chromium picolinate, an easily absorbed form of the mineral, or 9 grams (two teaspoons) of chromium-rich brewer's yeast.

It's true that chromium improves glucose tolerance, which is the body's ability to maintain normal levels of blood sugar after eating, only in people who are low in this trace mineral. But plenty of people fit that category, says Richard Anderson, Ph.D., lead scientist in the nutrient requirements and functions laboratory at the U.S. Department of Agriculture Beltsville Human Nutrition Research Center in Maryland and a leading chromium researcher. He found that most people get only 25 to 30 micrograms a day, which is much less than the Daily Value of 120 micrograms. You'd need to eat at least 3,000 calories a day to get 50 micrograms of chromium and 7,200 calories a day to get 120 micrograms, Dr. Anderson figures.

"No one knows how many people with diabetes are low in chromium, and there's no good way to assess chromium status," admits Kathleen Wishner, M.D., Ph.D., past president of the American Diabetes Association. Foods high in chromium include broccoli, bran cereals, whole-grain cereals and breads, green beans, and various fruits. Eating sugar uses up the body's chromium supply.

If you have diabetes and you want to try chromium supplementation, you should do so only under your doctor's supervision. He may need to adjust your insulin dosage as your blood sugar level drops.

B Complex May Help Nerves

It's old news that the B-complex vitamins—niacin, thiamin, folic acid, vitamin B_6, and others—are essential for your body to convert sugar and starches to energy. These vitamins are involved in many of the chemical reactions necessary for this process, which is known as carbohydrate metabolism.

A shortage of any one of the B-complex vitamins can cause problems. Vitamin B_6 deficiency, for instance, has been linked to something called glucose intolerance, which is an abnormally high rise in blood sugar after eating. This deficiency has also been linked to impaired secretion of insulin and glucagon. Both of these hormones are essential in regulating blood sugar levels.

Shortages of B vitamins can also lead to nerve damage in the hands and feet. Some studies indicate that people with diabetes experience less of the numbness and tingling of diabetes-caused nerve damage if they get supplemental amounts of B vitamins such as B_6 and B_{12}.

People with diabetes tend to be low in B vitamins, perhaps in part because the diabetes itself uses up B vitamins and because poorly controlled diabetes causes these nutrients to be excreted in the urine.

"In general, my recommendation is 100 milligrams of a B-complex vitamin daily," Dr. Eades says. "Then I'll determine whether someone may need bigger doses of particular B vitamins, such as thiamin, B_6 and B_{12} if there are symptoms of diabetic nerve damage."

In such cases, she may prescribe up to several hundred milligrams a day, or injections in the case of vitamin B_{12}, until symptoms wane, then cut back.

For vitamin B_{12}, she prescribes injections of 300 to 500 micrograms weekly until symptoms respond, then monthly doses of 500 micrograms indefinitely. (If you can't get B_{12} injections, she suggests 500 to 1,000 micrograms taken under the tongue. These supplements are available over the counter.)

Check with your doctor before taking an amount above the Daily Value of any B vitamin, since high dosages may lead to side effects. Doses of 200 milligrams or more of vitamin B_6 a day, for example, have caused nerve damage.

Some people may also benefit from taking biotin, another B vitamin, in amounts of up to 15 milligrams (15,000 micrograms) a day, Dr. Eades adds. A study by Japanese researchers found that this vitamin helps cells in muscle tissue use sugar more effectively.

Covering All the Bases

In addition to these particular vitamins, doctors may also recommend that people with diabetes take a multivitamin/mineral supplement that contains the Daily Value of every essential nutrient. That might not be such a bad idea. Research suggests that a multitude of nutrients—zinc, copper, manganese, selenium, calcium, vitamin D, and vitamin A—may be in short supply in people with diabetes.

Medical Alert

It's best to work with a doctor knowledgeable in nutrition when you're adding nutritional supplements to your diabetes treatment program. Your blood sugar and drug dosage need to be carefully monitored.

If you have diabetes and you want to try chromium supplementation, you should do so only under your doctor's supervision. He may need to adjust your insulin dosage as your blood sugar level drops.

People who have heart or kidney problems should talk to their doctors before beginning magnesium supplementation.

It's a good idea to talk to your doctor before taking more than 600 international units of vitamin E daily. If you are taking anticoagulants, you should not take vitamin E supplements.

Diarrhea

Battling through the Storm

It is the subject of jokes and slang terms, but suffering with diarrhea is no laughing matter. It can leave you feeling nauseated, dehydrated, and downright rotten, possibly for days.

Physicians talk about diarrhea in technical terms relating to stool. Normal stool weighs somewhere around 100 grams, of which about half is water weight. Moderate diarrhea is about 400 grams, with water accounting for the added weight. Severe diarrhea is anything higher than that and can result in a person losing as much as 4 pints of fluid a day, says Peter Holt, M.D., chief of the division of gastroenterology at St. Luke's–Roosevelt Hospital Center and professor of medicine at Columbia University College of Physicians and Surgeons, both in New York City.

You may never know exactly what caused a particular case of diarrhea. "There are a million and one causes," says Joel B. Mason, M.D., assistant professor of medicine and nutrition at Tufts University School of Medicine in Boston. "Acute infectious diarrhea, what people call gastrointestinal flu, is usually related to a viral or bacterial infection. It is self-limiting and usually runs its course in several days to a week. The only immediate danger is the loss of fluids and electrolytes, including sodium, magnesium, potassium, and calcium."

In the Belly of the Beast

Diarrhea can occur from either the colon or small intestine, Dr. Holt says. Diarrhea in the colon is not particularly troublesome. It usually only results in malabsorption of potassium and occasionally sodium, since little else of importance is absorbed there. When diarrhea strikes in the small intestine, however, malabsorption of many macronutrients and micronutrients—including vitamins as well as calcium, magnesium, potassium, and other electrolytes—can occur, he says.

"Diarrhea that comes as a result of a small-bowel disease can affect the absorption of many substances, since the small bowel is where these nutrients are digested," Dr. Holt says. If the diarrhea is prolonged, nutritional deficiencies and depletions can occur. The same is true with serious stomach or small-intestine operations or with diseases such as celiac sprue (an illness where gluten causes damage to the lining of the small intestine), ulcerative colitis (a condition of chronic inflammation and ulceration of the lining of the colon and rectum), Crohn's disease (a chronic inflammation of any part of the gastrointestinal tract), and HIV (human immunodeficiency virus).

"The issue of diarrhea most of the time is 'What's the diagnosis?'—not what vitamin or mineral should a person take," Dr. Holt says. That's because if the illness causing the diarrhea is cured, the diarrhea goes away, too. In cases where there is no known or expedient remedy for the disease that is causing the diarrhea, doctors must determine where in the small intestine the problem is taking place because the location helps pinpoint which nutrients are being lost.

The next step is to fortify the patient's body with the missing nutrients through shots, supplements, or some other intervention. Chronic replacement of specific nutrients depends on the type of ailment and location of affected intestinal tissue, Dr. Holt says. For example, people who have had operations to remove the part of the small intestine called the ileum must have monthly vitamin B_{12} shots because they no longer have the ability to absorb the nutrient.

Doctors can determine where a chronic diarrhea problem is coming from by running a series of tests. Some tests check to see what nutrients aren't being absorbed. This is done by examining blood, stool, or small-intestine fluid samples. Other ways to examine the condition include x-ray and colonoscopy. Biopsies of the small intestine or colon also may be called for to determine what is causing the diarrhea.

Surviving the Short Term

Events of acute diarrhea that are caused by common viruses and bacteria are usually over within 12 to 72 hours. They aren't a real cause for alarm, Dr. Holt says. Only very young children, very old people, and those who are very ill to begin with are at any risk of harm during these brief stints. "Short-lived events of diarrhea rarely result in deficiencies or depletions of any essential vitamins or minerals in healthy adults," Dr. Holt says.

When you do come down with a case of acute diarrhea, here are a few simple things that you can do to ensure against nutrient depletion and to encourage a speedy recovery, says Dr. Holt.

If you are nauseated and vomiting, don't try fluids or foods just yet. Wait out the storm, then try drinking some fluids.

Since you are losing so much fluid in your diarrhea, you need to prevent dehydration. Drinking just water probably isn't enough, Dr. Holt says. You also need to replace electrolytes, the nutrients responsible for regulating many essential body functions, including muscle movement, blood pressure, heart rate, and nerve impulses. Because your needs for electrolytes—especially sodium and potassium—are higher when you have diarrhea, drinking sports drinks like Gatorade can help replenish your stores. Start by slowly sipping about four ounces of a sports drink an hour. Some patients have difficulty tolerating these drinks, Dr. Holt says. He recommends diluting the beverage with water.

"The classic recommendation for people who had diarrhea was Coca-Cola because it has some potassium in it," Dr. Holt says. If you are drinking Coke, take it in the same way you would the sports drink.

If you have been sipping your fluids faithfully for about a day and the diarrhea seems to have slowed down, it's probably all right to try to eat something again, says Dr. Holt. Stick with carbohydrates that are mild, like plain pasta, bananas, white bread, or apple-sauce and keep the portions very small. If the runs stay away, gradually increase your portions. Once you can eat normal amounts again, it's probably okay to go back to your regular diet.

Medical Alert

If diarrhea lasts for more than 12 to 24 hours in an in-fant or an older person, you should seek medical help.

If you're an otherwise healthy adult, you should see your doctor if diarrhea persists for more than three days, if it is accompanied by fever or lethargy, if there is blood or pus in the stool, or if any signs of dehydration continue despite efforts to replace fluid.

Endometriosis

Living without Pain

Picture a puffy white dandelion that has gone to seed blowing in the wind, with all of the tiny para-chuted seeds spawning new dandelions across your front lawn. Now picture yourself trying to get rid of all of those deep-rooted weeds that crop up again and again and again, even after being pulled, mowed, and sprayed. Think also of how your whole body hurts after a day spent on your knees wrestling with these yellow devils.

By now you have a pretty clear picture of what endometriosis is all about: easily spread, hard as heck to get rid of, and downright painful.

Of course, endometriosis is a whole lot harder to live with than a lawn full of dandelions—almost impossible for many women whose menstrual cycles become monthly nightmares of extreme cramping and bleeding. But help may be on the horizon, say the experts, and it may be as close as your local supermarket.

"We've found that adopting a healthy lifestyle goes a long way in preventing and relieving the symptoms of endometriosis," says Susan M. Lark, M.D., author of *Fibroid Tumors and Endometriosis: A Self-Help Program*, director of the PMS and Menopause Self-Help Center in Los Altos, California, and a physician specializing in women's health. As part of her practice, Dr. Lark helps women with endometriosis live pain-free through a wide variety of dietary regimens and herbal and nutritional supplements.

Before you start stocking your pantry, it will help to understand what causes endometriosis and how it affects your body.

Strange Tissue in Strange Places

Endometriosis is simply tissue growing where it doesn't belong. During normal menstruation, cells from the uterine lining, the endometrium, break off and are flushed out through the vagina. In someone with endometriosis, these cells back up into the fallopian tubes. From there, they flow into the pelvic cavity and, like dandelion seeds, implant themselves in places you'd rather they not be, such as the cervix and the bowels. Being uterine tissue, these implants respond to hormone stimulation, swelling and bleeding each month just as they would if they were still inside the uterus. Except this blood doesn't have the vagina for an escape route. It gets trapped in the pelvic cavity, where it can cause pain, inflammation, cysts, scar tissue, and even structural damage and infertility.

No one knows why these implants occur in some women but not others. Some researchers believe excessive circulating estrogen may be to blame. Others say that an impaired immune system is likely at fault.

Bad Times Call for Good Nutrition

That's why nutrition is so important, say the experts. Whether estrogen or immunity is to blame, all of your body's systems need to be operating at maximum efficiency to properly regulate your hormones, maintain your immunity, and keep endometrial implants at bay.

This is not to say that medical treatments such as estrogen-blocking hormones and surgical removal of endometrial growths aren't effective, says Dr. Lark. They are. But too often endometrial implants recur even after surgical removal.

"Nutritional plans are particularly successful for women who have recently undergone traditional treatment," says Dr. Lark. "I don't suggest that women not use medications, because hormone treatments can really help lessen endometriosis. But to prevent the pain from recurring, nutritional programs work very well."

The following are nutrients that many experts recommend for controlling endometriosis.

Note: Because the required doses are high and vary from woman to woman, be sure to consult your doctor before starting a nutritional regimen. Because getting the Daily Values of all of the essential nutrients is important if you have endometriosis, doctors who use nutritional regimens recommend starting with a general multivitamin/mineral supplement and adding additional supplements as needed.

B Vitamins Lower Estrogen Levels

If you're looking for a natural way to keep your estrogen levels low and thus reduce recurrent episodes of endometriosis, try boosting your intake of B-complex vitamins, say the experts.

"The liver is responsible for breaking down and disposing of excess estrogen," explains Dr. Lark. "The B vitamins are important in regulating estrogen because they promote a healthy liver. Studies dating back to the 1940s show that if you remove B vitamins from animals' food, they can no longer metabolize estrogen." Studies have also shown that B vitamin supplementation helps alleviate other symptoms of excess estrogen, such as premenstrual syndrome and fibrocystic breasts, she says.

Some women apparently find that supplements alone do the trick for them. Dian Mills, for example, a nutrition consultant in London and author of *Female Health: The Nutrition Connection*, became a strong advocate of B vitamin supplements through personal experience.

"I was in absolute crawl-around-the-house agony. And none of the traditional treatments was taking the pain away," recalls Mills. Her doctor even recommended a hysterectomy, advice she flatly refused. "So I went to doctors of nutritional medicine in London, and I've been pain-free ever since."

Mills's supplement regimen included B vitamins, particularly thiamin, riboflavin, and vitamin B_6. Not only did her pain disappear, but she was so inspired by her success with the nutrition program that she went on to study clinical nutrition at the Institute of Optimum Nutrition in London and is now pursuing her master's degree in health education at the University of Brighton in England.

Dr. Lark recommends that women with endometriosis take considerably more than the Daily Values of the B vitamins. She suggests approximately 50 milligrams each of thiamin, riboflavin, niacin, and pantothenic acid, 30 milligrams of vitamin B_6, 50 micrograms of vitamin B_{12}, 400 micrograms of folic acid, and 200 micrograms of biotin.

You can also fortify your diet with B vitamins by eating whole-grain cereals, pastas and rice, fish, legumes, and green leafy vegetables.

Antioxidant Onslaught

Another way to thwart the effects of endometriosis is by upping your intake of these antioxidant nutrients: vitamins C and E, beta-carotene (which converts to vitamin A in the body), and the mineral selenium. Antioxidants are best known for their ability to fight free radicals, the naturally occurring unstable molecules that cause tissue damage in the body by stealing electrons from healthy molecules to balance themselves. Doctors know that antioxidants can also build immunity, lessen cramping, and reduce excessive menstrual bleeding. All of these are useful functions in treating endometriosis.

"While you can't just pop these supplements and expect instant relief from acute pain, I have found that doses of antioxidants, along with dietary changes, can treat the chronic problem of endometriosis," says Dr. Lark.

Dr. Lark recommends a daily regimen of 1,000 to 4,000 milligrams of vitamin C, 25,000 to 50,000 international units (IU) of beta-carotene, 400 to 2,000 IU of vitamin E, and 25 micrograms of selenium. These are dosages at which she has arrived during her many years of treating women's health problems.

Because the recommended doses of vitamin C and vitamin E are many times the Daily Values of these nutrients, you should check with your doctor before trying this therapy. Vitamin C can cause diarrhea when taken in doses exceeding 1,500 milligrams a day.

And just because symptoms improve, that doesn't mean that you can stop taking supplements, cautions Dr. Lark.

Antioxidants can have a dramatic effect on the regulation of bleeding as well as on the reduction of pain and cramps that may accompany endometriosis, says Dr. Lark. "Vitamin C is good for controlling excessive bleeding," she explains. "Vitamin A has also been shown to lessen profuse menstrual bleeding. And vitamin E has antispasmodic effects, which help in pain management."

To get more antioxidants in your diet, start by hitting the farmers' market. Broccoli, spinach, and cantaloupe are excellent sources of vitamin C and beta-carotene; cabbage, celery, and cucumbers are great sources of selenium. For more vitamin E, try sautéing these veggies in sunflower oil or safflower oil. Or reach for a handful of almonds, another good source of vitamin E.

Medical Alert

If you have symptoms of endometriosis, you should see a doctor for proper diagnosis and treatment.

Doses of vitamin C exceeding 1,500 milligrams a day may cause diarrhea.

Before taking the amount of vitamin E recommended here, you should discuss it with your doctor. Doses of vitamin E exceeding 600 international units a day can cause side effects in some people. If you are taking anticoagulant drugs, you should not take vitamin E supplements.

Epilepsy

Quieting a Short-Circuited Brain

Like all nerve tissue, our brains rely on electrical impulses to receive and send messages. Electrical currents that enter our brains through the spinal cord or optic nerves allow us to process billions of pieces of information and react to our environment, scratching an itch here, swerving to avoid a confused groundhog there, or adding a comma here, or is it there?

Normally, electrical currents move through the brain in an orderly and limited fashion. In epilepsy, however, the currents get short-circuited or out of sync for a variety of reasons. The result is a burst of electrical activity that causes a seizure, which can be anything from a staring spell, called an absence seizure, to a full-fledged grand mal, complete with jerking arms and legs and loss of consciousness.

People can become seizure-prone for many different reasons. "An injury to the brain from an accident, a stroke or lack of oxygen during birth, alcohol abuse, poisoning, a severe bacterial or viral infection such as meningitis or encephalitis, and high fever may all cause seizures," says James Neubrander, M.D., a doctor in private practice in Hopewell, New Jersey, with a special interest in epilepsy and nutrition.

Nutrients Can Play a Role

Less commonly, seizures are the result of a metabolic disease, an inherited disorder that results in an inability to properly utilize a particular nutrient in the body, such as a vitamin or an amino acid. "Seizures associated with metabolic disorders usually begin soon after birth and rarely start after age six," says Robert J. Gumnit, M.D., president of the Minnesota Comprehensive Epilepsy Program and director of the Epilepsy Clinical Research Center at the University of Minnesota, both in Minneapolis.

In about half of these cases, the metabolic disorder can be figured out. "A specialist, a pediatric neurologist, may consider 20 to 80 different metabolic disorders that are most commonly associated with seizures," Dr. Gumnit says. Sometimes seizures can be controlled by a diet that restricts certain foods. Children with a condition called phenylketonuria, for instance, need to avoid the amino acid phenylalanine, found in large amounts in aspartame (a sugar substitute).

Adding more of a nutrient may help others. Children who develop seizures because their bodies have a hard time using vitamin B_6, for instance, may take 25 to 50 milligrams of B_6 each day, an amount large enough to overcome metabolic roadblocks.

If you think your child has seizures because of a metabolic disorder, see a specialist for a diagnosis, Dr. Gumnit urges. Don't try to treat a metabolic disorder on your own.

Seizures can also be caused by nutritional deficiency. "Most doctors, however, think that nutritional deficiency is only rarely the cause of repeated seizures," Dr. Gumnit says. Shortages of magnesium, thiamin, vitamin B_6, and zinc have been reported to be associated with seizures in some individuals. These nutrients, among numerous others, are needed for normal chemical reactions in the brain.

Nutritional support for people with seizure disorders involves correcting metabolic problems and nutritional deficiencies. In some cases, it may also involve taking larger amounts of certain nutrients to help protect against drug-related damage and, in theory at least, against damage caused by the seizures themselves.

"There's absolutely no reason that optimum nutritional support can't be combined with traditional treatment," Dr. Neubrander says.

Here's what seems to be helpful.

Vitamin E Helps Prevent Seizures

There is good reason to believe that vitamin E could be helpful for some kinds of seizures. Animals given vitamin E are more resistant to seizures induced by pressurized oxygen, iron, and certain chemicals. And clinical studies show that people taking antiseizure drugs have reduced blood levels of vitamin E.

That's why researchers at the University of Toronto decided to test vitamin E in 24 children with epilepsy whose seizures could not be controlled by medication.

They found that the frequency of seizures was reduced by more than 60 percent in 10 of 12 children taking vitamin E supplements. They took 400 international units (IU) a day for three months in addition to their regular medication. Six of them had a 90 to 100 percent reduction in seizures. By comparison, none of the 12 children who took placebos (inactive substances) along with their medication improved significantly.

What's more, when the children who were taking placebos were switched to vitamin E, seizure frequency was reduced 70 to 100 percent in all of them. The researchers noted that there were no adverse side effects.

"Vitamin E apparently has no direct anti-epileptic action," says Paul A. Hwang, M.D., the study's main researcher, associate professor of neurology in the University of Toronto Department of Pediatrics and Medicine, and director of the epilepsy program at the Hospital for Sick Children in Toronto. In other words, once a seizure is taking place, vitamin E can't help. "But it may act as a scavenger of free radicals in some forms of epilepsy, such as post-traumatic seizures, and so help protect the membranes of brain cells."

Free radicals are unstable molecules that are generated by chemical reactions involving oxygen. These molecules are potentially harmful because they grab electrons from the healthy molecules embedded in cell membranes, damaging the protective membranes. Free radical scavengers called antioxidants, such as vitamin E, offer free radicals their own electrons and so save cell membranes from harm, Dr. Hwang explains.

In animals, seizures can be induced by chemicals that produce free radicals (ferrous chloride, for instance). Iron from blood that gets into the brain after a head injury may cause seizures in the same way, Dr. Hwang says. "And the seizure itself generates more free radicals, possibly setting up a cycle that leads to frequent seizures," he adds.

Dr. Hwang and his colleagues continue to use vitamin E with good results in their patients with seizures who don't respond to standard anticonvulsant drugs. "It's not a cure-all, but it can be very helpful," he says. "If someone is going to be helped by vitamin E, the benefits will be apparent in about three months."

He has found that 400 IU daily of d-alpha-tocopherol acetate, the most biologically active form of vitamin E, is safe and effective even in children as young as age three. (Nutrition experts say that infants under age one should not be given more than 50 IU daily.) Most adults can safely take up to 600 IU without problems, but don't take more than this amount daily without medical supervision. These high amounts are not easily available from foods, says Dr. Hwang.

"It's important to work with a doctor on this," Dr. Hwang adds. "In some cases, under medical supervision, it may be possible to reduce the dosages of some seizure drugs."

Selenium May Stop Seizures

The mineral selenium, another nutrient with antioxidant properties, also appears to help control seizures in some children, says Georg Weber, M.D., Ph.D., assistant professor in the department of pathology at Harvard Medical School and a researcher at the Dana-Farber Cancer Institute in Boston.

Dr. Weber has found that some children with severe, uncontrollable seizures and repeated infections have low blood levels of glutathione peroxidase, a selenium-dependent antioxidant enzyme.

"We've found that giving these children 50 to 150 micrograms of selenium a day significantly reduces their seizures," Dr. Weber says. "We believe that these children have a metabolic problem that prevents them from using selenium properly and that the problem may be far more frequent than has been believed."

Talk to your doctor if you're thinking about taking selenium supplements yourself and especially if you're considering giving them to your child with epilepsy, Dr. Weber says. Although he has found amounts up to 150 micrograms a day to be safe for children with severe deficiency, children's needs can vary greatly depending on the amount of deficiency they have, and giving too much selenium could be detrimental to their health.

For adults with epilepsy, experts who use nutritional therapy recommend 50 to 200 micrograms of selenium daily to control seizures. But be sure not to take more than 100 micrograms daily without medical supervision. You can get more selenium from foods if you eat lots of garlic, onions, whole grains, mushrooms, broccoli, cabbage, and fish.

Fill Up on Folic Acid

Deficiency of folate (the naturally occurring form of folic acid) isn't thought to often play a role in the development of seizures. But some antiseizure drugs deplete this B-complex vitamin, sometimes leading to abnormalities in red blood cell formation.

"Folate deficiency can also lead to serious birth defects called neural tube defects," explains Dr. Gumnit. "These birth defects happen very early in the pregnancy, often before a woman knows she is pregnant."

That is why any woman of childbearing age who's taking antiseizure drugs should also take 1,600 micrograms of folic acid a day, Dr. Gumnit says. And any woman who's taking antiseizure drugs and planning to become pregnant should also take three milligrams (3,000 micrograms) of folic acid every day for three months before she stops using birth control, he says. (That high amount requires a prescription supplement.)

Other people taking antiseizure drugs should simply take 400 micrograms, the amount of folic acid found in ordinary multivitamin/mineral supplements, Dr. Gumnit says. A few doctors recommend up to 5,000 micrograms a day for adults.

Make sure that you are under a doctor's supervision when taking more than 400 micrograms, because high amounts of folic acid can mask the symptoms of vitamin B_{12} deficiency, also known as pernicious anemia.

Some experts say that children ages 5 to 15 may safely take up to 2,500 micrograms of folic acid daily, but it's best to talk to a doctor about this first, Dr. Gumnit says.

Many doctors also recommend a multivitamin/mineral supplement for their patients with epilepsy, and that's probably not a bad idea. Some research suggests that deficiencies of vitamin B_6, zinc, and magnesium may also play roles in seizure disorders.

Medical Alert

If you have been diagnosed with epilepsy, you should be under a doctor's care.

Make sure that you are under a doctor's supervision when taking more than 400 micrograms of folic acid daily. High amounts can mask the symptoms of vitamin B_{12} deficiency, also known as pernicious anemia.

Don't take more than 100 micrograms of selenium daily without medical supervision.

Don't take more than 600 international units of vitamin E daily without medical supervision. Infants under one year of age should not be given more than 50 international units daily. If you are taking anticoagulant drugs, you should not take vitamin E supplements.

Fatigue

What to Do When You're Running on Empty

What do all doctors' waiting rooms have in common, besides outdated magazines?

Lots of tired people.

Surveys show that fatigue is one of the most common reasons that we consult our family doctors. And that's not surprising when you consider the

number of conditions, both major and minor, that have
fatigue as a symptom. Stress, depression, thyroid problems, anemia, and food allergies can all cause persistent
tiredness, says Susan M. Lark, M.D., author of *Chronic
Fatigue and Tiredness*, director of the PMS and
Menopause Self-Help Center in Los Altos, California,
and a physician specializing in women's health. Many
women also have premenstrual fatigue or fatigue that's
related to menopause.

And while it may seem obvious, many of us simply
don't get enough sleep. "While a small minority of
people can get by on four to five hours a night, most
people need six to nine hours," says Peter Hauri, Ph.D.,
director of the insomnia program at the Mayo Clinic
Sleep Disorders Center in Rochester, Minnesota. The
real test of whether you're getting enough sleep is how
you feel and function during the day.

Fortunately, there are a number of vitamins and
minerals that play roles in helping keep you fatigue-free.

Iron: The Usual Suspect

One of the most common causes of fatigue is iron-deficiency anemia, says Dr. Lark. She estimates that 20 percent of women who menstruate are anemic because of
the blood they lose each month. "Women with heavy
menstrual flow have the greatest risk," she adds. Anemia
is also common among teenagers, pregnant women,
and women nearing menopause.

If you suspect that you may be anemic, the first
step is to make an appointment with your doctor, says
Dr. Lark. It's the only way to find out for sure.

But even if you're not anemic, a slight iron deficiency can affect your energy level, and you may benefit from getting more iron in your diet, says Dr. Lark.

Experts who recommend iron to combat fatigue generally suggest between 12 and 15 milligrams a day. The best source of iron is animal products, so go for lean meats, oysters, and clams. Some vegetables such as spinach as well as legumes such as green beans, lima beans, and pinto beans are also rich in iron, but the type of iron found in them is not as easy to absorb as the iron found in animal sources.

If you're a vegetarian, drinking some orange juice or taking a vitamin C supplement of at least 75 milligrams along with iron-rich vegetables will help your body absorb more iron from your food, says Dr. Lark. Many commercial breads and breakfast cereals are also fortified with iron.

Potassium and Magnesium: A Potent Combination

Two other minerals that may be beneficial for people with persistent fatigue are potassium and magnesium, says Dr. Lark. "In studies where potassium and magnesium were given together, 90 percent saw improvements in their energy levels," says Dr. Lark. She recommends trying between 100 and 200 milligrams of each mineral for up to six months to see if they alleviate fatigue. It's safe for anyone in good health, she says, although people with heart or kidney problems or diabetes shouldn't take these minerals without consulting a doctor first.

Rev Up with Vitamin C

While more research needs to be done, some older studies suggest that low vitamin C intake can also contribute to fatigue. A 1976 study of 411 dentists and their wives found that those with low vitamin C intakes reported twice as many fatigue symptoms as those who got the most vitamin C. And studies of adolescent boys showed that even those with slight vitamin C deficiencies had more stamina after taking vitamin C supplements for three months.

Dr. Lark recommends about 4,000 milligrams of vitamin C a day for people with persistent fatigue. She warns that this high dose can cause temporary diarrhea in some people. "If this happens," she says, "just cut back on the dose to the point where the diarrhea goes away."

Medical Alert

People with heart or kidney problems should consult their doctors before taking supplemental magnesium.

People with kidney problems or diabetes should consult their doctors before taking supplemental potassium.

High doses of vitamin C may cause diarrhea in some people.

Gallstones

Clearing Out the Gravel Pit

The woman was about 20 pounds overweight. Nevertheless, she downed pizza, fries, and a milkshake with barely a pause to breathe, then topped it off with cheesecake.

Three hours later, she was in the emergency room, a sharp pain boring into the upper right quarter of her abdomen.

The diagnosis? One nasty little gallstone about the size of a pea, stuck in a duct that connects the gallbladder to the bowel. And it was there to stay until it would somehow squeeze through to the bowel or drop back into the gallbladder or until a surgeon would go in and yank it out—along with her gallbladder.

Eat and Squirt

Whether or not a doctor has ever looked you in the eye and announced the presence of a pea-size pellet wandering through your digestive system, there's a good chance that you have at least one. Close to 30 million Americans do. Most of them are over age 40, most of them are women, and most of them don't even know that the gallstones are there.

The stones are formed when a grain or two of calcium arrives in the gallbladder and hangs around long enough to become coated with either cholesterol or bilirubin, a substance that is part of the hemoglobin in your blood. Eighty to 85 percent of all stones are coated with layer upon layer of waxy-looking cholesterol, although many stones are coated with both substances. A few are made exclusively of yellowish green bilirubin.

Exactly what causes this buildup of cholesterol or bilirubin on the calcium is not totally clear. Normally, the gallbladder is a storage compartment for the somewhat slimy bile that your body needs to digest fat. You eat fat, the stomach sends it through to the bowel, and your gallbladder squirts some bile onto the food to break up the fat. Your body then finishes its digestive process, and everything heads for the exit.

But occasionally, your body screws up. Something breaks down during the eat-squirt-exit process, and the gallbladder's sludgelike contents crystallize. This provides the opportunity to layer thicker and thicker coats of cholesterol or bilirubin around a calcium speck, thus forming a gallstone.

Naturally occurring female reproductive hormones are known to encourage that process by delaying gallbladder emptying, such as during pregnancy and dieting. What's more, birth control implants that contain progesterone may do the same, while birth control pills containing estrogen seem to increase the cholesterol content of bile—not a helpful situation either.

Blame Your Genes and Diet

All told, hormones, pregnancy, dieting, and birth control may help explain why two-thirds of all gallstones belong to women. But aside from being a woman, what else puts you at risk for gallstones? (After all, many men get them, too.)

"Diet and genetics," replies Henry Pitt, M.D., vice chairman of surgery at Johns Hopkins University School of Medicine in Baltimore. And it's difficult to sort out which is responsible for what. So far, many scientific studies of populations only add to the confusion.

In Chile, for example, 60 percent of people have gallstones by the time they're 80 years of age. Yet in Africa, gallstones affect only 1 to 2 percent of the population.

Is that diet or genetics?

It could be one or the other or both, says Dr. Pitt. Studies of ethnic groups who rarely get gallstones indicate that when they move from a geographic location in which they have consumed a low-fat, low-cholesterol diet to a location in which they consume a high-fat, high-cholesterol diet, they start getting gallstones.

Aside from lowering calories and fat, another dietary factor may have an impact on gallstone formation, and it involves a mineral: calcium.

The Calcium Controversy

A low-fat, low-cholesterol diet may help prevent gallstones, agrees Alan Hofmann, M.D., Ph.D., professor at the University of California, San Diego, but the most important aspect of the diet is that it doesn't have too many calories, so a person stays slender. But Dr. Hofmann also feels there is reason to believe that supplementing the diet with calcium may act to prevent gallstones.

"In addition to helping your bones, calcium has a good effect on bile acid metabolism," explains Dr. Hofmann. "What has been found is that large doses of oral calcium form calcium phosphate in the gut." This sets off a chain of chemical events that eventually lowers the amount of cholesterol in the gallbladder, thus reducing the possibility that gallstones will form, he explains.

It also seems to explain why a study of 872 Dutchmen between the ages of 40 and 59 found that the more calcium the men consumed over a 25-year period, the fewer gallstones they were likely to have.

In fact, one study in the Netherlands revealed that men who had more than 1,442 milligrams of calcium in their diets every day had a 50 percent lower prevalence of gallstones.

"Since most individuals have stopped drinking much milk by the time they're 45 years old, it makes good sense to take calcium supplements," says Dr. Hofmann. Nonetheless, the view that large doses of supplemental calcium can prevent gallstones has not yet been tested experimentally. Normal doses of calcium do not increase the risk of kidney stones, however, and are likely to be good for both bones and bile. Studies are needed to prove this point as well as to prove that there are no important risks associated with long-term use of oral calcium supplements, says Dr. Hofmann.

Experts who recommend calcium to help prevent gallstones suggest aiming for the Daily Value, which is 1,000 milligrams. But before you race out to the drugstore, Dr. Pitt suggests that you take a moment to check with your physician, especially if you're a woman.

"Calcium may have something to do with the origin of most of the gallstones in this country," says Dr. Pitt. "It's at the center of almost every stone we find. And in our animal studies, diets with high calcium seem to enhance the formation of pigment stones," the stones made of bilirubin.

And keep in mind all of the hormonal factors that affect women, says Dr. Pitt. It may turn out that calcium prevents gallstones in men but actually contributes to their formation in women.

So while men can feel comfortable taking calcium supplements, women should ask their family physicians to help evaluate individual risks and benefits, particularly in light of their family medical histories, says Dr. Pitt.

"If all of the women in your family get gallstones and none of them gets osteoporosis, then I'd stay away from calcium," he advises. But if all of the women get osteoporosis and only an occasional stone rolls down someone's duct, then calcium should be okay, he adds.

Medical Alert

If you have a gallstone, you should be under a doctor's care.

Dr. Hofmann considers calcium supplementation to be fine for men. Calcium may contribute to the formation of some kinds of gallstones in women, however. He suggests that women discuss supplementation with their physicians.

Gingivitis

Exploring the Role of Vitamin C

hat if you floss and brush until you're blue in the face and you still have bleeding, receding gums?

You're dealing with a stubborn case of what's known as gingivitis. And it is cause for concern. Left for even a short time along your gum line, food particles and bacteria combine to form plaque, which hardens on your teeth and irritates your gums. Irritated gums bleed and eventually start to recede, creating pockets next to your teeth that collect even more junk. Before long, the plaque starts attacking the roots of your teeth and your jawbone; this is the point at which gingivitis turns into a more serious gum problem known as periodontal disease. If periodontal disease progresses too far without proper medical intervention, you might even lose some teeth.

When it comes to healthy gums, most dentists rightly focus on clearing out the crud with frequent flossing and brushing. But there's no doubt that diet also plays a role.

"After all, the mouth is attached to the rest of the body," says Cherilyn Sheets, D.D.S., a spokesperson for the Academy of General Dentistry and a dentist in Newport Beach, California. "Anything that improves health overall and the body's ability to resist disease will affect the mouth positively." Eat badly enough, or indulge in damaging behaviors such as smoking and excessive drinking, and your whole body suffers, including your mouth, says Dr. Sheets.

Take Vitamin C and See Improvement

"Certainly, vitamin C is the one nutrient that has been shown to have quite a positive effect on the mouth when in adequate levels in the body and a negative effect on the mouth when in low levels in the body," says Dr. Sheets. People with vitamin C deficiencies can have some of the worst gum and dental problems that dentists see.

To measure the effect of vitamin C deficiency on gum health, researchers at the University of California, San Francisco, School of Dentistry for 14 weeks fed 11 men rotating diets that purposely excluded fruits and vegetables. Vitamin C, in the form of a supplement dissolved in grape juice, was added to their diets only during certain weeks. At the end of the study, researchers found that as vitamin C levels in the men went down, their gums bled more. When they received more vitamin C, their gums bled less.

Further research with laboratory animals confirmed that vitamin C deficiency causes gum swelling, decreased mineral content of the jawbone, and loose teeth.

Why the damage? As it turns out, vitamin C is vital for production of collagen, the basic protein building block for the fibrous framework of all tissues, including gums, explains Mary Dan Eades, M.D., medical director of the Arkansas Center for Health and Weight Control in Little Rock. "Vitamin C strengthens weak gum tissue and makes the gum lining more resistant to penetration by bacteria," she says.

Dr. Eades recommends using vitamin C in two ways—as a mouthwash and as a supplement—to fight gingivitis. "Mix half a teaspoon of crystalline vitamin C with a sugar-free citrus beverage, swish the mixture in your mouth for one minute, then swallow, twice daily," she advises. Follow each rinse with plenty of fresh water.

Crystalline vitamin C is also called powdered pure ascorbic acid and is available in health food stores and through vitamin supply houses. Your doctor could help you find a supply.

You can also take 500-milligram slow-release vitamin C capsules, one or two in the morning and one or two in the evening, says Dr. Eades. Meanwhile, keep on brushing and flossing.

Medical Alert

If you have gingivitis, you should be under a dentist's care.

Chewable and powdered vitamin C have been found to erode tooth enamel, so it's best to use the crystalline form in a mouth rinse. This is a big problem and can also cause tooth sensitivity. Some dentists prefer using the oral rinse for three to five days at a time. Follow the rinse with plenty of fresh water.

Vitamin C can also cause diarrhea in doses exceeding 1,500 milligrams.

Glaucoma

Easing the Pressure

Thomas Goslin had the classic symptoms of glaucoma: a steady buildup of fluid in the eyeballs, creating excessive pressure and some loss of peripheral vision.

At his ophthalmologist's instruction, Goslin, a retired Presbyterian minister from Wildwood Crest, New Jersey, reluctantly began using prescription eyedrops, one of the most common treatments. He was reluctant because he has a history of allergic reaction to medication, and sure enough, by the end of the first day of using the drops, he was ready to try just about anything else.

That's when he was referred to Ben C. Lane, O.D., director of the Nutritional Optometry Institute in Lake Hiawatha, New Jersey. Dr. Lane had done research on nutrition and eye diseases at Columbia University in New York City before founding the institute.

"Dr. Lane told me that over the years, he had been successful in treating normal glaucoma based primarily on nutrition and diet, so I thought I'd give it a try," says Goslin. After doing a thorough eye exam and nutritional analysis, including a blood test and diet history, Dr. Lane made some specific recommendations for Goslin that included taking supplements of vitamin C and the mineral chromium.

It was a year before Goslin saw measurable improvement, but since then he has even regained the peripheral vision that he thought had been lost forever. "The proof is in the pudding," he says. "I would certainly attribute my improvement to Dr. Lane and his recommendations."

Goslin says he took oral chromium supplements until Dr. Lane discovered that his body wasn't absorbing them properly because of interference from other nutrients that were taken at the same time. He now takes two drops of aqueous chromium every day, under the tongue, either 30 minutes before a meal or more than three hours after a meal but not at the same time as vitamin C.

The Diet Connection

To fight glaucoma, which can cause blindness in its advanced stage, most ophthalmologists prescribe eyedrops or use surgery to relieve pressure inside the eyeballs.

Prescription eyedrops and surgery may be necessary in some glaucoma cases, Dr. Lane says, but nutritional evidence suggests that many people can experience some improvement through measures as simple as changing what they eat.

"It's not going to help everyone," he says. "But if they get the right nutrients over a period of a few years, many people with glaucoma are able to be weaned off medication or to use much less medication."

Taking a Shine to Chromium

Aside from making sure that your reading prescription is up-to-date, one of the best ways to lower pressure inside the eyeballs is with a mineral called chromium, says Dr. Lane.

In a study done at Columbia University, Dr. Lane asked more than 400 people with eye disease to detail the foods that they had eaten during the previous two months. Then they took tests to measure the vitamin and mineral content of their blood. Among the findings: Those people who didn't get enough chromium and who ate too many vanadium-containing foods were at higher risk for glaucoma. (Vanadium is another common mineral that occurs naturally in many foods, including kelp, dulse, and other seaweed as well as large marine fish.)

"What set of muscles do we use more today than ever before in recorded history? The focusing muscles in our eyes," says Dr. Lane. "And what nutrient helps facilitate the ability of our eye muscles to focus? The bottom line is that most of us need more chromium, especially if we have been eating refined and sugar-supplemented foods." Adequate chromium levels are necessary to help deliver needed energy to your eye-focusing muscles, he says.

And what's the connection between eye muscles and glaucoma? When you perform tasks that require prolonged intense focus, such as reading, too much fluid can be produced inside the eyeballs, Dr. Lane explains. In some people, he says, the fluid doesn't drain properly and pressure builds, contributing to glaucoma.

People who suffer from Type II (non-insulin-dependent) diabetes seem more likely to develop glaucoma, says Dr. Lane. And that's not surprising, he says, because both people with diabetes and those with glaucoma have been found to be low in chromium.

The best sources of chromium include egg yolks, brewer's yeast, and most unrefined foods rich in energy content. Consequently, ripe fresh sweet and starchy fruits and vegetables also contain more than adequate chromium, says Dr. Lane.

The Daily Value for chromium is 120 micrograms.

If you want to try chromium supplementation, discuss it with your doctor. This is especially important if you have diabetes, since chromium may cause your blood sugar level to drop and reduce your need for insulin. Your doctor should monitor your insulin level carefully while you're taking supplements.

Dr. Lane also notes that many people make the mistake of taking chromium at the same time that they take vitamin C. Vitamin C interferes with the uptake of chromium.

Vitamin C Lets Up on Pressure

Like chromium, vitamin C also seems to reduce intraocular pressure, but by a different method. Studies show that it apparently raises the acidity of the blood, explains Dr. Lane. "That in and of itself seems to help normalize intraocular pressure," he says. (Intraocular pressure is the pressure inside the eyeballs. In people with glaucoma, the pressure is too high, which hinders the blood supply to the eye.)

Vitamin C delivers yet another benefit for your eyes. It increases the efficiency of fuel utilization by the eye muscles, says Dr. Lane. Between 750 and 1,500 milligrams of vitamin C daily seems to work best. Any more than that increases the risk that the jellylike substance in your eye may gradually become more liquefied, causing it to be pulled away from the retina and related structures at the back of the eye, says Dr. Lane. (The retina contains a light-sensitive layer of cells that receives images.) Taking more than 1,500 milligrams of vitamin C daily, however, can cause diarrhea in some people.

Take part of your vitamin C with juice before breakfast in the morning, then allow at least one meal to go by before taking the rest, advises Dr. Lane. Vitamin C has a tendency to block the absorption of other nutrients such as copper and chromium, he says.

Medical Alert

Nutritional therapy for glaucoma is not commonly practiced, nor is it for everyone. It is important to remain under a doctor's care if you have glaucoma and to continue using whatever medication your doctor prescribes. But do discuss your concerns with your doctor.

If you want to try chromium supplements, discuss it with your doctor. This is especially important if you have diabetes, since chromium may affect your blood sugar level. Also, many people make the mistake of taking chromium at the same time that they take vitamin C. Vitamin C interferes with the uptake of chromium.

Taking more than 1,500 milligrams of vitamin C daily can cause diarrhea in some people.

Heart Arrhythmia

Subduing Electrical Storms of the Heart

Day in and day out, our hearts have the seemingly endless task of pumping blood through the 62,000 miles of arteries, veins, and capillaries in our bodies. Seventy or so beats a minute, 4,200 beats an hour, 100,800 beats a day—it adds up fast, and most of us never give it a moment's thought.

If your *lub-dub* becomes a *lub-lub-a-dub* or *lub-a-dub-dub*, however, it's going to attract attention—either yours or your doctor's. Such irregular heartbeats, called arrhythmia, occur when nerves that regulate the contraction of the heart go haywire.

Normally, a heartbeat is a highly coordinated event, directed by the sequential firing of nerves that signal each chamber of the heart to contract. When all goes well, the atrial chambers and the ventricular chambers of the heart work in sequence, pumping blood to the lungs and the rest of the body. When things go awry, the nerve signals may be delayed, or the nerves may fire more often than necessary. The chambers may not pump in proper sequence. The end result is that the heart pumps blood less efficiently.

In the case of Joel Levine of Pine Brook, New Jersey, blood flow was so disturbed that he would faint during episodes. "My arrhythmia kept getting worse, despite changes in medication," he says. "Finally, it got so bad that I was having an attack a day." This was inconvenient, to say the least. But it speaks for his skill as a home furnishings salesman that he did not lose his job despite occasionally ending up on the floor. "He would try to lie down if he knew he was going to faint," explains his wife, Anne. "There was no hiding the fact that something was wrong."

Arrhythmia comes in all sorts of variations. Some types, such as atrial fibrillation (chaotic, quivering contractions), the kind Joel Levine had, may be upsetting. But since they rarely cause serious symptoms, they're not likely to kill you. Other types, such as ventricular fibrillation, are deadly.

"People with serious arrhythmia are usually under a doctor's care," says Michael A. Brodsky, M.D., associate professor of medicine at the University of California, Irvine, and director of the Cardiac Electrophysiology/Arrhythmia Service at the University of California, Irvine, Medical Center. Indeed, it's often a doctor who discovers the problem, since arrhythmia frequently has no apparent symptoms, he adds.

What makes the heart get out of sync? In serious cases, disease of the coronary arteries or heart muscle is the most likely cause, Dr. Brodsky says. But in some cases, and often in conjunction with heart disease, mineral imbalances interfere with the heart's normal nerve function.

Nutritional therapy for arrhythmia focuses on two minerals in particular: magnesium and potassium. Nerve cells make use of both to help fire off messages, and a shortage of either one can cause life-threatening problems.

Doctors have known for some time just how vital potassium is for normal heartbeat. Magnesium is an entirely different story, however. "Apparently, many doctors still don't realize how important a role this mineral can play in some heart patients," says Carla Sueta, M.D., Ph.D., assistant professor of medicine and cardiology at the University of North Carolina at Chapel Hill School of Medicine. "We see patients referred by doctors from all over our state, and magnesium levels have not been routinely checked."

Here's what research has to say about these two heart-healthy minerals.

Magnesium Helps Hearts Stay Regular

Several studies have shown that when it comes to certain types of arrhythmia, magnesium can save lives.

One study, by Dr. Sueta and her colleagues at the University of North Carolina at Chapel Hill, found that the risk of developing potentially fatal ventricular arrhythmia was reduced by more than half in people with heart failure who received large intravenous doses of magnesium compared with those who did not receive the mineral.

"This is important, because ventricular arrhythmia can progress to ventricular fibrillation, which can result in sudden death," Dr. Sueta explains. The study showed that magnesium reduced the incidence of several types of ventricular arrhythmia by 53 to 76 percent.

Joel Levine, for instance, found that his attacks stopped completely within 24 hours of his first dose of 400 milligrams (the Daily Value).

Intravenous magnesium, says Dr. Sueta, is now considered standard therapy for two types of arrhythmia: torsades de pointes, an unusual type of ventricular arrhythmia, and ventricular arrhythmia induced by digitalis, a commonly prescribed heart drug.

And researchers are doing preliminary work to see if people with heart disease who take oral magnesium supplements can reduce their chances of developing arrhythmia. "Right now we're trying to establish a dosage that raises people's blood levels of magnesium enough to do some good," Dr. Sueta says.

In the meantime, both she and Dr. Brodsky test all of their heart patients for magnesium deficiency. They prescribe oral magnesium supplements or intravenous magnesium when blood levels are low and sometimes oral supplements when blood levels are normal but symptoms suggest it might help. "If blood levels are low, you can be pretty sure someone is deficient," Dr. Brodsky says. "But people can have low tissue stores of magnesium and still have normal blood levels."

One thing on which more doctors than ever apparently agree is that a fair number of people with heart problems can benefit from getting enough magnesium. "I'd say that 50 to 60 percent of the people I see have at least mild magnesium deficiencies," Dr. Brodsky says.

Getting Enough Magnesium

Studies have shown that 65 percent of all people in intensive care units and 11 percent of people in general care sections of hospitals are deficient in magnesium, according to Dr. Sueta. So are 20 to 35 percent of people who have heart failure. "This is much more common than most people realize," she adds.

Magnesium deficiency can be induced by the very drugs meant to help heart problems. Some types of diuretics (water pills) cause the body to excrete both magnesium and potassium, as does digitalis. And magnesium deficiency is often at the bottom of what's called refractory potassium deficiency, Dr. Brodsky adds. "The amount of magnesium in the body determines the amount of a particular enzyme that determines the amount of potassium in the body," he explains. "So if you are magnesium-deficient, you may in turn be potassium-deficient, and no amount of potassium is going to correct this unless you are also getting enough magnesium."

If you have arrhythmia, talk to your doctor about the possibility of magnesium supplementation, Dr. Brodsky suggests. Have your blood level of magnesium checked, and if you start taking magnesium supplements, have your blood levels of magnesium and potassium checked regularly, especially if you are taking large amounts of either of these minerals.

"How much magnesium you need to take depends on the results of your blood tests," Dr. Brodsky says. "Not everyone needs to take the same amount."

Both Dr. Brodsky and Dr. Sueta give their patients supplements of magnesium lactate. Both magnesium lactate and magnesium gluconate are easily absorbed and are less likely to cause diarrhea than magnesium oxide and magnesium hydroxide, the other forms of magnesium. (Magnesium hydroxide is found in Phillips' Milk of Magnesia, Mylanta, and Maalox.)

"I generally give my patients either Slow-Mag or

MagTab, up to about six tablets—about 450 milligrams—a day," Dr. Brodsky says.

He has found that magnesium can help heart medications such as digoxin work better. "Most people won't be able to go off their drugs completely, but they may be able to cut their dosages," Dr. Brodsky says. It's important to cut dosage slowly, over time, with your doctor's supervision, he adds. Stopping abruptly could make your heart problems worse.

Although magnesium is considered to be a fairly safe mineral, even in high doses, don't take supplemental magnesium without medical supervision if you have kidney or heart problems. Your heart or breathing could slow down too much.

Studies have shown that men get about 329 milligrams of magnesium daily, while women average 207 milligrams. The highest concentrations of magnesium are found in whole seeds such as legumes, nuts, and unmilled grains. Bananas and green vegetables are also good sources.

Potassium Powers Healthy Hearts

There's no doubt that potassium is just as important as magnesium for regular heartbeat. And doctors know it. In heart patients, low potassium levels are likely to be recognized and quickly corrected. Heartbeat irregularities, along with muscle weakness and confusion, are among the classic signs of potassium deficiency.

"Unlike magnesium, potassium levels are carefully regulated in the kidneys, and the body normally conserves potassium," Dr. Brodsky says. People who have normal kidney function and healthy hearts usually have adequate blood levels of potassium, even if they eat only a serving or two of fruits and vegetables a day.

People run into severe potassium deficiency that causes heart arrhythmia only when something interferes with the kidneys' potassium-hoarding tendency. "People who take thiazide diuretics or digitalis, who have poorly functioning kidneys, or who are alcoholics often become low in potassium unless they take supplements," Dr. Brodsky says. Prolonged diarrhea or vomiting and laxative abuse can also cause dangerously low potassium levels.

Here again, the amount of potassium each person should take depends on blood levels of this mineral. Too much potassium is as bad as too little, which is one reason potassium supplements containing more than 99 milligrams per tablet (the amount found in a bite or two of potato) are available only by prescription. Potassium supplements should not be taken by those with diabetes or kidney disease or by those using certain medications, including nonsteroidal anti-inflammatory drugs, potassium-sparing diuretics, ACE inhibitors, and heart medications such as heparin.

"Even though doctors may advise their patients to eat more potassium-containing foods, if they're on high-dose diuretics there's no way that they're going to get all of the potassium they need from foods alone," Dr. Sueta says.

The Daily Value for potassium is 3,500 milligrams. Studies show that among the general population, intakes vary widely—anywhere from 1,000 to 3,400 milligrams a day. Eating lots of fruits, vegetables, and fresh meats and drinking juices is the way to pack in the most potassium. A medium banana supplies 451 milligrams of potassium; one cup of cubed cantaloupe, 494 milligrams; and one cup of cooked cabbage, 146 milligrams.

Medical Alert

If you have been diagnosed with a heart arrhythmia, you should be under a doctor's care.

Mineral balance is important to a beating heart, but people with irregular heartbeats should take mineral supplements only under medical supervision. That's because the amounts of minerals they need to take depend on their blood levels, which must be carefully monitored.

People with kidney problems should check with their doctors before taking supplemental magnesium.

Potassium supplements should not be taken by those with diabetes or kidney disease or by those using certain medications, including nonsteroidal anti-inflammatory drugs, potassium-sparing diuretics, ACE inhibitors, and heart medications such as heparin.

Heart Disease

The News Is Simply FABB-ulous

For a variety of reasons, men are more likely to die of heart disease than anything else. It accounts for nearly half of all American male deaths, killing roughly half a million men every year. Before age 65, men suffer heart attacks at almost three times the rate of women.

You can cut your risk by not smoking; eating a low-fat, high-fiber diet; exercising at least three days a week; and effectively managing your stress levels. But if you're interested in tilting the odds even further in your favor, consider supplementing smartly with vitamins and minerals.

Be advised that not all experts in the field are ready to give supplementation blanket approval. "We do not yet have a clear consensus on supplements and won't until clinical trials prove their effectiveness. There is clear agreement, however, that eating a balanced diet with at least five servings of fruits and vegetables a day is important for heart health," says Ronald Krauss, M.D., head of the molecular medicine department, Lawrence Berkeley National Laboratory at the University of California, Berkeley, and chairman of the American Heart Association's Nutrition Committee.

Still, many experts are ready to give supplements the green light. One of the reasons is because heart disease risk doesn't just ride on your cholesterol and triglyceride numbers. "Lipids are still an important factor in coronary artery disease, but there are other nutritional factors that can influence and help prevent disease as well," says Robert M. Russell, M.D., associate director of the Jean Mayer U.S. Department of Agriculture Human Nutrition Research Center on Aging at Tufts University in Boston.

The Homocysteine Chapel

The most exciting noncholesterol research relating to heart disease centers around one little amino acid in the blood called homocysteine. What makes amino acids important is that they are the building blocks of protein. But in the case of homocysteine, too much can mean trouble. It can be toxic to the blood vessel wall, allowing plaque to form, Dr. Russell says. In several studies, high blood homocysteine levels were strongly associated with higher risks for coronary artery disease.

Although researchers don't know exactly what causes elevated levels of homocysteine in the blood, they have made some interesting findings. Studies have drawn a connection between high homocysteine in the blood and inadequate levels of several B-complex vitamins. An examination of 1,401 men and women from the Framingham Heart Study found that when blood concentrations of folic acid, vitamin B_6, and vitamin B_{12} were low, homocysteine levels were higher. And moderate to high concentrations of the vitamins corresponded to lower homocysteine levels. Further, inadequate blood levels of one or more of these B vitamins appeared to contribute to 67 percent of the cases of high homocysteine.

While some people may be genetically susceptible to high homocysteine, many may simply have their diets to blame. "Research has shown us that if any or all of these vitamins are low in the body, then homocysteine will build up. And when you give these vitamins back to people with high levels, their homocysteine levels drop," Dr. Russell says. "A few years ago, no one would have ever suspected that water-soluble vitamins, such as folic acid, vitamin B_6, and vitamin B_{12} would play a role in the prevention of heart disease. But now we have evidence that they play a role through the homocysteine mechanism."

The Beatles may have been the Fab Four, but to

protect your heart, you should remember the "FABB" Three: Folic Acid, B_6, and B_{12}.

"Folic acid seems the most likely candidate for lowering homocysteine, but since some people are responsive to vitamin B_6 and some to vitamin B_{12}, it's difficult to determine which B vitamin is at the root of the problem. I, as a general measure, recommend taking all three," says James Anderson, M.D., professor of medicine and clinical nutrition at the University of Kentucky in Lexington.

The Framingham Heart Study suggests that when folic acid levels drop below the Daily Value of 400 micrograms a day, homocysteine levels rise.

"If you are eating a healthy diet that includes at least five servings of fruits and vegetables a day, you should be able to reach homocysteine-lowering levels of the nutrient. If not, you should consider taking a multivitamin containing 100 percent of the Daily Value for folic acid," Dr. Russell says. Multivitamins also will give you levels of vitamins B_6 and B_{12} that are slightly higher than the Daily Value (2 milligrams and 6 micrograms, respectively), which seems to be all you need to have an effect on homocysteine.

Dr. Anderson suggests that if heart disease runs in your family, or if you have already been diagnosed with hardening of the arteries, your daily intake should be more. These individuals, he advises, should take 1 milligram (1,000 micrograms) of folic acid, 25 milligrams of vitamin B_6, and 10 milligrams of vitamin B_{12} daily. One caution: Check with your doctor before supplementing folic acid above 400 micrograms because it can mask signs of a vitamin B_{12} deficiency.

The B-complex vitamins aren't the only players in the heart protection game. Research shows that vitamins E and C as well as beta-carotene may help keep your ticker ticking longer. Here's what you should know.

Vitamin E: Neutralizing Cholesterol

Vitamin E helps keep your heart healthy in two ways: Its antioxidant powers help prevent low-density lipoprotein (LDL, or "bad") cholesterol from oxidizing into plaque-forming substance on your artery walls, and the nutrient also serves as an anticoagulant. "It may work by having some interaction with the platelets in the blood, which are the cells that cause blood clotting. Vitamin E also works with vitamin K, which is necessary for the synthesis of various clotting factors," Dr. Russell says.

Regardless of which way vitamin E is working to lower heart disease risks, research from all over the world shows that it does the job effectively. Even in a study of more than 11,000 older people, ages 67 to 105, conducted by researchers at the National Institute on Aging, use of vitamin E was associated with roughly a 40 percent reduction in coronary disease deaths, compared with nonuse of the supplement. That's after variables such as smoking history and use of alcohol were factored into the picture.

"Almost all the research that has been done on vitamin E points to much higher dosages than are possible with just a healthy diet," Dr. Russell says. Since a beneficial effect has been shown only with much higher amounts than the Daily Value of vitamin E—30 international units (IU)—supplementation is necessary, he says. That means that doctors and patients have to treat vitamin E like an over-the-counter medication, not a nutrient, says Dr. Russell.

Supplementation of 100 to 400 IU a day is considered effective and safe, Dr. Russell says. "If you are on another anticoagulant medication, like warfarin sodium (Coumadin) or aspirin, and plan to take more than 400 IU daily, you need to make your physician aware of it," he says. In very high doses (more than 800 IU), Dr. Russell warns that vitamin E appears to interfere with the body's metabolism of vitamin K—a nutrient necessary for the synthesis of blood-clotting materials.

Dr. Anderson recommends 800 IU of vitamin E to people who are at high risk for or who have evidence of heart disease. Check with your doctor before supplementing vitamin E above 600 IU daily. But don't think that popping vitamin E supplements is enough, he warns. It's effective only as part of a total lifestyle program that includes, among other things, healthy eating habits and regular exercise.

"I think that vitamin E is becoming a much more common physician recommendation and someday might be just as common as exercise. I tell my patients about it so that they can make up their own minds. I also have recommended in several cases to take supplements of vitamin E," Dr. Russell says.

Beta-Carotene: Preventing Heart Attacks

The antioxidant beta-carotene, a precursor to vitamin A, was hailed as a very promising nutrient in research circles after several studies found that it was linked to reduced risk of heart disease. But it was dropped like a hot potato after several studies on humans using extremely high doses revealed either no effect on coronary artery disease or, as in the case of one Finnish study, even increased risk for heart disease and cancer. While some experts have backed off recommending supplements of any kind since, others are calling these studies a minor setback in the search for beta-carotene's potential.

"I think that some of the problems that those studies found with beta-carotene stem from the kinds of dosages the subjects were given," Dr. Anderson says, adding that the extremely high supplemental doses used in those trials, nearly 17 times the Daily Value given every other day, resulted in far higher blood levels of beta-carotene than his recommendations do.

Dr. Anderson generally suggests that people get 10,000 IU of beta-carotene daily, the same amount he takes himself. By consuming five or more servings of fruits and vegetables a day, you should be able to meet that easily—one raw carrot alone puts you over the mark.

If you don't eat nutritiously, consider taking a multivitamin or beta-carotene supplement that meets these requirements.

Additional data indicate that beta-carotene and other carotenoids may prevent second heart attacks in people who have already survived one, Dr. Russell says.

Vitamin C: The Antioxidant Attack Ship

Although the research is less persuasive, vitamin C may be beneficial in the fight against heart disease, says Dr. Anderson. How it works is still unclear, but it seems that vitamin C might protect vitamin E from damage within the body.

"It appears that vitamin C can also raise high-density lipoprotein (HDL, or "good") cholesterol levels, but we don't know if it will lower the risk of coronary artery disease in and of itself," Dr. Russell says.

"I think that vitamin C is where we will see the next major breakthrough in terms of increased Recommended Dietary Allowances," Dr. Anderson says. He advises that every adult get 250 milligrams of vitamin C twice daily, 500 milligrams twice daily if you have or are at high risk for coronary artery disease.

Medical Alert

If you have heart disease, you should discuss vitamin and mineral supplementation with your doctor.

If you are taking anticoagulant drugs, you should not take vitamin E supplements.

High Blood Pressure

Get Down with Minerals

For decades, sodium and high blood pressure have gone together like salt and pepper. If you had high blood pressure, the doctor would tell you to go easy on the salt (also known as sodium chloride). Like most things in life these days, though, it's not that simple anymore.

Sure, sodium may still be a factor for some people with high blood pressure. But the latest research shows that other minerals play key roles in the equation that equals 120/80 and below (healthy blood pressure readings) or 140/90 and above (potentially dangerous levels).

Just a quick refresher if you haven't had your blood pressure checked lately: The first number, the systolic blood pressure, is a reading that measures the maximum force going away from the heart. The second number, the diastolic pressure, measures the minimum force of blood at the end of the heartbeat. These figures are important tools in determining your risk for stroke, heart attack, and kidney disease, so you should have your physician check your blood pressure at least once a year, says Edward Saltzman, M.D., medical director of the Obesity Center at the New England Medical Center and scientist at the Jean Mayer U.S. Department of Agriculture Human Nutrition Research Center at Tufts University School of Medicine in Boston. If your numbers are on the high side—formally known as hypertension—minerals may help you control them. Here's what you need to know.

Sodium: The Misunderstood Mineral?

Because of how your body handles it, if you take in too much sodium, your body will hold on to more liquid to give the sodium something to swim in. This excess liquid makes the blood swell to a greater volume, and that causes your heart to work overtime, trying to pump all the blood through your system.

Even though some research has questioned

whether salt is really to blame for hypertension in our diets, most experts agree that too much of it is bad news for sodium-sensitive individuals. "Sodium is one mineral that has shown a definite connection to hypertension in that too much can raise blood pressure," says Ronald Krauss, M.D., head of the molecular medicine department, Lawrence Berkeley National Laboratory at the University of California, Berkeley, and chairman of the American Heart Association's Nutrition Committee.

But there are generally two schools of thought when it comes to who needs to watch their sodium, says Dr. Saltzman. One school believes that everyone should have a low-sodium diet. That's because, regardless of whether a person actually develops high blood pressure with sodium, the mineral tends to elevate levels. Dr. Saltzman says that physicians in this corner of the debate feel that the lower your blood pressure, the less likely you are to have a stroke or a heart attack. So everyone should limit sodium intake to 2,400 milligrams or less per day—period.

The other school of thought believes that only those people whose intakes of sodium seem to signal elevated blood pressure should care about how much sodium they eat or drink. The rest of the population doesn't need to be so careful. There's just one catch: The only practical way to identify a sodium-sensitive person is to limit his sodium consumption and see if his blood pressure comes down. "Often, when a person comes in and is newly diagnosed as hypertensive, the first thing he is told to do is lose any excess weight and decrease his dietary salt," Dr. Saltzman says. If the patient follows those instructions, it may not be clear if the shed pounds or the reduced salt did the trick, at least in the beginning.

Magnesium's Magic

Magnesium has shown moderate benefits in lowering high blood pressure in some studies, says Dr. Saltzman. One such study was conducted in Sweden on 71 people with mildly elevated blood pressures who were not taking any hypertension medications. Researchers found that giving magnesium supplements to folks who had low levels of the mineral appeared to reduce their blood pressure readings by several points.

A few points are enough to make a difference to a borderline hypertensive person, but they are not a big deal to someone with a bigger blood pressure problem, Dr. Saltzman says. "While some trials have shown benefits from taking magnesium supplements, it's just too early to know if there is any consistency to these findings," he says.

The American Heart Association is not ready to advocate magnesium, or any other mineral, as a significant factor in lowering blood pressure, Dr. Krauss says.

Dr. Saltzman suggests that getting your Daily Value's worth (400 milligrams) is a good idea, however. Dark green leafy vegetables, whole grains, fish, legumes, and nuts are good sources of magnesium. Adults seem to be able to get enough of this mineral from their diets, so supplements aren't necessary.

The Power of Potassium

To keep sodium levels from getting too high, the body also needs other minerals. One such nutrient is potassium, which helps clear your bloodstream of excess sodium. To make matters worse, a shortage of potassium can cause your body to hold on to more sodium. "In studies where diets of people who have lower blood pressures are assessed, they tend to be higher in potassium as well as magnesium and calcium," says Dr. Saltzman. While some believe that potassium supplements may lower blood pressure, results of intervention trials have shown only moderate and inconsistent effects, he says.

"If you have a low dietary intake, or a deficiency, you are more likely to reap the benefit from increasing your potassium supplies than someone who gets enough of the mineral already," Dr. Saltzman says. The Daily Value for potassium, 3,500 milligrams, is all you need to keep you out of the deficiency doghouse. All the epidemiological studies supporting potassium as a blood pressure reducer have examined food intake, not supplements, says Dr. Saltzman. So sticking with food is your best bet. These foods include bananas, potatoes, yams, raisins, and a host of other fruits and vegetables and dairy products.

Apart from people on medications that lower potassium, supplements have not proved to be worth investing in, says Dr. Saltzman. Megadosing on potassium supplements is definitely out of the question. "If you exceed your body's ability to excrete potassium, it can cause fatal heart arrythmias," he cautions. People who have diabetes or kidney problems, or who are taking anti-inflammatory drugs, potassium-sparing diuretics (water pills), ACE (angiotensin converting enzyme) inhibitors, or heart medications should not supplement potassium without medical supervision.

The Role of Calcium?

Very preliminary research has indicated that calcium may have a role in keeping blood pressure in check. "It may work with potassium somehow, or there may even be an independent effect of calcium. These ideas are very sketchy, at best, at this point," says Dr. Saltzman. Even if the research isn't very strong, he notes, this just shows another good reason to get your bone-protecting 1,000 milligrams of calcium each day.

Medical Alert

If you have been diagnosed with high blood pressure, you should be under a doctor's care.

If you have heart or kidney problems, you should check with your doctor before taking supplemental magnesium.

People who have diabetes or kidney problems or who are taking anti-inflammatory drugs, potassium-sparing diuretics, ACE inhibitors, or heart medicines such as heparin should not supplement potassium without medical supervision.

High Cholesterol

High Noon in the Heartland

Today's topic: Is low-density lipoprotein, which goes by LDL for short, born to be bad? Or is it just the company it keeps?

It's the old question of nurture versus nature, applied to cholesterol. For years, LDL cholesterol has been the artery-clogging villain in the gunfight for your heart. Its brother, high-density lipoprotein, or HDL, has played the sheriff who keeps your arteries safe by running LDL cholesterol out of town. It turns out that it's not quite that black and white.

Both forms of cholesterol are soft, fatlike substances transported in the blood. In order to float through your bloodstream, cholesterol needs a coating of protein. This coating is called lipoprotein. LDL cholesterol only turns mean when it becomes oxidized in the blood. That process sets loose destructive molecules called free radicals, which damage the blood vessel and artery walls, making it easier for plaque to form on them. That's what clogs your arteries.

If you can prevent LDL cholesterol from oxidizing, you can prevent—and even reverse—hardening of the arteries, which, in turn, can lead to heart attacks and strokes, says James Anderson, M.D., professor of medicine and clinical nutrition at the University of Kentucky in Lexington. That's where antioxidants come in. And vitamins E and C are just what the doctor ordered, he says.

Vitamin E: Radical Action Hero

So what would LDL cholesterol be like if it didn't hang out with those rampaging free radicals? "If you can prevent the LDL cholesterol from being oxidized, it doesn't have as damaging a property," says Robert M. Russell, M.D., associate director of the Jean Mayer U.S. Department of Agriculture Human Nutrition Research Center on Aging at Tufts University in Boston. In effect, LDL might be a nicer cholesterol if it could be sheltered from oxidation. That's what vitamin E tries to do.

Studies on both animals and humans have shown that high levels of vitamin E in the blood have been strongly associated with reduced coronary artery diseases and deaths, Dr. Anderson says.

Vitamin E attacks the free radicals, destroys them, then lets the leftover particles wash away in the bloodstream, he says. This prevents a whole series of events that can lead to heart attacks and strokes.

"Alpha-tocopherol, a compound in vitamin E, is responsible for about 90 percent of the antioxidant factor that goes to work on LDL cholesterol in the blood," Dr. Anderson says. Other vitamin E compounds, such as gamma-tocopherol, are being investigated, but Dr. Anderson says that it's too early to know how effective they might be in the fight against heart disease.

It's next to impossible to get all the vitamin E you need from food. That's where supplements come into play. According to both Dr. Russell and Dr. Anderson, 400 international units (IU) of vitamin E—which is more than 13 times the Daily Value of 30 IU—is a safe and effective dose. If you already have heart disease, or are at very high risk for it, Dr. Anderson suggests taking 800 IU of vitamin E daily.

If you plan to take levels higher than 600 IU, discuss it with your doctor first. Doses above that mark can interfere with anticoagulating medications, and doses higher than about 800 IU can disturb your body's vitamin K metabolism.

Note: Supplementing with vitamin E isn't a cure-all. For total heart health, the American Heart Association recommends a lifestyle program that includes losing excess weight, quitting smoking, cutting down the fat (especially saturated fat) and cholesterol in your diet, increasing your dietary fiber intake, eating five to nine servings of fruits and vegetables a day, and exercising at least 30 minutes three times a week.

Vitamin C: Best Supporting Actor

If vitamin E gets an Oscar for its performance as a free-radical basher, the Academy Award for best supporting actor would have to go to vitamin C. Vitamin E is constantly being repaired by vitamin C in the blood. Because of this, vitamin E can work effectively at controlling LDL cholesterol oxidation, Dr. Anderson says.

Vitamin C might have cholesterol-tapping functions of its own, too. Researchers measured levels of vitamin C in the blood (from either foods or supplements) in 827 men and women participating in the Baltimore Longitudinal Study on Aging. The study was conducted by the National Institute on Aging in Bethesda, Maryland, to find out how vitamin C affects HDL cholesterol levels. The study found that, up to a certain dietary level, the more vitamin C people got, the higher their HDL levels were. In women, 215 milligrams a day seemed to be the optimum amount. In men, 346 milligrams appeared to be the maximum.

"It appears that vitamin C can raise HDL cholesterol levels, but we don't know if it will lower the risk of coronary artery disease in and of itself," Dr. Russell says. Until further evidence regarding this nutrient is found, exercise remains the best proven way to raise your HDL levels. The Daily Value for vitamin C is 60 milligrams. That's enough to prevent the deficiency disease scurvy, says Dr. Anderson; but it does nothing to provide cholesterol benefits. He recommends that people consume a healthy diet with lots of vitamin C–rich fruits and vegetables and that they take a 250-milligram supplement twice daily. If you have high cholesterol or heart disease already, Dr. Anderson recommends that you take 500 milligrams of vitamin C twice daily. At these levels, the water-soluble vitamin is considered quite safe.

Medical Alert

If you have been diagnosed with high cholesterol, you should be under a doctor's care.

If you are taking anticoagulant drugs, you should not take vitamin E supplements.

Immunity

Fortifying the Troops

If you wanted to learn how to wage war, you could examine the battlefield strategies of history's great generals.

Or you could study your immune system, a mind-boggling array of internal defenses designed to protect your body from the assault of disease-causing trouble-makers.

Your immune system carries on a never-ending battle against a relentless horde: airborne microscopic spike-covered cold and flu viruses trying to attach themselves to your nose and throat. Cancer-causing particles sucked into your lungs. Fungus clinging to your feet after a shower at the gym. Even bacteria breeding on your unrefrigerated roast beef sandwich.

Your own standing army of immune system defenders fights a continuing battle. Is there anything you can do to help the troops fight the good fight? Yes, a great deal!

Soldiers Need Their Rations

Medical researchers have long recognized the connection between good nutrition and the strength of your immune system. They know, for example, that in impoverished countries, millions of children die each year from measles, pneumonia, and diarrhea because they don't get enough vitamin A to keep their immune systems up to par.

While they're usually less extreme, nutritional deficiencies present an immune system problem in America as well. Some experts believe that subtle vitamin and mineral deficiencies as well as enhanced nutrient requirements at different stages of life can cause your immune system to falter in its important work.

"We know that in many older folks, for example, immune response is compromised," says Adria Sherman, Ph.D., professor and chair of the department of nutritional sciences at Rutgers University in New Brunswick, New Jersey. "It's not clear whether this is an inevitable characteristic of aging, a physiological process, years of nutritional depletion, poor eating habits, or increased needs. But in my opinion, it's probably some combination of all of these." Dr. Sherman is certainly not alone in this opinion.

"Several surveys show that almost one-third of apparently healthy elderly people have reductions in the intake of several nutrients," according to Ranjit Kumar

Chandra, M.D., research professor at Memorial University of Newfoundland and director of the World Health Organization's Center for Nutritional Immunology, also in Newfoundland. "The most common deficiencies are those of iron, zinc, and vitamin C. Correction of these deficiencies by following nutritional advice or by taking dietary or medicinal supplements results in a significant improvement in immunity."

While the whole story isn't yet in, researchers are slowly identifying the roles that specific nutrients play in helping your immune system keep you free of disease and infection.

Vitamin A: Immunity Enhancer

Vitamin A seems to top the A-list of nutrients that are vital for a strong immune system.

While studying the effects of vitamin A in children, Dr. Chandra observed that even a moderate deficiency can weaken the immune defenses of a child's respiratory tract. Vitamin A deficiency causes damage to the naturally protective mucous membrane barrier of the respiratory tract, and it's thought that bacteria and viruses take advantage of that damage.

How might that affect a child's health? After a flu virus attacks, for example, the lining of a normal throat will repair itself. Not so in those who are vitamin A–deficient. "Instead, you might get that once-healthy cell replaced by an abnormal cell," says Charles B. Stephensen, Ph.D., associate professor in the department of international health at the University of Alabama in Birmingham. "That may predispose you to having a more severe episode of an infection or having another infection on top of a viral infection."

"The link between vitamin A deficiency and the

severity of respiratory disease is very well established,"
agrees Susan Cunningham-Rundles, Ph.D., associate professor of immunology at Cornell University Medical
Center in New York City and editor of *Nutrient Modu-
lation of the Immune Response*.

Such deficiencies are common in poorer countries, where foods high in vitamin A, such as green leafy
vegetables and fortified milk, are not readily available or
are not utilized. And as a result, health officials in those
countries routinely prescribe vitamin A supplements to
prevent measles and other infections, particularly diarrhea, from becoming life-threatening. This strategy has
cut deficiency-related deaths by 30 percent in some
countries.

Many experts believe that immune-compromising
vitamin A deficiencies are also widespread among children in the United States. Some 28 percent of children
in the United States may be vitamin A–deficient, according to Martha Rumore, Pharm.D., associate professor at the Arnold and Marie Schwartz College of Pharmacy and Health Sciences in Brooklyn. In a published
review of vitamin A research, Dr. Rumore found that vitamin A deficiency has been correlated with decreased
resistance to pneumonia, tuberculosis, whooping
cough, and infectious diarrhea.

Another study, this one of 20 U.S. children with
measles, showed that half were vitamin A–deficient.

How could children in a land so well-supplied with
milkshakes and salad bars be vitamin A–deficient? For
one thing, measles actually depletes vitamin A. And for
another, many people, especially kids, just don't eat
foods that contain vitamin A.

"There's no doubt about it. All of the continuing
food consumption survey studies have shown that vi-

tamin A intakes are low among children, especially in poverty areas," says Adrianne Bendich, Ph.D., a clinical research scientist in the human nutrition research department at Hoffmann–La Roche in Nutley, New Jersey.

How much vitamin A is enough? The Daily Value for vitamin A is 5,000 international units (IU).

Beta-Carotene: Immunity Booster

Beta-carotene is the pigment that helps turn carrots, cantaloupe, and other fruits and vegetables orange or yellow. But researchers are discovering that this nutrient does a lot more than add color to your favorite produce.

In fact, studies have shown that beta-carotene does quite a bit of immune-boosting work of its own.

Researchers in one study found that the number of T-helper cells in male volunteers jumped 30 percent after the men took 180 milligrams—almost 299,000 IU—of beta-carotene a day for two weeks. (T-helper cells are important components of the immune system.)

In another study, this time at the University of Arizona in Tucson, groups of men and women were given daily doses of 15 milligrams (about 25,000 IU), 30 milligrams (about 50,000 IU), 45 milligrams (about 75,000 IU), or 60 milligrams (almost 100,000 IU) of beta-carotene for two months, according to Ronald R. Watson, Ph.D., research professor at the University of Arizona College of Medicine. An enhanced immune response was noticeable at 30 milligrams and above, with increased numbers of both natural killer cells and activated lymphocytes, which are also important immune system components.

In studies of AIDS patients and in studies of older patients with precancerous oral lesions, a similar immunological effect was seen with 30 milligrams of beta-carotene a day during a three-month period. The effect declined after the three months, however.

Levels being tested in clinical trials are between 50,000 and 100,000 IU a day. These dosages are considered safe as well as potentially effective in preventing both cancer and heart disease.

No toxic level of beta-carotene has been shown in research so far. A potential side effect is discoloration of the skin, which fades as the dosage is decreased.

Most research has found that smokers benefit the most from beta-carotene supplementation, as lung cancer usually shows the strongest association with low levels of beta-carotene. And lung cancer risk is reduced the most in smokers who consume high levels of beta-carotene–containing foods or supplements. Most doctors and researchers, however, still recommend eating more fruits and vegetables and eliminating smoking.

There is no Daily Value for beta-carotene, but nutrition experts generally recommend getting 8,300 to 10,000 IU a day. Most people get 1,600 to 3,300 IU a day from foods.

B$_6$: You May Need More

Researchers at Tufts University School of Nutrition in Medford, Massachusetts, discovered that when healthy elderly people had vitamin B$_6$ almost completely taken out of their diets, immune response went down. Even more telling: The amount of B$_6$ needed to restore strength to the immune system was higher than the Daily Value of 2 milligrams. When the study participants were provided with 50 milligrams of B$_6$ daily, immunity was boosted to a level that was even better than before the study began.

"These data tell us two things," says Dr. Bendich. "One is that the Daily Value of vitamin B_6 is not high enough for optimum function in the elderly. The other is that taking a B_6 supplement enhances immunity."

Several other studies, in fact, have shown that older folks in general don't seem to eat enough vitamin B_6. One study of older residents of New Mexico showed that they eat barely one-fourth of the B_6 that they need each day.

Whether you're young or old, you can boost your vitamin B_6 intake by eating chickpeas (garbanzos), prune juice, turkey, potatoes, and bananas. A banana provides 33 percent of your Daily Value of B_6, while an eight-ounce glass of prune juice provides 28 percent.

Vitamin C Gets Votes

There is general agreement in the medical community that vitamin C is vital to the production of white blood cells, the foot soldiers of your immune system.

"The best experimentation that I've seen suggests that vitamin C is in some way or another stimulating the white blood cells to function better," explains Elliot Dick, Ph.D., professor of preventive medicine and chief of the respiratory virus research laboratory at the University of Wisconsin–Madison and one of the country's leading cold researchers. "White blood cells attack the infected cell, gather around it, destroy it, and then clean up."

By the same token, at least one study has shown that levels of vitamin C don't have to be very low, even in otherwise healthy men between ages 25 and 43, to cause a decline in immune function. During a three-month study, researchers at the U.S. Department of Agriculture Western Human Nutrition Research Center in San Francisco found that getting 20 milligrams or less of vitamin C a day caused a delayed reaction to a skin test designed to provoke an immune response, such as swelling or a rash. What's more, "the researchers could not bring the levels of vitamin C back up to where they were before the deficient diet until the volunteers were given 250 milligrams of vitamin C a day for three weeks," says study investigator Robert A. Jacob, Ph.D., research chemist in micronutrients at the Western Human Nutrition Research Center.

While the Daily Value for vitamin C (60 milligrams) is lower than the amounts used in many of these studies, many people don't get even that much.

"You'll find a significant number of people who do not get even 75 percent of the Daily Value of vitamin C, a vitamin that is very abundant, to say the least," says Vishwa Singh, Ph.D., director of the human nutrition research department at Hoffmann–La Roche. No one should be deficient in vitamin C, he maintains, not when so many fruits and vegetables have such high amounts. An eight-ounce glass of orange juice has 200 percent of the Daily Value, for example. And a half-cup of chopped raw red bell peppers provides 158 percent.

But is the Daily Value enough to keep your immune system functioning in tip-top form? That's the question. And researchers simply don't know the answer yet. Many nutrition experts, however, recommend that you get at least 500 milligrams a day.

Delivering Potential Benefits with Vitamin D

Vitamin D is also developing a reputation as a key player in a healthy immune system. When researchers at the

University of Wisconsin–Madison tested vitamin D–deficient laboratory animals, they found that the thymus gland was not doing its job of generating a sufficient number of immune system cells. And it took eight weeks of a diet with normal vitamin D levels to restore proper immunity.

The Daily Value for vitamin D is 400 IU. The nutrient is found in eggs and fortified milk. You even create your own supply as a natural reaction when sunlight touches your skin.

So who wouldn't get enough? Experts say people who avoid milk to bypass stomach problems or who stay out of the sun for fear of getting wrinkles could be putting themselves at risk for a shortage. "It could be more of a problem in the elderly than in the young," says Dr. Bendich. "What we're finding is that elderly people aren't able to make vitamin D in their skin as well as younger people. They don't go out in the sun as much. They use more skin protectors—sunscreens that block the formation of vitamin D. And they don't drink a lot of milk." The elderly need to get their Daily Value of vitamin D from a multivitamin/mineral supplement, according to Dr. Bendich.

Vitamin D is in most multivitamin/mineral supplements as well as most calcium supplements and is safe at the levels in these supplements, according to Dr. Bendich.

Vitamin E: A Well-Known Aid

The story on vitamin E and immunity is long and positive. For years, researchers have been finding dramatic immune-enhancing effects using vitamin E supplements, including increased levels of interferon and interleukin. Both of these biochemicals are produced by the immune system to fight infection.

In one study, Tufts University researchers divided older volunteers into two groups: 18 who took daily 800-milligram vitamin E supplements and 14 who took placebos (inactive look-alike pills). At the end of 30 days, the researchers found that the vitamin E takers had a 69 percent increase in levels of interleukin-2 and a decrease in levels of a substance called prostaglandin, which can reduce the number of white blood cell soldiers patrolling your body.

"The work at Tufts has very clearly shown that giving the elderly doses of vitamin E can improve immune response," says Dr. Singh.

Vitamin E also helps prevent oxidative damage in the body. This is a kind of damage that has been linked to lowered immune response. It seems that when immune system killer cells such as macrophages do their jobs of attacking and absorbing viruses, bacteria, and other foreign invaders, dreaded free radicals are created as a by-product. Free radicals are unstable molecules that steal electrons from healthy molecules to balance themselves, weakening or damaging cells in the process. Vitamin E tames these free radicals by offering them its own electrons, helping to shield healthy cells from abuse.

How much vitamin E is enough to create this immune-boosting effect? Experts generally recommend getting 400 IU a day.

Iron: Tops for Immunity

Not only is iron an important mineral for healthy immune system functioning, but iron deficiency is fairly common, says Dr. Sherman. The deficiency can be caused by not eating enough iron-containing foods such as red meat and green leafy vegetables. Menstruating women often have low iron stores because of the monthly loss of iron-rich blood. Stomach problems such as ulcers also cause the loss of blood, as do parasitic infections and, of course, serious injuries, she says.

Stored in the liver, spleen, and bone marrow, iron is used first and foremost to produce hemoglobin in the blood. You're not considered iron-deficient until your blood hemoglobin level begins to fall, according to Dr. Sherman.

The Daily Value for iron is 18 milligrams, which is considered enough to keep the immune system up to par. Many researchers urge caution in taking more. Getting too much can cause abdominal pain, diarrhea, and constipation.

Think Zinc

Like iron, zinc is crucial for making sure that the first wave of immune fighters, lymphocytes, has enough troops.

"When the body is exposed to a pathogen, one of the things that happens is that immune cells begin to proliferate. That is the beginning of all of the steps in killing the offender," says Dr. Sherman. "And both zinc and iron are involved in that process." Less zinc means that lymphocytes will respond more slowly to the foreign invader and that fewer will even make it to the battlefield.

Fortunately, serious zinc deficiencies are rare. Far more common, however, are moderate zinc deficiencies. Strict vegetarians are often at the greatest risk for zinc deficiency because they shun meats and seafood, the best sources of zinc.

Getting the Daily Value of zinc (15 milligrams) should be enough to keep the immune system functioning properly. And getting that amount shouldn't be a problem. Just three ounces of any lean red meat delivers about 32 percent of that amount, while six steamed oysters provide five times the amount of zinc that you need.

Taking Some Multivitamin Insurance

There's also a good deal of research that supports the idea of taking a multivitamin/mineral supplement every day. In a yearlong study of 100 elderly Canadians, for example, Dr. Chandra gave half of the group daily multivitamin/mineral supplements with extra vitamin E and beta-carotene. The other half simply received placebos each day. At the end of the study, Dr. Chandra found that the group taking supplements had half as many colds, flus, and other infection-related illnesses as the group taking placebos. And when they did get sick, those taking supplements recovered in half the time, on average.

Since then, another multivitamin/mineral study has produced similar results. Researchers used skin tests to measure immune responses to proteins from bacteria and fungi that cause tuberculosis, diphtheria, tetanus, and other ailments. After one year, the supplement takers in the study had significantly more virile immune systems than did the people who took placebos for the same amount of time, according to research leader John Bogden, Ph.D., professor in the Department of Preventive Medicine and Community Health at the University of Medicine and Dentistry of New Jersey/New Jersey Medical School in Newark.

Why would a simple multivitamin/mineral tablet make such a difference in the performance of your immune system? Dr. Bogden thinks he has the answer, at least for the elderly. "We think it may be either that older people have increased requirements or that the Recommended Dietary Allowances, or levels near the Recommended Dietary Allowances, are not adequate to support optimum immunity," he says.

Medical Alert

If you are taking anticoagulant drugs, you should not take vitamin E supplements.

Insomnia

Resetting the Sleep Clock

The late-night talk show hosts look more familiar than most of your relatives. You and the night cashier at the 7-Eleven are on a first-name basis. You can't remember the last time you paid full price for a long-distance call; in fact, you could use more friends in faraway time zones who would still be up when you are.

If you sometimes have trouble sleeping, you're far from alone. About 30 percent of adults have an occasional bad night that keeps them from functioning at their best the following day. That, by the way, is how the experts decide whether your insomnia is a problem.

"It is not how many hours you sleep but how you feel during the next day that's important," says Peter

Hauri, Ph.D., director of the insomnia program at the Mayo Clinic Sleep Disorders Center in Rochester, Minnesota. "Some people routinely sleep only four hours a night but feel fine during the day. They don't have insomnia."

But while an occasional bad night won't ruin your life, a whole string of them can pose some serious problems. Some of the worst industrial accidents of the century have been linked to errors made by sleep-deprived workers, according to Dr. Hauri. If you're among the 9 percent of Americans who have chronic insomnia, you know that sleepless nights make a big difference in the way you feel, the way you work, and the way you relate to other people.

Sleuthing beneath the Surface

"Insomnia is not a disease. It's just an indicator that something is wrong," says Dr. Hauri. In about half of all cases, the underlying problem is psychological. Depression, job stress, and marital problems can all lead to insomnia.

Sometimes the cause is physical, such as an allergy or chronic pain, says Dr. Hauri. If that's the case, finding an effective treatment for those symptoms should end insomnia as well.

Sleepless nights can also be caused by environmental factors (noise), bad sleep habits (sleeping late on weekends), and circadian rhythm problems (feeling sleepy at the wrong times).

Finally, a growing body of research shows that sleep can be affected, positively or negatively, by what you put in your mouth. "There are so many other factors—illness, stress, depression, lifestyle—that are likely to have much stronger effects on your sleep than nutrition would," says James G. Penland, Ph.D., head researcher with the U.S. Department of Agriculture (USDA) Grand Forks Human Nutrition Research Center in North Dakota. "But once those factors have been ruled out, our research suggests that getting more or less of certain nutrients can improve the quality of sleep."

Copper Gets a Medal

A study by the USDA found that low intake of copper was associated with poor sleep quality in premenopausal women. Women on a low-copper diet of less than 1 milligram daily took longer to fall asleep and felt less rested in the morning than women who consumed the same diet but also got a 2-milligram copper supplement daily, says Dr. Penland, who directed the study.

The Daily Value for copper is 2 milligrams—a tiny amount, but more than the average American is getting. Most of us get about 1 milligram of copper a day. That is not enough of a deficiency to cause obvious symptoms, but it may be enough to affect the way we sleep. The best food sources of copper are lobster and cooked oysters. Seeds, nuts, mushrooms, and dried beans also contain copper, but you'd have to eat several servings a day to meet the Daily Value, says Dr. Penland.

Iron Makes a Difference

Another mineral that seems to have an effect on sleep quality is iron. One study by the U.S. Department of Agriculture found that women who got only one-third of the Recommended Dietary Allowance for iron experienced more awakenings during the night and poorer sleep quality than those who got the full Recommended

Dietary Allowance. And while both low-iron and low-copper diets cause total sleep time to increase, that's not necessarily a good thing, says Dr. Penland. "When people are sick, they sleep more," he says. "Greater total sleep time often indicates that the body is trying to cope with some kind of challenge, which may be the case if you're not consuming enough copper or iron."

If you suspect that low copper or iron intake is affecting your sleep, a multivitamin/mineral supplement is a safe, easy way to correct the problem, says Dr. Penland. Just be sure that the supplement contains 2 milligrams of copper and the Recommended Dietary Allowance of iron, which is 15 milligrams for menstruating women and 10 milligrams for men and nonmenstruating women.

Aluminum Can Foil Sleep

Another mineral that seems to have an effect on sleep quality is aluminum. Dr. Penland and his colleagues compared the sleep quality of women who consumed over 1,000 milligrams of aluminum a day with the sleep quality of women who consumed only 300 milligrams of aluminum a day. The women who consumed more aluminum reported poorer sleep quality.

We all absorb small amounts of aluminum from air and water as well as from aluminum cooking utensils and some antiperspirants, but it probably isn't enough to cause a problem, says Dr. Penland. But if you regularly take an antacid, especially a liquid, you should be aware that many brands contain as much as 200 to 250 milligrams of aluminum per teaspoon. If you take an antacid and find yourself waking up during the night, try giving it up for a few weeks to see if your sleep improves, suggests Dr. Penland. You can also try switching to tablets, which are usually aluminum-free. Check the active ingredients on the label to be sure.

Keep an Eye on Magnesium

Some research suggests that a low magnesium level can also lead to shallower sleep and more nighttime awakenings. "Low magnesium status means that your magnesium intake is very low on a daily basis, probably less than 200 milligrams a day," says Dr. Penland. "It isn't uncommon, especially among people with reduced caloric intakes, such as the elderly and people on weight-loss diets."

Even if your magnesium intake is normal, certain medications can keep your body from absorbing the mineral efficiently. The most common are probably diuretics (water pills) prescribed for high blood pressure. If you're taking them, your doctor should keep an eye on your magnesium level. Just make sure your physician knows about any medications that you're taking, especially if you're being treated by more than one doctor.

The Daily Value for magnesium is 400 milligrams. If you opt for a supplement, this amount should be enough to prevent sleep problems, says Dr. Penland. If you have heart or kidney problems, be sure to consult your doctor before taking magnesium supplements.

Medical Alert

People with heart or kidney problems should consult their doctors before taking magnesium supplements.

Intermittent Claudication

Improving Circulation

The fight to save H. Stanley Andrews's left leg from intermittent claudication may not sound like a major medical battle—until you learn what happened to his right leg. Seeing little alternative, doctors removed it.

Andrews's wife, Gertrude, knew that there had to be a better way to fight the circulatory disease caused by impeded blood flow in the legs. Suffering from heart problems herself, she explored ways to keep both herself and her husband healthy and away from the surgeon's knife.

Today, pounds lighter and free of pain, these Valrico, Florida, residents practice a wellness strategy that includes low-fat eating and vitamins. And there's no doubt in their minds, or in the mind of their new doctor, Donald J. Carrow, M.D., a physician in private practice in Tampa, Florida, with a particular interest in nutritional therapy, that supplements of vitamin E and fish oil have helped both of them turn the corner on the road to better health.

"His leg was going cold," Gertrude Andrews says. "He doesn't have pain, but he did. At 82, he's out raking the yard right now."

Clogging Up the Works

It's rare that intermittent claudication costs someone his leg. More commonly, the condition creates mild to severe pain during exertion.

The same things that contribute to heart disease, such as smoking and too much dietary fat, also contribute to intermittent claudication. Fatty deposits build up along artery walls, impeding circulation and reducing the amount of blood reaching the legs.

If you have this condition, at first you might find that you are able to walk long distances and suffer only minor pain. But eventually, as blood flow continues to slow, even a short walk can cause difficulty. Skin becomes weak and susceptible to wounds from lack of proper amounts of blood, oxygen, and nutrients. Pain can develop in the hips, thighs, calves, and feet. People with advanced cases can develop sores on their toes and heels.

Vitamin E Helps Open Arteries

To help get the blood flowing again, more doctors are turning to a vitamin that first showed promise decades ago and that has captured the attention of modern researchers as well: vitamin E.

The rage for helping to prevent and treat heart disease, vitamin E also has quite a history of use for intermittent claudication. Back in 1958, Canadian researchers divided 40 men with intermittent claudication into two groups: one that received 954 international units (IU) of vitamin E a day and one that received placebos (blank pills). The study lasted 40 weeks.

Although only 17 men from each group completed

the study, 13 of the vitamin E takers were able to walk farther without experiencing pain than the placebo takers. The researchers who conducted the study noted one finding that they considered important: "We also found that there is a considerable delay before any response can be noted, and we conclude that therapy should be continued for at least three months before being abandoned."

A long-term study in Sweden, published in 1974, gave the Canadian theory a boost. For two to five years, the Swedish researchers tracked 47 men with intermittent claudication. Half of the group took 300 IU of vitamin E a day; the other half took drugs designed to increase blood flow to their legs.

After 4 to 6 months, 54 percent of the vitamin E takers were able to walk nearly a mile without stopping, while just 23 percent of those who took drugs were able to cover the same distance without stopping. Arterial blood flow also improved in the vitamin E group 12 to 18 months into the study, and by 20 to 25 months, they had a 34 percent increase in the amount of blood flowing through their legs.

Laboratory study seems to confirm the claims of those who advocate vitamin E for intermittent claudication, says Mohsen Meydani, Ph.D., associate professor of nutrition at the Jean Mayer USDA Human Nutrition Research Center on Aging at Tufts University in Boston. Researchers at Tufts have found that when the linings of arteries are bathed in vitamin E, plaque-forming cells are less likely to stick to them than to arteries without the vitamin E treatment, he says. "It's just my clinical observation, mind you, but it makes sense that vitamin E would be useful," says Dr. Meydani.

There are at least two more reasons that vitamin E seems to help improve intermittent claudication, experts say. Even though reduced blood flow prevents adequate oxygen from getting to muscles in the legs, vitamin E helps the muscles use what little oxygen they get more efficiently. It also helps muscles get by on less oxygen.

More important, vitamin E seems to reduce the ability of blood cells to stick together and form clots. Actually, it's a good thing that blood can form clots. "If I cut my finger and hold it in front of me, blood will stop pumping out of it before I die from loss of blood," says Dr. Carrow. "It's an inherent, built-in safety mechanism."

This same safety mechanism causes problems, however, after fatty deposits called plaque have built up along the walls of your leg's arteries. Sensing injury at the scene of the plaque, blood cells pile on like cars at a traffic accident, clotting and further decreasing the flow of blood.

By making your blood cells less sticky, vitamin E helps prevent any further decrease in blood flow and might even reverse some of the damage, says Dr. Carrow. "Most people with intermittent claudication learn that they can walk to the point of discomfort and then walk through it," he explains. "Now this is not true in the later stages, but when you use vitamin E and fish oil, it is almost always true."

Dr. Carrow generally advises taking between 1,600 and 4,000 IU of vitamin E a day, in three divided doses throughout the day, for a limited period of time.

Vitamin E is also recommended by Paul J. Dunn, M.D., a physician in private practice in Oak Park, Illinois, as part of a multifaceted treatment program for intermittent claudication. His prescription: about 400 IU of vitamin E daily for each 40 pounds of body weight.

For both doctors, a recommendation for vitamin E supplementation comes only after a diagnosis based on the results of a comprehensive medical history, thorough examination, and testing. "Based on all of that information, I design an integrated, multifaceted treatment program that includes lifestyle changes, diet, exercise, and supplements. If you come in with pain in the calves when you walk three blocks, I wouldn't just say, 'Here is some vitamin E,'" says Dr. Dunn. "Vitamin E is a helpful adjunct to treatment, but it's not the sole treatment."

Medical Alert

If you have intermittent claudication, you should be under a doctor's care.

It's best to check with your doctor before taking vitamin E in doses that exceed 600 international units daily. If you are taking anticoagulant drugs, you should not take vitamin E supplements.

Kidney Stones

Dissolving a Painful Problem

Take a look at a kidney stone under a microscope and you'll understand why the pain of passing a stone is unforgettable. Most stones are spiked with razor-sharp crystals. No wonder those who have gone through the experience say that the agony is equivalent to a knife in the back.

Kidney stones develop when urine concentrations of minerals and other dissolved substances get so high that the minerals can no longer remain dissolved. Stones can also form if the pH (acid-alkaline balance) of urine is too high or too low. In all cases, the minerals form insoluble crystals and precipitate, or drop out, of the urine, exactly the same way too much sugar drops to the bottom of a glass of iced tea. The crystals collect in the kidney ducts, slowly solidifying into stones.

Most doctors these days rely on both dietary measures and drugs, often diuretics (which decrease urinary calcium and increase urine flow), to keep kidney stones from coming back.

Know Your Stone

While some dietary changes seem to help prevent all kinds of kidney stones, a few work for only certain types of stones. So it's important to know the kind of stone that you have formed, doctors say. The only way to do that is with laboratory analysis of a captured stone. The most common type of kidney stone, made of calcium oxalate, is found in more than 80 percent of cases.

"It's also important to know why you're forming stones. The only way to do that is with urine and blood tests and measures of levels of some hormones, such as parathyroid hormone, which regulates body levels of calcium," explains Freda Levy, M.D., clinical associate professor at Methodist Medical Center in Dallas. "People form stones for lots of different reasons, including metabolic abnormalities and infections."

Check with your doctor to make sure you're selecting the best dietary changes for your specific condition before you try any of these measures, she adds.

Magnesium May Counterbalance Calcium

The chemistry behind kidney stone formation is complex. Some doctors believe that the ratio of calcium to magnesium, another essential mineral, in the diet is important. They recommend that people who've had one or more bouts of calcium oxalate stones make sure that they get at least the Daily Value of magnesium, 400 milligrams, through diet and supplements, if necessary.

Most kidney specialists believe that there's only a minor role, if any, for magnesium in the treatment of kidney stones. They might recommend supplemental magnesium to someone whose urine is low in magnesium and high in calcium, which is a rare condition, says Fred Coe, M.D., professor of medicine and physiology and chief of nephrology at the University of Chicago Pritzker School of Medicine.

But some researchers and some doctors with an interest in nutrition believe that magnesium's potential for preventing stones has not been fully appreciated. They maintain that getting an optimum amount can help prevent stones in many people.

"Doctors think it doesn't work because they don't try it," says Stanley Gershoff, Ph.D., professor of nutrition and dean emeritus at Tufts University School of Nutrition in Medford, Massachusetts.

In a study that Dr. Gershoff did years ago, 149 people who had had at least two stones annually for five years saw their stone formation drop dramatically when they started taking 300 milligrams of magnesium a day. (They also took 10 milligrams of vitamin B_6 a day, which is discussed below.) The people were followed for $4\frac{1}{2}$ to 6 years. Over 90 percent had no stones during that period, Dr. Gershoff says. Only 12 people continued to make stones, but with much less frequency, he adds. "I think magnesium is definitely worth a try," he says.

Studies also show that magnesium-deficient animals are more likely than normal to develop calcium oxalate crystals in their kidneys, making stones more likely.

In Dr. Gershoff's studies, urine from people taking supplemental magnesium was capable of holding more than twice as much calcium oxalate in solution compared with urine from people not taking magnesium. This finding held even when the pH and the amount of calcium in the urine were adjusted so that they were exactly the same for both groups.

"Magnesium helps prevent calcium oxalate from crystallizing, although exactly how it does that isn't known," Dr. Gershoff says. One theory, that magnesium competes with calcium to bind with oxalate and forms a soluble compound that can be excreted from the body, is intriguing but not proven, Dr. Gershoff says.

He recommends that anyone who has passed a calcium oxalate stone take 300 milligrams of supplemental magnesium a day. "That amount worked just fine in our study," he says. Some other doctors recommend taking 400 to 500 milligrams daily.

Studies show that most men get about 329 milligrams a day and most women get about 207 milligrams a day through foods.

Stick to the lowest dose that works for you and get medical supervision, especially if your kidneys have been damaged or if you have a heart problem, Dr. Gershoff says.

Good food sources of magnesium are green vegetables, nuts, beans, and whole grains.

Vitamin B$_6$ Provides Anti-Oxalate Protection

Along with magnesium, some doctors recommend vitamin B$_6$ to people who get kidney stones.

"A vitamin B$_6$ deficiency throws up a roadblock in the body's metabolism, so more oxalic acid is made, which means that high amounts get into the urine," Dr. Coe explains. Oxalic acid then combines with calcium to form insoluble calcium oxalate, the stuff from which stones form.

In one study, conducted in India, researchers found that people with a history of kidney stones who took 40 milligrams of vitamin B$_6$ a day were much less likely to form stones than they were prior to beginning the vitamin. (A few people required up to 160 milligrams a day before they stopped forming stones.)

Most kidney stone specialists, however, discount the idea that people in the United States could be so shortchanged when it comes to vitamin B_6 that they develop kidney stones as a result. "It might be given to someone whose urine is very high in oxalic acid, but in my opinion, most stone-formers aren't B_6-deficient," Dr. Coe says. People with stones are seldom tested for B_6 deficiency or asked about their intakes of B_6-rich foods such as fish, bananas, and nuts. (Studies show that in the United States, both men and women get less than the Daily Value of 2 milligrams of B_6. Men average 1.87 milligrams a day; women, 1.16 milligrams a day.)

If you're supplementing vitamin B_6, stick to no more than 50 milligrams a day without medical supervision, says Dr. Coe. In large doses, B_6 has been associated with nerve damage. Stop taking B_6 if you develop numbness in your hands or feet or unsteadiness in walking. Medical experts suggest that if you're taking B_6 supplements, make sure you're also taking a well-balanced multivitamin/mineral formula that includes the array of B-complex vitamins. (B vitamins work in harmony with each other.) But again, be sure that the two supplements combined give you no more than 50 milligrams of B_6 a day.

Protection with Potassium Power

Medical experts agree that eating grains, vegetables, and fruits helps avert kidney stones, and one reason for this may be that vegetarian fare offers lots of potassium. Low levels of this mineral can increase the risk of stone formation.

"People with low potassium levels, and especially

those on potassium-draining diuretics such as thiazides, are likely to be prescribed potassium supplements and to be told to get more potassium in their diets," explains Lisa Ruml, M.D., assistant professor of medicine and a researcher in the department of mineral metabolism at the University of Texas Southwestern Medical Center at Dallas. "Low potassium can lead to low urine citrate, which is the direct reason for increased stone risk."

Doctors who recommend potassium as a preventive for kidney stones generally suggest aiming for 3,500 to 4,500 milligrams daily. You can get this amount by eating at least five servings of fruits and vegetables, including plenty of citrus fruits and juices, every day.

One form of this mineral, potassium citrate, which is available by prescription, may be helpful not only for people with low blood levels of potassium but also for many who form calcium oxalate stones, Dr. Ruml adds.

In a study done by researchers at the University of Texas Southwestern Medical Center at Dallas, people cut their chances of forming new stones to close to zero during three to four years of daily potassium citrate therapy.

"Potassium citrate changes the pH of urine, making it able to hold more calcium oxalate without forming crystals because citrate is increased," Dr. Ruml explains. "Instead of forming stones, the calcium oxalate is excreted in the urine. We use potassium citrate now in most of our patients who get calcium stones."

Medical Alert

No supplement program dissolves kidney stones that have already formed.

If you have kidney or heart problems, check with your doctor before taking supplemental magnesium.

People taking potassium-sparing diuretics or who have kidney disease or diabetes should not use potassium supplements of any kind without first consulting their doctors.

Some doctors recommend taking no more than 50 milligrams of vitamin B_6 without medical supervision. Large doses have been associated with nerve damage. Stop taking B_6 if you develop numbness in your hands or feet or unsteadiness in walking.

Lupus

Fighting Off an Immune System Attack

Most of the time, your immune system is your best friend, fighting off invading microbes and keeping you healthy. But in certain cases—in someone with lupus, for example—the immune system gets confused about who the enemy is.

A painful and potentially life-threatening illness, lupus occurs when the immune system turns renegade and attacks the body's own tissues, causing inflammation and damage. Skin, kidneys, blood vessels, eyes, lungs, nerves, joints—just about any part of the body can be involved.

At the same time, in severe cases the immune

system sometimes shirks its normal protective duties, making infections of all sorts more likely. "No one knows what sets off the immune system in the first place, but a genetic tendency and exposure to some sort of outside trigger, perhaps a virus, may be involved," explains Sheldon Paul Blau, M.D., clinical professor of medicine at the State University of New York at Stony Brook and co-author of *Living with Lupus*.

Lupus affects about 1 in 2,000 people, mostly women between puberty and menopause (ages 13 to 48) and, more frequently, African-American women. Some get the more common form of the disease, systemic lupus erythematosus, which affects the entire body. Another form of the disease, discoid lupus erythematosus, can cause disfiguring skin problems. Both conditions can flare up, then subside.

Lupus may be treated with corticosteroid drugs, such as prednisone (Deltasone), which reduce inflammation and suppress the immune response. "But most people newly diagnosed with lupus don't need steroids," Dr. Blau says. "They may do well on nonsteroidal anti-inflammatory drugs such as aspirin or with some dietary changes."

It's still important to see a doctor, preferably a rheumatologist (one who specializes in arthritis and autoimmune diseases), for assessment and long-term follow-up, Dr. Blau says. One good reason: People with lupus can develop inflammation in their kidneys, blood vessels, and other organs but have no obvious symptoms until damage is severe. Your doctor can periodically check your kidneys with blood and urine tests.

Nutritional therapy for lupus involves correcting drug-induced deficiencies and eating a balanced diet to help prevent heart disease. Women with lupus are much more likely than normal to develop heart disease. People with kidney disease also need to follow special protein restriction guidelines.

In addition, some doctors recommend so-called antioxidant nutrients that may help reduce inflammation and protect against heart disease. "There's good evidence that vitamins C and E can help prevent heart disease, and since that's such a big risk, even in these young women, I feel that these vitamins are essential," Dr. Blau says.

Some doctors also recommend fish oil, which helps fight inflammation.

Here are the nutrients that may help the symptoms of this disease.

Antioxidants May Offer Protection

Inflammation produces unstable molecules called free radicals, which damage cells by grabbing electrons from healthy molecules in a cell's outer membrane. Antioxidants help stop a free radical free-for-all by generously offering up their own electrons.

There's no doubt that inflammation produces free radicals. And lupus creates inflammation, sometimes all over the body. Doctors who recommend vitamins C and E, the mineral selenium, and beta-carotene (the yellow pigment found in carrots, cantaloupe, and other orange and yellow fruits and vegetables) to people with lupus are hoping that over time these nutrients will help reduce the inflammation by mopping up some of the free radicals.

"Studies of animals with lupus do show that these nutrients can help stop the damage from inflammation," Dr. Blau says. "I give these nutrients to all of my patients, from day one."

He recommends a daily intake of 1,000 milligrams of vitamin C, 1,000 international units (IU) of vitamin E, 25,000 IU of beta-carotene, and a supplement that includes 50 micrograms of selenium and 15 milligrams of zinc, which is used by the body to produce a free radical–dousing enzyme. Dr. Blau urges all people with lupus to discuss any vitamin or mineral treatment with their doctors.

In two studies, people with discoid lupus, a form of lupus typically characterized by red, inflamed skin in a butterfly pattern on the nose and cheeks, who took more than 300 IU of vitamin E daily (most took 900 to 1,600 IU daily) saw clearing of their inflamed skin. And a British doctor reported that large doses of beta-carotene (50 milligrams, or 83,000 IU, three times daily) completely cleared up sun-induced skin rashes in three of his patients with discoid lupus.

Vitamins C and E and beta-carotene are considered safe, even in fairly large amounts. Both selenium and zinc have much smaller ranges of safety. It's best not to take more than 100 micrograms of selenium or 15 milligrams of zinc a day without medical supervision, experts say.

Bone Up with Calcium and Vitamin D

Frequently, people with severe lupus need to take corticosteroid drugs such as prednisone. These drugs get inflammation under control, but at a price. One side effect is bone loss.

"If these drugs are being given to women in their twenties and thirties, a time when they should be maintaining optimum bone mass, chances are that they will begin to develop osteoporosis fairly early in life, by their forties or fifties," says Joseph McCune, M.D., associate professor of rheumatology at the University of Michigan Hospitals in Ann Arbor. Osteoporosis, which literally means porous bones, can lead to painful, crippling fractures.

That's why doctors who treat lupus recommend that anyone taking corticosteroid drugs for the condition get at least 1,000 milligrams of calcium a day through foods and supplements, if necessary. They also keep an eye on vitamin D, aiming for the Daily Value of 400 IU, to help calcium absorption. Some doctors recommend supplements; others reserve vitamin D supplements for those who are already showing signs of osteoporosis on special x-rays that measure bone density. Vitamin D can be toxic in large doses, so supplements should be taken only when approved by your doctor.

A glass of 1 percent milk, a top source of calcium, offers 300 milligrams, so you'll need to drink slightly more than three glasses a day to reach 1,000 milligrams. That same amount of milk provides almost 400 IU of vitamin D. Egg yolks and fatty fish such as salmon are also excellent sources of vitamin D.

Medical Alert

Anyone with lupus should be taking vitamin and mineral supplementation only after discussing it with a physician.

Vitamin D can be toxic in large amounts, so supplements should be taken only under medical supervision.

It's a good idea to consult your doctor before taking vitamin E in doses exceeding 600 international units daily. If you are taking anticoagulant drugs, you should not take vitamin E supplements.

Memory Loss

Helping Your Brain Work Better

Y ou've heard of the tree of knowledge? Think of
your brain. Inside that four-pound organ sitting inside your skull is a root and branch system of truly
biblical proportions.

Hundreds of billions of brain cells called neurons
stretch toward each other with rootlike growths called
axons and dendrites.

Close as they might get, the tiny nerve endings of
one axon never touch those of the dendrites branching
toward it. Instead, memories and other thoughts have
to hurdle what are called synaptic gaps.

Without chemicals called neurotransmitters (such
as dopamine, norepinephrine, serotonin, and acetylcholine) bridging them, these tiny gaps may as well be
as wide as the Grand Canyon. Information just can't get
from one neuron to the other. And that means memories, though stored throughout your brain, are just out
of reach.

"You know that if you have a phone, I can call
you," says Michael Ebadi, Ph.D., professor of pharmacology and neurology at the University of Nebraska College of Medicine in Omaha. "But if you don't have a
phone, there's nothing I can do. That's the way it is

with neurotransmitters. In order for things to occur, you know you need transmitters. In the absence of transmitters, biological function is halted."

Turning Memories into Mush

If neurotransmitters are the stuff that helps transmit memories, then what makes neurotransmitters? Although the brain's primary fuel is glucose, experts believe that key vitamins and minerals supply the raw material for many of these neurotransmitters.

And that may be what's at the heart of many memory loss problems. Although Americans eat a lot of food, they don't always choose the right kinds. As a result, many of us just don't get enough brain-boosting nutrients. And even if you are among the few who are getting the Daily Values of these essential nutrients, you may not be home free as far as memory is concerned.

Some doctors wonder whether the Daily Values are set high enough to meet all of the body's needs. Not only that, but it's possible to consume all of the nutrients in all of the right amounts and still be shortchanged if your body isn't doing a good job of absorbing the nutrients. This is a situation most likely to develop among older people, precisely the population that is most likely to be beset by memory problems.

Malabsorption of vitamin B_{12}, which means that your body can't get sufficient B_{12} from foods no matter how much you eat, is thought to affect at least one in five older adults, says Sally Stabler, M.D., associate professor of medicine at the University of Colorado Health Sciences Center School of Medicine in Denver.

Mix already poor nutrition with improper or impaired nutrient absorption and you have a recipe for memory loss.

Benefits of B$_6$

It's one thing to occasionally misplace your car keys. It's another to forget where you parked your car—especially when it's in the garage, where you usually keep it. Yet that's what some research shows could happen if you don't get proper amounts of vitamin B$_6$, also called pyridoxine.

One study showed that more than 80 percent of the healthy, independent-living, middle-income elderly surveyed in Albuquerque, New Mexico, had vitamin B$_6$ intakes below three-fourths of the Daily Value (the Daily Value for B$_6$ is 2 milligrams).

A group of researchers in the Netherlands decided to see what would happen if they added vitamin B$_6$ to the diets of healthy older men. First the men were given a mental test that included things such as being able to remember different objects flashed on a screen and the names and occupations of people in a list. Then one group took 20 milligrams of B$_6$ a day, while the others took placebos (blank pills).

At the end of three months, the men were tested again. The memories of those in the vitamin B$_6$ group showed "modest but significant" gains, especially in long-term memory. The bottom line: The researchers felt that their study made a strong case for taking B$_6$ supplements.

There's a good reason why vitamin B$_6$ helps memory. Remember those all-important neurotransmitters with the long names? Vitamin B$_6$ apparently helps create dopamine, serotonin, and norepinephrine, says Dr. Ebadi.

The Daily Value of 2 milligrams should be sufficient to help keep your memory in good working order. You can easily get this amount as part of a B-complex supplement that supplies the Daily Values of all B vitamins. You should never take B_6 by itself without medical supervision, as amounts above 100 milligrams can be toxic.

Boosting the Brain with B_{12}

In one study, when 39 people were treated for neurological symptoms related to vitamin B_{12} deficiency—things such as memory loss, disorientation, and fatigue—all of them improved, sometimes dramatically. "B_{12} deficiency causes problems in the nervous system, including burning points in the feet and mental problems such as difficulty with recent memory and the ability to calculate, that sort of thing," says Dr. Stabler. A B_{12} deficiency has even been known to change brain wave activity, she says.

Nearly one-third of people over age 60 can't extract the vitamin B_{12} they need from what they eat. That's because their stomachs no longer secrete enough gastric acid, the stuff that breaks down food and helps turn it into fuel for your brain and body.

And taking supplements won't help, because they are also broken down in the stomach. So doctors who suspect vitamin B_{12} deficiencies in people with memory problems give them B_{12} shots, thus bypassing the faltering digestive system.

Vitamin B_{12} deficiency caused by diet is rare when the digestive system is in good working order. That's because eating just small portions of dairy products or animal protein gives you enough of this vital nutrient. About the only eating plan that seems to put you at risk is diets that completely eliminate meats and dairy products. But even then you have to adhere to such a diet for at least several years before a deficiency develops, says Dr. Stabler.

Virtually all animal products, such as milk, cheeses, yogurt, and lean beef, contain vitamin B_{12}. The Daily Value for B_{12} is 6 micrograms.

Fortification at Its Finest

Both thiamin and riboflavin, other important B vitamins, are routinely added to most flours, cereals, and grain products.

Even mild deficiencies of these vitamins can have an impact on your thinking and memory. While checking brain function and nutrition status of 28 healthy folks over age 60, a U.S. Department of Agriculture (USDA) study showed that those with low thiamin registered brain activity impairment. On the other hand, the folks with adequate thiamin had better memories.

Thiamin deficiencies have also been found to cause mood changes, vague feelings of uneasiness, fear, disorderly thinking, and other signs of mental depression—symptoms that researchers say often affect memory.

Fortunately, it doesn't take much thiamin to make a difference. One study showed that women who were restricted to 0.33 milligram of thiamin a day became irritable, fatigued, and unsociable. These symptoms improved with just 1.4 milligrams of thiamin a day.

The Daily Value for thiamin is 1.5 milligrams, while the Daily Value for riboflavin is 1.7 milligrams.

The Lecithin-Choline Connection

As a doctoral candidate overwhelmed by the vast amounts of information she had to study, Florence Safford took lecithin supplements to help keep her memory sharp—and she told her friends about the benefits.

Her friends don't have to just take her word for it any longer. Twenty years later, Dr. Safford, now professor of social work and gerontology at Florida International University in Miami, has conducted two studies that help shed light on how lecithin and choline, a B vitamin, can actually boost memory.

Lecithin is a common food additive; it's used in ice cream, margarine, mayonnaise, and chocolate bars to help wed the fat in these foods with water. It has healthful qualities as well, such as mildly increasing the amount of choline in your brain. And more choline means more acetylcholine, an important neurotransmitter that you need for your memory to function.

In one study, 61 volunteers between ages 50 and 80 were divided into two groups: 41 took two tablespoons of lecithin a day, while 20 were given placebos (inactive substances). At the end of five weeks, the volunteers who took lecithin had "significant improvement" in memory test scores and fewer memory lapses than those who took the placebos, says Dr. Safford.

In another study, 117 volunteers were divided into three groups according to their ages: 35 to 50, 50 to 65, and 65 to 80. These groups were then subdivided, with half taking 3.5 grams of a form of lecithin a day and the other half taking placebos. At the end of three weeks, those who took the lecithin recorded almost half as many memory lapses on average, says Dr. Safford.

"The fascinating thing about lecithin is that when it helps, it's right away," says Dr. Safford. "It's one of the few substances like alcohol, which crosses the blood-brain barrier and produces an immediate reaction." (In a bid to prevent harmful substances from reaching your brain, you're equipped with what is called the blood-brain barrier. Like an armed guard at a checkpoint, your blood-brain barrier allows only certain chemicals in your blood to pass into your brain.)

Dr. Safford recommends two tablespoons of lecithin granules a day. Just mix it in with foods such as yogurt, applesauce, and cereals.

Iron and Zinc to Help You Think

While researchers have established the importance of iron and zinc in the mental development of infants, you have to dig into the scientific literature before you'll find studies showing that these minerals help make for better memories in adults as well.

In one small preliminary study, researchers measured the effects of mild zinc or iron deficiency on short-term memory in 34 women between ages 18 and 40, a group at risk for low levels of both minerals.

For eight weeks, researchers gave the women either 30 milligrams of zinc, 30 milligrams of iron, or both—or supplements containing other micronutrients. A mental test found that the short-term memories of those taking zinc or iron improved by 15 to 20 percent, says Harold Sandstead, M.D., professor in the department of prevention medicine and community health at the University of Texas Medical Branch at Galveston.

Those who took iron supplements had better

short-term verbal memory, while visual memory, or the ability to remember pictures, was improved by both zinc and iron.

Although the women received supplements during the study, Dr. Sandstead says that foods are much better sources of these nutrients. Steamed clams and oysters, Cream of Wheat cereal, soybeans, and pumpkin seeds are all good sources of iron, while whole grains, wheat bran, wheat germ, seafood, and meats are top sources of zinc.

Women who menstruate need between 2 and 2.5 milligrams of iron a day to offset loss of the mineral, explains Dr. Sandstead. (The Daily Value for iron is much higher—18 milligrams—because your body doesn't absorb all of the mineral that you take in.) "If they have heavy menstrual loss, the level goes up even more," he adds. Men need about 1 milligram of iron a day.

And how does iron help memory? Experts believe that pumping up your iron intake helps build those all-important brain neurotransmitters, among other things.

For a closer look at zinc's role in helping you to think, researchers at the USDA Grand Forks Human Nutrition Research Center in North Dakota fed 10 men living at the center meals containing 1, 2, 3, 4, or 10 milligrams of zinc every day for five weeks each.

At the end of the 25-week study, researchers noted that the week the men ate 10 milligrams of zinc a day, they were better able to remember shapes and responded faster to simple motor tasks, says James G. Penland, Ph.D., head researcher at the center and author of the study. "There was a very clear improvement at 10 milligrams versus the other amounts, with the others being more or less the same," he says.

And how does zinc help memory? Apparently, vitamin B_6 can't do its job without zinc pitching in, says Dr. Ebadi. "In the absence of zinc, active B_6 is not formed properly in the brain, and as a result, neither are key neurotransmitters," he says. Not only that, but large amounts of zinc have been found in the brain's memory center, the hippocampus.

Some experts say that some elderly people may get less than half of the zinc that they need (the Daily Value for zinc is 15 milligrams).

Menopausal Problems

Reinventing the Change of Life

Some women have a miserable time at menopause. Others barely notice that it's happening.

Either way, as the century turns, more women all over the world will go through "the change" than at any other time in history.

Menopause is not really a single event but rather a process that can last a decade or longer. The average woman has her last period between the ages of 48 and

52, but menopausal changes actually begin much earlier. Women often notice changes in their cycles when they're in their early forties or even before then. Periods may be shorter or longer, lighter or heavier; they may come closer together or farther apart.

The Estrogen Connection

It's during this time, known as perimenopause, that the ovaries gradually slow their production of the female hormone estrogen and that a woman begins to notice the effects this has on her body. So why do some women experience such discomfort at menopause, while others never have so much as a single hot flash?

It may be because some women experience more drastic drops in their estrogen levels than others do, says Margo Woods, D.Sc., associate professor of community health at Tufts University School of Medicine in Boston. Dr. Woods is doing research on the effects of soy on menopausal symptoms. Asian women, who have lower estrogen levels before menopause than Western women, experience less drastic drops in estrogen, which may be one reason why they report fewer menopausal symptoms, says Dr. Woods. Many researchers feel that diet may influence menopausal symptoms.

And some lucky women, about 25 to 30 percent, don't entirely stop producing estrogen, says Susan M. Lark, M.D., director of the PMS and Menopause Self-Help Center in Los Altos, California, author of *Menopause: Self-Help Book*, and a physician specializing in women's health. Even after their ovaries stop producing estrogen, their adrenal glands and one small area of each ovary called the stroma continue to produce small amounts of this hormone. These glands don't produce enough estrogen to promote menstruation, but they do produce enough to keep the most bothersome symptoms of menopause at bay, explains Dr. Lark.

"Some women are just good estrogen producers," she says. "We don't know why."

The amount of estrogen that the body continues to produce is out of a woman's hands, adds Dr. Lark. But there are plenty of other factors that a woman can control that can reduce menopausal discomfort. "Women who avoid stress, who don't overdo caffeine, and who get regular exercise have a much easier time of it than women who don't do those things," she says.

"There isn't much hard evidence to prove it, but it has been my experience that women who have a history of premenstrual syndrome and bad menstrual cramps also have more hot flashes and other symptoms of menopause," says Dr. Lark. And here again, lifestyle factors come into play. "These women tend to have very stressful lives, poor diets, and poor coping skills," she maintains.

Finally, nutrition apparently plays an important role in determining whether your menopause will be an endurance contest or a walk in the park. Here's what experts say you can do to make the transition as comfortable as possible.

Vitamin E Snuffs Out Hot Flashes

A hot flash—that sudden, intensely hot feeling in your face and neck that makes you wish for a walk-in refrigerator—can happen anytime, anywhere: at home, at work, while you're driving in traffic, or even while you're sleeping.

Caused by hormonal surges, hot flashes usually last for three to five minutes, but they can feel like an eternity. Some women get flushed, sweat profusely, and even have heart palpitations. Other women have flashes so mild that they barely notice them. About 80 percent of all women going through menopause have hot flashes at one point or another.

Studies show that thin women are more prone to hot flashes than heavier women. This is because even after the ovaries slow their hormone production, fat cells continue to produce small amounts of estrogen. So women with a lot of fat cells go through less drastic estrogen withdrawal than their leaner sisters.

While hot flashes can be relieved by hormone replacement therapy, there may be another, less drastic option: a daily vitamin E supplement.

Vitamin E can act as an estrogen substitute, explains Dr. Lark. Studies have shown that it can relieve hot flashes, night sweats, mood swings, and even vaginal dryness. "Vitamin E is really an essential part of a supplement program for women during the menopause years," she says.

If vitamin E is so effective, why hasn't your doctor recommended it? Chances are she has never heard of it, or if she has, she's waiting to see some hard scientific proof that it works. And sad to say, there isn't any. While a number of studies were done in the 1940s on vitamin E and menopause, the connection hasn't been investigated recently. A number of doctors who use nutritional therapies as part of their medical practices recommend it, however, and find that it often works.

If you get hot flashes and would like to try vitamin E, Dr. Lark recommends a fairly high dose: about 800 international units (IU) a day. And while vitamin E is nontoxic at this level, she says, women should get their doctors' okay before taking this high amount, especially if they have diabetes or high blood pressure.

Reduce Bleeding with Nutrients

Many women approach menopause expecting menstrual flow to taper off and finally stop. But for a good percentage, periods during perimenopause are heavier than ever.

Besides the inconvenience—perimenopausal bleeding is often so irregular that women have to be prepared anytime, anywhere—frequent heavy bleeding can seriously endanger a woman's iron stores, says Dr. Lark.

Heavy bleeding can be treated effectively with nutrients, says Dr. Lark. "Some studies have shown that besides replenishing the iron lost through bleeding, a daily iron supplement may actually reduce the amount that a woman will bleed during future periods," she says.

Women with heavy bleeding also benefit from loading up on vitamin C and bioflavonoids, she says. Bioflavonoids are chemical compounds related to vitamin C; they're found in many citrus fruits and included in many supplements.

"Both vitamin C and bioflavonoids reduce bleeding by strengthening the capillary walls, which are at their weakest just before and during the menstrual period," says Dr. Lark. And since bioflavonoids have many of the same chemical properties as estrogen, they can also be helpful in controlling hot flashes, night sweats, and mood swings. She recommends a daily supplement that includes at least 1,000 milligrams of vitamin C and 800 milligrams of bioflavonoids.

Because vitamin C helps the body absorb iron more efficiently, Dr. Lark recommends taking these two nutrients together. If you take a multivitamin/multimineral supplement, check to make sure that it contains both vitamin C and iron. Another option is to take an iron supplement, about 15 milligrams, with a glass of orange juice. If you have a juicer, juicing the white pulp of the orange along with the rest of the fruit guarantees an abundant dose of bioflavonoids, Dr. Lark adds.

B Complex Battles the Blahs

Depression is also common around the time of menopause, though nobody knows for sure how much of it results from hormonal fluctuations and how much is triggered by the everyday stresses that women face at midlife.

Regardless of what's causing it, emotional stress can deplete the body of B vitamins, leaving a woman feeling tired, anxious, and irritable, says Dr. Lark.

"High levels of estrogen can also deplete vitamin B_6 and cause depression," says Dr. Lark. "Women who take the Pill or hormone replacement therapy sometimes have this, and some perimenopausal women go through a period of having very high estrogen levels." B_6 also plays an important role in helping the liver regulate estrogen levels, says Dr. Lark.

Vitamin B_6 should always be taken as part of the B complex, says Dr. Lark. She suggests a B-complex supplement containing 50 milligrams each of thiamin and niacin and 30 milligrams of B_6.

Coping with Surgical Menopause

While most women experience the gradual progression of natural menopause, others go through "the change" much more abruptly. Each year thousands of women undergo hysterectomy, the surgical removal of the uterus and sometimes the ovaries because of conditions as varied as pelvic infection, endometriosis, and cancer.

In most cases, the woman's ovaries are left intact; they continue to produce estrogen until the woman goes through normal menopause. But if a woman's ovaries are removed along with her uterus in what is called a complete hysterectomy, she'll experience surgical menopause, with the same symptoms as any other woman who is going through natural menopause.

Women who experience surgical menopause may actually have more severe symptoms because they go through menopause so abruptly, says Dr. Lark.

A woman who undergoes a hysterectomy can benefit from the same nutritional strategies that help women who are going through natural menopause, says Dr. Lark. "As far as your body is concerned, it's the same process," she says.

Medical Alert

If you're considering taking vitamin E in doses that exceed 600 international units a day, you should discuss it with your doctor first.

If you are taking anticoagulant drugs, you should not take vitamin E supplements.

Menstrual Problems

Nutrients to Ease Monthly Distress

Imagine you were moving to the North Pole for five years. How would you prepare for your new life? Most likely, you'd learn everything you could about coping with the cold. And if there was anything you could eat or any supplement you could take to make the experience more pleasant, of course you'd want to know about it. It's five years of your life, after all. You might as well be comfortable.

Maybe you never thought about it, but if you add it up—month after month, year after year—you have your period for about five years of your life. And if you're like most women, you'd do anything to sail through those days without feeling crampy and exhausted and swollen up like a baby beluga.

Why You Feel So Bad

Most women have some degree of menstrual discomfort at some point in their lives, says Susan M. Lark, M.D., director of the PMS and Menopause Self-Help Center in Los Altos, California, author of *Men-*

strual Cramps: A Self-Help Program and *PMS: Self-Help Book*, and a physician specializing in women's health.

Most menstrual pain is classified as either spasmodic or congestive. Doctors know that spasmodic pain is caused by the female hormones estrogen and progesterone and by prostaglandins, hormonelike substances that control muscle tension. Women with spasmodic cramps generally have an excess of a certain type of prostaglandins called 2 series prostaglandins, which are responsible for contraction of the smooth muscles, including the uterus. Prostaglandin production increases toward the end of your cycle, resulting in cramps that are sometimes accompanied by nausea, constipation, or diarrhea.

Probably the best thing that can be said about spasmodic pain is that it tends to improve with age. It's usually most severe in women in their teens and twenties. Spasmodic pain often improves after a woman has children, says Dr. Lark.

The other type of menstrual pain is known as congestive. Women with congestive pain also tend to suffer from bloating, water retention, headaches, and breast pain. In addition, they often notice a worsening of their cramps when they eat certain foods, such as wheat and dairy products, or when they drink alcohol, says Dr. Lark. Unfortunately, congestive pain tends to get worse with age, whether or not a woman has children.

While monthly cramps aren't pleasant, they are normal, says Dr. Lark. She cautions that in some cases, the pain can be a symptom of a health problem that requires medical attention, such as endometriosis. "You should always discuss unusual menstrual symptoms with your doctor," she advises.

But most of the time, the cause of cramps is simply menstruation itself. And in such cases, some doctors maintain that a few prudent nutritional changes can do wonders to improve your quality of life during your period, says Dr. Lark. The following nutrients have been shown to help soothe menstrual symptoms.

Calcium and Manganese: A One-Two Punch for Cramps

Scientists at the U.S. Department of Agriculture Grand Forks Human Nutrition Research Center in North Dakota have found that getting enough of certain minerals all month long can make a significant difference in how a woman feels during her period.

In one study, a group of menstruating women were fed a number of different diets over several months and questioned about how they felt at different points in their menstrual cycles. One of the diets was unusually low in calcium and manganese, a trace mineral that's found in nuts, tea, whole-grain cereals, and dried peas and beans. The same women also tried a diet that was supplemented with both minerals.

When the researchers analyzed the women's premenstrual symptoms, they noticed a clear pattern: Most women reported much less severe symptoms when they followed the diet high in both calcium and manganese.

It's interesting to note that the diet the researchers considered low in calcium, the one that produced the most uncomfortable menstrual periods, included about

587 milligrams of calcium per day. The high-calcium diet had about 1,336 milligrams of calcium, which is close to the amount experts recommend to prevent osteoporosis, the brittle bone disease.

Just how these minerals fend off menstrual discomfort isn't clear. Researchers know that calcium is involved in the production of prostaglandins. "It may be calcium's role in prostaglandin metabolism that's responsible for the mineral's effect on pain," says James G. Penland, Ph.D., head researcher at the Grand Forks Human Nutrition Research Center.

Manganese's role is even more mysterious. "We do know that manganese is involved in blood clotting, and some research shows that a low intake is associated with a heavier menstrual flow," says Dr. Penland. "This is definitely an area that needs more study."

While researchers continue to try to figure out exactly how these two minerals work their magic on menstrual symptoms, a daily multivitamin/mineral supplement that includes the recommended levels of both calcium and manganese makes good sense for women who want to minimize menstrual discomfort, says Dr. Penland. The Daily Value for manganese is 2 milligrams. Because women of all ages have trouble getting enough calcium through diet, Dr. Penland recommends increasing your intake of low-fat, high-calcium foods such as low-fat yogurt and skim milk. If you still need more calcium, he suggests taking 500 to 1,000 milligrams of supplemental calcium a day.

Vitamin B₆ Keeps Cramps at Bay

The whole B complex is essential for good health, but when it comes to relieving monthly symptoms, vitamin B₆ and niacin are the stars, says Dr. Lark.

Vitamin B_6 plays a key role in the production of 1 series prostaglandins, the "good" prostaglandins that relax the uterine muscles and keep cramps under control, according to Dr. Lark. But a woman's B_6 stores are easily depleted. Stress and certain medications, such as oral contraceptives, can easily cause a shortage. As a result, your body may not manufacture enough of the right kind of prostaglandins, leaving you feeling tied up in knots when your period comes. And if you're bothered by water retention or monthly weight gain, B_6 can ease those symptoms, too, Dr. Lark says.

Dr. Lark recommends taking vitamin B_6 as part of a B-complex supplement. Look for a B-complex supplement that contains no more than 200 to 300 milligrams of B_6. Large doses can be toxic, she says. It's a good idea to check with your doctor before taking doses of more than 100 milligrams daily.

Equally important in staving off cramps is niacin. "Some research shows that niacin is about 90 percent effective for relieving cramps," says Dr. Lark. To head off cramps before they start, she suggests taking between 25 and 200 milligrams of niacin a day, beginning 7 to 10 days before your period is due and stopping the day that your period starts. This treatment can be repeated every month to prevent menstrual cramps.

Because niacin can cause slight flushing in some women, start with 25 milligrams a day for the first month. "If it doesn't seem to help, you can always increase the dose the following month until you find the level that's right for you," she advises. Women with liver disease should use niacin only under medical supervision, cautions Dr. Lark.

Nutrients to Lessen Bleeding

Next to cramps, heavy bleeding is probably the most common complaint of menstruating women, says Dr. Lark. Besides being inconvenient, heavy bleeding can deplete a woman's iron stores and can even lead to anemia.

It isn't surprising, then, that doctors recommend iron supplements to women with heavy bleeding. What is surprising is that getting extra doses of this mineral doesn't just replace the iron that has been lost. It may actually reduce the amount of bleeding in the future, says Dr. Lark.

"Women need only a small amount of iron. But what they need they really need," she says. She recommends a daily supplement of about 15 milligrams.

Women with heavy bleeding also need plenty of vitamin C and bioflavonoids, says Dr. Lark. Bioflavonoids are chemical compounds related to vitamin C; they're found in many citrus fruits and included in many supplements. Both vitamin C and bioflavonoids reduce bleeding by strengthening the capillary walls, which are at their weakest just before and during the menstrual period, says Dr. Lark. She recommends a daily supplement that includes at least 1,000 milligrams of vitamin C and 800 milligrams of bioflavonoids.

Because vitamin C helps the body absorb iron more efficiently, Dr. Lark recommends taking these two nutrients together.

Medical Alert

Do not take niacin in doses exceeding 100 milligrams without medical supervision. Women with liver disease should use niacin only under medical supervision.

Vitamin B$_6$ can cause side effects when taken in doses of more than 100 milligrams daily, so it's a good idea to talk to your doctor before supplementing the amount recommended here.

Migraines

Ending the Pain

The hammering inside your head is utterly horrendous, as if someone were using your brain for a bongo. For what it's worth, you're not the only one with a built-in percussion section: Roughly 45 million Americans reportedly experience headaches each year.

Although tension headaches are by far the most common, chronic migraines are much more likely to send a desperate individual to the doctor seeking relief. "I use the term *victim* when I refer to chronic headache sufferers, because it's a very wicked syndrome," says Burton M. Altura, M.D., professor of physiology and medicine at the State University of New York Health Science Center at Brooklyn. "Besides the agonizing pain, these folks often have tremendous sensitivity to light and noise. Just snapping your fingers or clapping around them can be excruciating."

The one-sided, throbbing headache known as a migraine is actually more common in women; roughly 75 percent of those who get migraines are female. But what migraines lack in gender equality they make up for in severity. Some migraines are so extreme that they cause limb numbness, hallucinations, nausea, and vomiting.

The good news is that medical research has come up with several vitamin and mineral therapies that might prove helpful for people who have been unable to find relief elsewhere.

"B" Headache-Free

Fifty-two quarts of chocolate syrup. Nine hundred bowls of cornflakes. These might prevent a migraine— if they weren't guaranteed to give you a stomachache first. They add up to a super-high dose of riboflavin, which research hints may ward off the someone's-put-a-soccer-ball-in-my-head pain.

Fortunately for the 49 people in a Belgian headache study, they were able to take supplements to get the necessary 400 milligram daily dose. The migraine-prone people in the study received this high dose (it's about 235 times the Daily Value) every day for three months. In addition to the riboflavin, 23 of the people in the study took one low-dose aspirin a day.

By the end of the study, migraine severity decreased by nearly 70 percent in both groups compared with what it had been at the study's start. Aspirin had no added value.

Why would something like riboflavin work? Researchers have noticed a deficit in certain energy generators in the brain cells of some people with migraines. They suspect that flooding the system with riboflavin could indirectly help regenerate this flagging energy system and somehow short-circuit migraine pain.

What's attractive about riboflavin, if rigorous scientific studies support these preliminary findings, is that it's likely to have fewer side effects than current headache preventives (although no one knows for sure what the long-term effects of this much riboflavin might be).

"I wouldn't use it as the first line of attack, because we have other agents of proven value," says Seymour Solomon, M.D., professor of neurology at Albert Einstein College of Medicine in New York City. "But since this appears to be a relatively harmless treatment, it would be worthwhile to explore it with patients who haven't responded well to standard therapy."

Although riboflavin generally is quite harmless, it's a good idea to check with your doctor before supplementing with such a high amount.

Making the Magnesium-Migraine Link

An increasing number of doctors believe that a fairly large percentage of the most severe cases of migraines may actually be caused by an imbalance of key minerals such as magnesium and calcium.

"Not all headaches are produced by this imbalance, but we now know that 50 to 60 percent of migraines are magnesium-linked. And that's probably why no prescription therapy on the market successfully treats headaches across the board. They're simply not treating the cause," says Dr. Altura.

"Of the 17 people we've treated with magnesium, 13 have had complete improvement," says Herbert C. Mansmann Jr., M.D., professor of pediatrics and associate professor of medicine at Jefferson Medical College of Thomas Jefferson University in Philadelphia.

The magnesium-migraine link still is not commonly accepted by headache experts. In fact, Dr. Altura says that one of his magnesium studies was rejected by a prominent medical journal at the suggestion of a top headache researcher. (Shortly thereafter, the study was published by another journal.)

But the weight of evidence for magnesium's use in the treatment of migraines is building. "There's no question that the literature strongly supports it," says Dr. Mansmann. "The so-called headache experts don't believe the data because they don't know anything about the development of magnesium deficiencies within cells."

To understand why magnesium might do the trick, it helps to take a look at how migraines happen.

Migraines are thought to be caused by vascular changes, or changes in the blood vessels, that reduce blood or oxygen flow in the scalp and brain. What causes these vascular changes? Things such as muscle contractions during times of stress and biochemicals called catecholamines and serotonin, which are circulating in the blood. Too much serotonin can cause blood flow to slow; too little can cause blood to move through too rapidly, explains Dr. Altura.

While mainstream researchers have long known that changes in serotonin and catecholamine levels cause migraine pain, stopping these changes has been a hit-or-miss proposition, says Dr. Altura. Aspirin, for example, temporarily inhibits the effects of serotonin but does nothing to prevent a migraine from coming back, he says.

Dr. Altura says that he's the first to prove that loss of magnesium from the brain is behind the problem. Without enough magnesium, serotonin flows unchecked, constricting blood vessels and releasing other pain-producing chemicals such as substance P and prostaglandins, he says. Normal magnesium levels not only prevent the release of these pain-producing substances but also stop their effects, says Dr. Altura.

It's very likely that magnesium deficiency is a widespread cause of migraines, maintains Dr. Mansmann. Studies show that many people don't even come close to getting the Daily Value of magnesium, which is 400 milligrams. "On a daily basis, 30 to 40 percent of American people take less than 75 percent of the Daily Value of magnesium," says Dr. Mansmann.

What's more, several different things, from the caffeine in just two cups of coffee a day to the chemicals in most asthma medications, remove some magnesium from your system. "We know that intake is low for a lot of people. We know that a lot of medications, such as diuretics (water pills) and a variety of cardiovascular medications, can increase magnesium losses. We know that people with diabetes who have high blood sugar lose a lot more magnesium in the urine and, as a result, run the risk of magnesium deficiency," says Karen Kubena, Ph.D., associate professor of nutrition at Texas A&M University in College Station. Even stress, a frequent cause of migraines, can remove magnesium from your system, says Dr. Mansmann.

Based on his records, Dr. Altura says that about 50 to 60 percent of his migraine patients have low magnesium levels. But once they begin treatment, he says, they often experience immediate relief. "We can say that 85 to 90 percent of these patients are successfully treated, and that's pretty miraculous," says Dr. Altura.

Can getting more than your share of magnesium every day prevent migraines? Dr. Altura says it's still unclear. "I'd like to be able to answer that question. I can't at this point, but my guess is that it would," he says.

In Dr. Mansmann's experience, a magnesium gluconate supplement works best. "The advantage is that dose for dose, magnesium gluconate causes one-third of the amount of diarrhea that magnesium oxide produces and one-half of the frequency of diarrhea that magnesium chloride produces," he says. It's also absorbed more quickly, he says.

The difference: Magnesium gluconate is more biologically active. "The active form of magnesium is ionized magnesium. When a substance is chemically bound, it's sort of neutralized. When it's ionized, it is available to do what it is supposed to do, which in this case is possibly prevent constriction of blood vessels in your brain and scalp," explains Dr. Kubena.

Dr. Mansmann's migraine patients take two 500-milligram magnesium gluconate tablets at lunch, two in the afternoon, and two at bedtime, upping the dosage each week until their stools become soft, an indication that there is enough magnesium in the body.

If you decide to give this therapy a try, you should be working with a doctor who is willing to monitor your progress. (People who have kidney or heart problems should supplement magnesium only under medical supervision.)

The Calcium Connection

Even if you monitor your magnesium level like a maniac, you're still at risk for migraines if your calcium level is out of whack. The reason: Magnesium and calcium interact with each other.

It seems that higher than normal blood levels of calcium cause the body to excrete the rest, which in turn triggers a loss of magnesium.

"Let's say you have just enough magnesium and too much calcium in your blood. If calcium is excreted, the magnesium goes with it. All of a sudden, you could be low in magnesium," says Dr. Kubena.

In fact, says Dr. Altura, people who have low magnesium and elevated calcium levels are among those who are most successfully treated with magnesium.

Medical Alert

The recommended doses of magnesium and riboflavin are extremely high. If you wish to try these supplements to treat migraines, you should discuss it with your doctor.

People who have kidney or heart problems should supplement magnesium only under medical supervision.

Mitral Valve Prolapse

Easing Symptoms of a Troubled Heart

Normally, the valves that regulate blood flow through the heart close neatly, snapping shut with the *lub-dub* sound that we recognize as a heartbeat.

In mitral valve prolapse, however, an additional click—*lub-dit-dub*—is added to the heartbeat. The extra sound occurs because the valve between the two left chambers of the heart is pushed out of shape by high blood pressure in the compressing heart. The valve pops upward, almost like a parachute being snapped in the wind. The condition happens when one of the fibrous cords that hold the valve in place stretches out too far or when either of the two leaflets that make up the valve is elongated, thickened, or floppy. If the valve does not seal perfectly, blood may leak backward, causing the swishing noise that's known as a heart murmur.

"Mitral valve prolapse syndrome is considered a hereditary disorder," explains Kristine Scordo, R.N., Ph.D., assistant professor at Wright State University in

Dayton, Ohio, director of the Mitral Valve Prolapse Program of Cincinnati, and author of *Taking Control: Living with the Mitral Valve Prolapse Syndrome*. "People with the disorder—and there are three times as many women as men—are often tall and slender, with long arms and fingers and thin chests."

Although mitral valve prolapse usually causes no life-threatening problems, it has been associated with an array of disturbing symptoms, including heart palpitations, chest pain, shortness of breath, dizziness, fatigue, anxiety, headaches, and mood swings. Doctors refer to these collectively as mitral valve prolapse syndrome. "These symptoms aren't caused by the valve itself," Dr. Scordo says. "But they are often part of the package."

These symptoms seem to be caused by disturbances in the body's autonomic nervous system. That's the nervous system that works without conscious control and governs the glands, the heart muscle, and the tone of smooth muscles, such as those of the digestive system, the respiratory system, and the skin.

"People with mitral valve prolapse often have overreactive autonomic nervous systems," explains Sidney M. Baker, M.D., a general practitioner in private practice in Weston, Connecticut, with a special interest in mitral valve prolapse. "Their bodies have a hard time adjusting to changes in the environment. They may be sensitive to light and noise, for instance."

"The symptoms are believed to be caused by a number of physiological changes and can often be helped by dietary changes. In fact, dietary changes are often all that's needed to alleviate symptoms," Dr. Scordo says.

Here's what is recommended.

Magnesium Plays a Role

There's no doubt that minerals play important roles in a properly beating heart. Both the nerves that coordinate the heartbeat and the muscles that contract to move blood through the heart need magnesium in order to do their jobs.

One mineral that has gotten some attention when it comes to mitral valve prolapse is magnesium. Several studies have found that a high percentage of people with mitral valve prolapse have lower than normal magnesium levels.

And one study by researchers at the University of Alabama School of Medicine in Birmingham found that supplemental magnesium relieved many of the symptoms associated with this disorder.

The study, of 94 people with mitral valve prolapse, found that 62 percent of them had low red blood cell levels of magnesium. Those people were also more likely to have additional symptoms: muscle cramps, migraines, and a condition called orthostatic hypotension, in which their blood pressure dropped when they first stood up, making them light-headed.

Fifty of the 94 people took 250 to 1,000 milligrams of magnesium daily, in addition to their regular treatment, for four months to four years.

Overall, there was a 90 percent decrease in muscle cramps, a 47 percent decrease in chest pain and a definite decrease in blood vessel spasms in the people taking magnesium, reports the study's main researcher, Cecil Coghlan, M.D., professor of medicine at the University of Alabama School of Medicine. Palpitations also were markedly less, and a certain kind of heart arrhythmia called premature ventricular contraction was reduced by 27 percent. People taking magnesium also reported fewer migraines and less fatigue.

Magnesium deficiency can be induced by the very drugs meant to help heart problems, such as digitalis and some types of diuretics (water pills). These drugs cause the body to excrete both magnesium and potassium, leaving people in short supply of these nutrients.

Others most likely to come up short on magnesium, in Dr. Scordo's opinion, are those who drink a lot of soft drinks or alcohol, those under stress, and anyone eating a poor diet with lots of calories from sugar or fat. "The consensus among magnesium watchers is that it is one of the most prevalent and important deficiencies in North America," according to Dr. Baker. Poor diet is to blame.

"We tell people to make sure that they are getting the Daily Value of magnesium, 400 milligrams, through either foods or supplements," Dr. Scordo says. But because people employ a number of dietary changes to relieve their symptoms, "it's very hard for us to know if the magnesium is helpful or not," she adds.

Dr. Baker recommends from 200 to about 800 milligrams of magnesium a day, along with nutrients that work with magnesium, such as vitamin B_6. "People who are going to respond will begin to see improvement in their symptoms within a few days," he says.

Although magnesium is considered to be a fairly safe mineral, even in high doses, people with heart problems or kidney problems should take supplements only under medical supervision. Too much magnesium could cause a dangerous buildup of the mineral in the blood.

Note that people can have normal blood levels of magnesium and still have inadequate supplies in their tissues. If you are severely deficient, you may benefit by initially getting intravenous magnesium or high oral doses, Dr. Baker says. This treatment, of course, would have to be administered by your doctor.

Studies show that men get about 329 milligrams of magnesium daily, while women average 207 milligrams. Meats are a good source of magnesium, but if you want heart-healthy sources, try steamed or broiled halibut and mackerel, rice bran, nuts, seeds, tofu, and green leafy vegetables such as spinach and Swiss chard.

"And since the magnesium that's found in plants depends on the amount of magnesium in the soil, I recommend organically grown produce, which contains a better balance of minerals than produce grown with potassium-rich inorganic fertilizers," Dr. Baker adds.

Unlike magnesium, vitamin B_6 can be toxic in large doses.

Medical Alert

If you have been diagnosed with mitral valve prolapse, you should be under a doctor's care.

People with heart or kidney problems should take magnesium only under medical supervision.

Take B_6 supplements in excess of 100 milligrams per day only under the supervision of your doctor.

Osteoarthritis

Slowing Joint Wear and Tear

Check out a chicken drumstick the next time you bake a bird. You'll note that the knobby end of the thighbone is covered with a tough, rubbery coating. That's cartilage, a tissue designed to cushion joints and ensure smooth motion.

In osteoarthritis, cartilage breaks down. It becomes frayed, thin, perhaps even completely worn away in areas. The underlying bone disintegrates, while painful bone spurs may grow around the edges of the joint. A formerly smooth, quiet joint may feel like it's grinding. It might even sound rough, like crinkling cellophane, when it's moved.

No one really knows why cartilage breaks down. Heavy use of a joint is sometimes a contributing factor. Also, a joint injured in the past tends to develop osteoarthritis sooner than a normal joint, perhaps because misalignment causes cartilage wear.

Osteoarthritis usually develops slowly, over many years. Some people never have more than a mild ache. Others develop crippling pain, and a few even end up trading in a creaky old hip or knee for a shiny new titanium-alloy model.

Many doctors who treat osteoarthritis consider it pretty much an unavoidable part of growing older. In fact, more than half of people ages 65 and older can expect to have at least a touch of osteoarthritis. Those same doctors think there's not a whole lot that can be done for this disease, except to nurse aching joints with mild painkillers such as acetaminophen or aspirin, heat, and a careful balance of exercise and rest.

The relatively few doctors who treat osteoarthritis with nutritional therapy take a different stance, however. They contend that osteoarthritis is a metabolic disorder, a breakdown in the body's ability to regenerate bone and cartilage. Although they concede that the breakdown is partly the result of old age, they also believe that providing the proper nutrients, in proper amounts, can help stop the process of deterioration and reduce pain and swelling.

Unfortunately, while there is some sketchy evidence that certain nutrients can help osteoarthritis, the kind of large scientific studies that would confirm these benefits have yet to be done.

Until then, here's what doctors say may be helpful.

B$_{12}$ Gives Bones a Boost

Vitamin B$_{12}$ is best known for its role in maintaining a healthy blood supply. In the bone marrow, B$_{12}$ stimulates stem cells, a certain type of bone cell, to make red blood cells. When B$_{12}$ levels are low, people develop anemia.

But that's not the only role that vitamin B$_{12}$ plays in bone. A few years ago, researchers at the University of Southern California School of Medicine in Los Angeles discovered that B$_{12}$ also stimulates osteoblasts, another type of bone cell that generates not red blood cells but bone. That could be important to people with osteoarthritis because underneath degenerating cartilage, bone also deteriorates, causing additional pain and further cartilage erosion.

This finding about vitamin B_{12} led researchers at the University of Missouri in Columbia to try giving B_{12} to people with osteoarthritis in their hands. They found that people who took 20 micrograms of B_{12} (3.3 times the Daily Value of 6 micrograms) and 6,400 micrograms of folic acid, another B vitamin that works in concert with B_{12}, for two months had fewer tender joints and better hand strength and took less medicine for pain than people not getting this B vitamin combo. (This amount of folic acid is 16 times the Daily Value and should be taken only under medical supervision, as excess folic acid can actually mask signs of B_{12} deficiency.)

"This doesn't necessarily prove that vitamin B_{12} deficiency causes osteoarthritis or that getting extra B_{12} will cure it, but I'd say that it is definitely worth discussing with your doctor," says Margaret Flynn, R.D., Ph.D., a medical nutritionist at the University of Missouri–Columbia School of Medicine, the study's main researcher. She notes that the people in her study were not B_{12}-deficient. They were getting enough of the vitamin in their diets, and they had blood levels that are considered normal. Still, they benefited from getting more.

"Older people often have trouble absorbing vitamin B_{12}, and that accounts for about 95 percent of B_{12} deficiencies in the United States," she says. Taking large doses of vitamin B_{12} supplements may help overcome the absorption problem. Or your doctor may recommend B_{12} injections, she says.

Vitamin E Eases Painful Joints

Joints damaged by osteoarthritis don't get as hot and swollen as joints hit with rheumatoid arthritis, but they are somewhat inflamed. That's one reason why doctors sometimes recommend vitamin E for osteoarthritis. Vitamin E fights inflammation by neutralizing the biochemicals that are produced during inflammation. These biochemicals, released by immune cells, contain free radicals, unstable molecules that grab electrons from your body's healthy molecules, damaging cells in the process. Vitamin E offers up its own electrons, protecting cells from damage.

In a study by Israeli researchers, people with osteoarthritis who took 600 international units (IU) of vitamin E every day for 10 days had significant reductions in pain compared with when they were not taking vitamin E. "Vitamin E also apparently stimulates the body's deposit of cartilage-building proteins called proteoglycans," says Joseph Pizzorno Jr., N.D., a naturopathic physician and president of Bastyr University in Seattle.

Doctors recommend 400 to 600 IU of vitamin E, amounts that are considered safe, says Jonathan Wright, M.D., a doctor in Kent, Washington, who specializes in nutritional therapy and is the author of *Dr. Wright's Guide to Healing with Nutrition*. These large amounts are available only by supplementation. To get some vitamin E from foods, try sunflower oil, almond oil, and wheat germ. Most people get about 10 IU a day.

Selenium, a mineral that increases the effectiveness of vitamin E, is often added to the osteoarthritis formula in amounts of about 200 micrograms a day. "That amount is considered safe, but you won't want to take more than that without medical supervision," says Dr. Wright.

Vitamin C Stimulates Cartilage Repair

Most of us know vitamin C as an infection fighter and an immunity builder. But vitamin C is also used throughout the body to manufacture a variety of tissues, including collagen. Collagen forms a network of protein fibers that lay down the structural foundation for many tissues, including cartilage, bone, tendons, and muscles, all necessary to keep joints strong and operating smoothly.

"It's well-known that animals deficient in vitamin C develop an array of health problems associated with collagen breakdown, including joint pain and cartilage breakdown," Dr. Pizzorno says.

Guinea pigs, one of few animals besides humans that can't make vitamin C in their bodies, show the classic symptoms of osteoarthritis—cartilage erosion and inflammation—when put on a diet containing only a small amount of vitamin C.

And one study suggests that large amounts of vitamin C encourage the growth of cartilage cells (chondrocytes) by stimulating synthesis of these cells' genetic material, report researchers at the State University of New York at Stony Brook.

"Although there are no human studies confirming a benefit, there's enough evidence out there, I think, to include vitamin C in a program to slow osteoarthritis," Dr. Pizzorno says. And there's some evidence that vitamins C and E work together to protect cartilage from breakdown. You can get sufficient vitamin C for this purpose in a multivitamin/mineral supplement, he says.

Niacinamide Could Be Worth a Try

You may not have heard of niacinamide. It's a form of niacin, one of the B-complex vitamins.

Some nutrition-oriented doctors have been recommending large doses of niacinamide for osteoarthritis since the 1940s, when William Kaufman, M.D., Ph.D., a pioneer in nutrition research for the treatment of osteoarthritis, found it helpful in relieving swelling and joint pain and improving muscle strength.

"I've treated more than 1,000 patients for joint dysfunction using niacinamide alone or combined with other vitamins," says Dr. Kaufman, now retired, of Winston-Salem, North Carolina. Improvement is usually noticeable after the first few weeks and becomes even more pronounced with continued treatment, he says. Very severely damaged arthritic joints respond slowly, or don't respond at all, to niacinamide treatment, however.

No one really knows why niacinamide seems to help osteoarthritis, Dr. Kaufman admits. "The vitamin is thought to somehow improve the metabolism of joint cartilage," he says. No further studies of niacinamide have been published since Dr. Kaufman's work, but reports of its clinical use remain positive.

"As a practitioner who has been doing this for more than 20 years, I can tell you that niacinamide is extremely effective in a large majority of cases at taking the pain out of osteoarthritis and in most cases at taking out the swelling, too, and apparently stopping the process," Dr. Wright says.

Niacinamide is often recommended as an alternative to niacin because it produces fewer side effects. This is one remedy, however, for which medical supervision is essential. The large amounts of niacinamide used in this treatment, from 500 milligrams twice a day to 1,000 milligrams three times a day, have the potential to cause liver problems.

"Anyone taking more than 1,500 milligrams of niacinamide a day should have a blood test for liver enzymes after three months of treatment, then annually thereafter," Dr. Wright says. "If the levels are elevated, the dose should be reduced." Nausea is an early warning sign of stress on the liver.

If you have liver disease, you should not use this treatment.

Adding a Bit of Insurance

Doctors who treat osteoarthritis make an additional recommendation that's designed to cover all bases. They recommend a multivitamin/mineral supplement that provides the Daily Values of all of the essential vitamins and minerals.

That recommendation might not be such a bad bit of advice. There's a scattering of evidence that a host of nutrients—pantothenic acid, vitamin B_6, zinc, and copper and other trace minerals—play roles in maintaining healthy bones and cartilage. "And these nutrients interact in many ways that we still don't understand," Dr. Wright points out.

Medical Alert

If you have symptoms of osteoarthritis, you should see your doctor for proper diagnosis and treatment.

High amounts of folic acid should be taken only under medical supervision, as excess folic acid can actually mask signs of vitamin B_{12} deficiency.

Large amounts of niacinamide can cause liver

problems. Doses significantly above 100 milligrams a day require careful medical supervision. If you have liver disease, you should not use this treatment.

Selenium doses of 200 micrograms exceed the Daily Value for this mineral. While some doctors consider this dosage to be safe, you may want to talk to your physician before taking suplements.

If you are taking anticoagulant drugs, you should not take vitamin E supplements.

Osteoporosis

Walking Tall into Your Golden Years

Imagine a bank that never let you know how much (or how little) money you have in your account. Unless you were a diligent bookkeeper, chances are that sooner or later, you'd start bouncing checks. Well, your bones are that bank, only instead of money, you're withdrawing calcium.

Essentially, that's what happens when people get osteoporosis, a disease causing porous bones: Their skeletons become bankrupt. Their bodies have withdrawn more calcium from the bones than has been deposited over the years, and all that's left is a fragile shell.

Osteoporosis is responsible for 1.5 million fractures each year, most notably fractures of the vertebrae (these cause the hunched appearance often seen in elderly women), forearms, wrists, and hips (these are often crippling and sometimes fatal).

That's the bad news. The good news is that osteoporosis is both preventable and treatable.

"There is no reason that this disease should exist. It's so preventable just through nutrition and exercise, if a woman starts young enough," says Ruth S. Jacobowitz, former vice-president of Mount Sinai Medical Center in Cleveland, a member of the board of trustees of the National Council on Women's Health, and author of *150 Most-Asked Questions about Osteoporosis*. "It is never too early and never too late to build bone. Even very elderly women can still build some amount of bone density."

Making Deposits into the Bone Bank

The first step in building bone is understanding how bones work. Even after we've stopped growing, our bones undergo constant remodeling. *Remodeling* is the actual term that doctors use to describe the body's ongoing process of removing old bone and forming new bone. Generally, the formation of new bone stays ahead of, or even with, the removal of old bone during the first 20 to 30 years of our lives.

Sometime after age 30, our bones begin operating in the red, and both men and women lose slightly more bone than they form—that is, until women hit menopause and stop producing estrogen, one of the hormones that regulate remodeling. Then they lose significantly more bone than men, up to 2 to 5 percent a year during the first five to seven years after menopause. For this reason, osteoporosis is much more common among women, though it does occur in elderly men.

That is why it's particularly important for women to build and maintain peak bone mass, the maximum amount of bone that you can form during your lifetime. And you form peak bone mass by taking in calcium and getting plenty of exercise, explains Clifford Rosen, M.D., director of the Maine Center for Osteoporosis Research and Education at St. Joseph's Hospital in Bangor. The earlier you start, the better, because the majority of peak bone mass is achieved by your mid-twenties, though some researchers believe that you can build bone until age 35.

Does that mean you're doomed if you're already past age 30 and just learning what peak bone mass is? "Absolutely not," says Dr. Rosen. Calcium and exercise can prevent the bone loss that occurs in your thirties and forties. "And slowing bone loss is enough to keep you from having osteoporosis, no matter how low your peak bone mass," he says.

One of the most effective ways of preventing bone loss and osteoporotic fractures is hormone replacement therapy, says David Dempster, Ph.D., director of the Regional Bone Center at Helen Hayes Hospital in West Haberstraw, New York, and associate professor of clinical pathology at Columbia University in New York City. Hormone replacement therapy is not appropriate for all women, however. You should discuss the pros and cons of this treatment with your doctor.

And medical experts agree that for both women and men, a healthy diet plays an important role in preventing and treating osteoporosis.

In addition to calcium, the nutrients shown by research to have the best bone-building potential include vitamin D, boron, magnesium, fluoride, manganese, copper, zinc, and vitamin K. This is what we know so far.

Straight from the Cow

Mom always said, "Drink your milk, or you won't have strong teeth and bones." As usual, she was right.

"Far and away, the biggest problem with osteoporosis is a lack of calcium in people's diets," explains Paul Saltman, Ph.D., professor of biology at the University of California, San Diego.

Calcium, a mineral abundant in milk, is essential for strong, healthy bones. In fact, 99 percent of the body's calcium is stored in the skeleton. But you also need a stable level of serum calcium (calcium in your blood) for normal heartbeat, nerve and muscle function, and blood coagulation. It's your bones that suffer when there isn't enough to go around.

Maintaining enough calcium in the blood is the body's ultimate priority, explains Dr. Rosen. "If it doesn't have enough, it goes to the reservoir and takes it," he says. The reservoir, in this case, is your bones.

To keep that reservoir full and calcium-rich, Dr. Saltman recommends that all people, beginning in their teens, take supplements and eat a good diet to ensure that they receive between 1,200 and 1,500 milligrams of calcium daily.

According to researchers at the University of California, San Diego, every little bit of calcium counts. Of the 581 60- to 79-year-old women they studied, those who had drunk one or more glasses of milk daily as adolescents and young adults had significantly higher bone mineral density at the mid-forearm (3 to 4 percent), spine (5 percent), and hip than those who had not. The effect of drinking milk on bone mineral density was even greater at the hip (4 percent) and spine (7 percent) for adults ages 20 to 50.

Calcium can also be helpful in treating osteoporosis once the disease has developed. Investigators at Winthrop-University Hospital in Mineola, New York, studied 118 women past the age of menopause. Over a three-year period, they gave the women 1,700 milligrams of calcium, 1,700 milligrams of calcium plus the female hormones estrogen and progesterone, or placebos (medically ineffective pills). Though the calcium-hormone mix was most effective, calcium alone significantly slowed bone mineral loss. Researchers measured bone mineral loss in the upper thighbone, noting a 0.8 percent decline a year in the women taking calcium versus a 2 percent decline a year in those taking the placebos.

When it comes to getting enough calcium, however, drinking more milk is by no means the final word. Calcium from dairy products can be difficult to absorb, and many people have difficulty digesting dairy products, says Neal Barnard, M.D., president of the Physicians Committee for Responsible Medicine in Washington, D.C., and author of *Eat Right, Live Longer*. He recommends foods such as beans, broccoli, and fortified orange juice as calcium sources instead. Other calcium-rich foods include collard greens, kale, mustard greens, butternut squash, tofu, and sweet potatoes.

The Daily Value for calcium is 1,000 milligrams. And the National Institutes of Health in Bethesda, Maryland, recommends the following intakes:

◆ Men, ages 25 to 65: 1,000 milligrams

◆ Women, ages 25 to 50: 1,000 milligrams

◆ Pregnant and nursing women: 1,200 to 1,500 milligrams

◆ Women at menopause (ages 51 to 65) who are taking estrogen: 1,000 milligrams

◆ Women at menopause (ages 51 to 65) who are not taking estrogen: 1,500 milligrams

◆ Men and women over age 65: 1,500 milligrams

Since many people fall short of getting these amounts from foods, doctors often recommend supplements of between 500 and 1,200 milligrams of calcium per day to make up the difference.

Play in the Sunshine for Vitamin D

Often referred to as the sunshine vitamin, vitamin D is a must if you want all of that calcium to do any good. Vitamin D, which your skin makes whenever it's exposed to sunlight (except during the winter at northern latitudes), helps your body absorb calcium and build good bones.

There are no conclusive studies pointing to vitamin D deficiency as a direct cause of osteoporosis. It is well-documented that vitamin D deficiency causes osteomalacia, or soft bones, in adults, which could contribute to fractures.

Vitamin D might also be useful as an osteoporosis treatment. In one study, Finnish researchers found that 341 elderly people (mostly women ages 75 and older), given annual large-dose injections of vitamin D during a five-year period, experienced fewer fractures than 458 people who did not receive the vitamin.

"Research here in Boston and in Europe has found that up to 40 percent of elderly men and women with hip fractures are vitamin D–deficient," says Michael F. Holick, M.D., Ph.D., director of the General Clinical Research Center and chief of the Section of Endocrinology, Nutrition, and Diabetes, both at Boston University Medical Center, and director of the Vitamin D, Skin, and Bone Research Laboratory at Boston University School of Medicine.

Unfortunately, your skin's ability to manufacture vitamin D decreases with age, says Dr. Holick. Matters are even worse for those living where the days are short and the winters are long. You can't make any vitamin D in the wintertime at northern latitudes such as Boston. "During the months from November through February in Boston, even if you exposed your entire body to sunlight from sunrise to sunset, you would not be able to make enough vitamin D to satisfy your body's requirement," Dr. Holick says. And the closer your abode to the polar ice caps, the longer that stretch.

"This problem is compounded by the use of sunscreen in the summer," adds Dr. Holick. "Sunscreen with an SPF (sun protection factor) of eight is enough to markedly diminish your ability to make vitamin D. Clothing completely prevents it."

Although it's okay to drink fortified milk, you shouldn't count on it as your primary source of vitamin D, notes Dr. Holick. "It is difficult to fortify milk with vitamin D, and our research has shown that only 30 percent of milk samples contain the amount of vitamin D shown on the label. That percentage is even lower in skim milk samples."

That makes it rather difficult to get adequate amounts of vitamin D from your diet alone. Fortunately, the answer to the vitamin D dilemma is as close as your local drugstore, especially if you walk there on a sunny day.

Vitamin D can be toxic in large doses. For that reason, you should never take supplements in excess of 600 international units (IU) daily unless your doctor specifically recommends it. Many multivitamin/mineral formulas contain adequate amounts of vitamin D, however. "Taking a multivitamin/mineral supplement that contains 400 IU of vitamin D essentially guarantees that you get at least the adult Daily Value of vitamin D, which is also 400 IU," says Dr. Holick. "We also recommend that people, particularly the elderly, go outside for 5 to 10 minutes, two or three times a week, during the spring, summer, and fall for sun exposure on their hands, faces, and arms. It is casual exposure to sunlight that provides us with more vitamin D."

Take Magnesium to Regulate Calcium

Magnesium, an essential mineral used to treat almost everything from depression to heart attack, is also crucial to bone health. Magnesium helps calcium get into the bones and also converts vitamin D to its active form in the body. Nearly half of the body's magnesium is found in the skeleton.

"We don't have enough research, but if I had to guess which nutrient is most important to bone health, I would say magnesium," says Alan Gaby, M.D., endowed chairman of therapeutic nutrition at Bastyr University in Seattle and author of *Preventing and Reversing Osteoporosis*.

Magnesium may also help in the treatment of osteoporosis. Researchers in Israel studied 31 women with osteoporosis who were past the age of menopause. They gave the women daily magnesium supplements of 250 to 750 milligrams for 6 months and then 250 milligrams for 18 months. At the end of that period, 22 women increased their bone density by 1 to 8 percent, and 5 women experienced decreases in their rates of bone loss. Conversely, bone density decreased markedly in 23 women who did not receive magnesium supplements during the same period.

Here in the United States, the U.S. Department of Agriculture continues to study magnesium's role in osteoporosis, says Forrest H. Nielsen, Ph.D., director of the U.S. Department of Agriculture–Agricultural Research Service Grand Forks Human Nutrition Research Center in North Dakota. "Based on what we know about magnesium regulating calcium, we can say that an adequate magnesium diet is necessary to maintain healthy bones," he says.

The Daily Value for magnesium is 400 milligrams. Since many Americans lack sufficient magnesium in their diets, doctors who recommend magnesium supplements advise taking 200 to 400 milligrams daily. (If you have heart or kidney problems, you should talk to your doctor before taking magnesium supplements.) Magnesium-rich foods include wheat germ, sunflower seeds, seafood, nuts, dairy products, and green leafy vegetables.

Boron Plugs the Calcium Leak

Researchers have speculated that boron, a trace mineral found mostly in fruits and vegetables, may reduce urinary excretion of both calcium and magnesium and therefore help prevent osteoporosis.

"It's still too early to tell how much of a benefit boron is," says Curtiss Hunt, Ph.D., a research biologist at the Grand Forks Human Nutrition Research Center. In one study, Dr. Hunt and his fellow researchers found marginal differences in the amounts of calcium and magnesium excreted in the urine of 12 women past the age of menopause who were given first a low-boron diet and then daily supplements of three milligrams of boron.

"So far, we've found that boron has a slight effect in decreasing urinary excretion of calcium and magnesium as well as in increasing the production of estrogen and testosterone, but the results haven't been dramatic," says Dr. Hunt. "It's still important to eat a boron-rich diet, however. Beyond a shadow of a doubt, boron affects bone and mineral metabolism, especially in animals. But it would be foolhardy to take boron supplements at this time. People should eat their fruits and vegetables. You can get 0.5 milligram of boron just by eating one good-size apple."

Something in the Water Could Help

Fluoride, the electrically charged form of fluorine, has long been touted for its cavity-fighting ability. Now some researchers believe it can build bones as well.

"The women in our study had a 70 percent reduction in spinal fractures over a 30-month period and close to a 5 percent increase in spinal bone density every year for almost three years," says Khashayar Sakhaee, M.D., professor of internal medicine at the

Center for Mineral Metabolism and Clinical Research of the University of Texas Southwestern Medical Center at Dallas.

In the study, Dr. Sakhaee gave 48 women who were past menopause 25 milligrams of slow-release fluoride and 800 milligrams of calcium (as calcium citrate) twice a day for three 12-month cycles, with a 2-month break from fluoride between cycles. With this new method of delivery, Dr. Sakhaee says, fluoride treatment is safe and effective.

"Other researchers used to use a rapid-release fluoride that went right to the skeleton, and the patients were getting toxic levels," says Dr. Sakhaee. The rapid-release formula did create dense bones, he explains, but the bone material it formed was brittle and weak. The new slow-release formula is creating strong bones.

Researchers remain leery about rapid-release sodium fluoride. Very high doses of fluoride, from 2,500 to 5,000 milligrams, can be fatal, though amounts needed for bone health are nowhere near that level, says Dr. Sakhaee.

"People really aren't getting enough fluoride to do their bones any good," says Dr. Sakhaee. He notes that soil and well water are rich in fluoride, but in towns and cities where the water is fluoridated, government standards prohibit more than 1 milligram of fluoride per liter of water. And many communities don't have fluoridated water at all.

Fluoride supplements are available only with a doctor's prescription. If you want to try fluoride, you'll have to discuss these supplements with your doctor. If your water isn't fluoridated, good food sources of fluoride include tea, mackerel, and canned salmon with bones. Daily intake of up to 10 milligrams of fluoride from foods and water is considered safe for adults.

Zinc, Copper, and Manganese: Working Together for Stronger Bones

For years, researchers have looked for connections between osteoporosis and the minerals zinc, copper, and manganese. While it's well-documented that deficiency of any one of these nutrients has a negative impact on bone health, research shows that they may work best when taken together.

"The diets of many elderly people are lacking in essential nutrients, including zinc. And certainly, zinc deficiency leads to problems with bone metabolism," says Joseph Soares, Ph.D., professor of nutrition in the nutritional sciences program at the University of Maryland at College Park. It's not known, however, whether zinc deficiency plays a role in the development of osteoporosis, he says.

The story is the same for copper. Experiments with copper deficiency in animals have been reported to produce bone abnormalities, and severe copper deficiency has been reported to result in osteoporosis in malnourished premature infants, says J. Cecil Smith, Ph.D., research chemist at the U.S. Department of Agriculture phytonutrients laboratory in Beltsville, Maryland. "But there are no conclusive studies on copper and osteoporosis," he says.

Manganese is also essential to bone formation, and manganese deficiency has been reported in women with osteoporosis. Dr. Nielsen maintains that like zinc and copper, manganese probably works best in concert with other vitamins and minerals.

Recognizing the importance of each of these minerals, investigators at the University of California, San Diego, studied the effects of zinc, copper, and manganese when taken together. During a two-year study of 59 women past the age of menopause, the researchers found that 1,000 milligrams of calcium slowed spinal bone mineral loss. Adding a "mineral cocktail" of 15 milligrams of zinc, 2.5 milligrams of copper, and 5 milligrams of manganese, however, actually stopped bone mineral loss in these women.

"For the best results, I recommend that people take a multivitamin/mineral supplement that supplies 100 percent of the daily requirements of zinc, copper, and manganese as well as a separate calcium supplement," says Dr. Saltman, a leading investigator in the study.

The Daily Value for zinc is 15 milligrams; for both copper and manganese, it's 2 milligrams. Since too much zinc can block the absorption of copper, it is important to keep them in balance.

Vitamin K: The Unsung Hero

If you were to tell someone to get vitamin K, their response would probably be "Vitamin what?" Yet vitamin K, abundant in the food chain and produced by intestinal bacteria, plays a key role in bone formation. And vitamin K deficiency, which was previously thought to be very rare, may be a factor in osteoporosis.

"Research shows that people with osteoporosis have low blood levels of vitamin K," says Dr. Gaby, who believes that vitamin K deficiency may not be all that rare. When medical scientists deemed vitamin K deficiency a rarity, they were using crude measuring techniques, he says. "And our overuse of antibiotics today may be inhibiting intestinal vitamin K production," he adds.

One study done in the Netherlands, in fact, showed that vitamin K may help protect the body's calcium stores. Seventy women past the age of menopause were given one milligram (1,000 micrograms) of vitamin K daily for three months. They experienced "significant" decreases in urinary calcium loss.

The Daily Value for vitamin K is 80 micrograms, and it's easy to get this vitamin in your diet. Fruits, leafy greens, root vegetables, seeds, and dairy products are all good sources. For those who wish to take supplements, 100 micrograms daily is a safe limit, says Dr. Gaby, although he often prescribes larger amounts in specific cases.

The Grab Bag

In addition to these vitamins and minerals, some doctors have suggested the possible benefits of vitamin C, vitamin B_6, and folic acid. Researchers don't recommend individual supplements of these nutrients for osteoporosis, but they don't hesitate to recommend a little multivitamin/mineral insurance.

"It wouldn't hurt to take your calcium supplement as well as a multivitamin/mineral to make sure that you're getting the Daily Values of all of the essential vitamins and minerals," advises Dr. Saltman.

Medical Alert

If you have been diagnosed with osteoporosis, you should be under a doctor's care.

If you have heart or kidney problems, you should talk to your doctor before taking magnesium supplements.

Phlebitis

Staying Out of Deep Trouble

You might think you've been kicked in the leg or you've pulled a muscle, but you can't for the life of you remember just when or where or how it happened. That's because it didn't happen. That painful knot you feel in your calf isn't a bruise or a muscle injury. It's phlebitis, a swollen, inflamed vein that can be caused by anything from staying put too long to birth control pills.

Phlebitis is not uncommon. And it's not necessarily that serious when it occurs in a superficial vein, since these veins are numerous enough to permit your body to rechannel the flow of blood, bypassing the inflamed vein.

Phlebitis that occurs in deep veins, called thrombophlebitis, is a serious matter. It usually involves formation of a blood clot in the vein, and it can lead to life-threatening circulation problems. "If the clot breaks free, it can travel to the brain, lungs, or heart and cause devastating damage," explains Robert Ginsburg, M.D., director of the cardiovascular intervention unit at the University of Colorado Health Sciences Center in Denver.

Thrombophlebitis doesn't always have clear symptoms, but it can be detected with ultrasound. It must be treated promptly with blood-thinning medication. Superficial phlebitis, which is most likely to occur in varicose veins, responds to a judicious combination of exercise and resting with your feet elevated. "Stopping smoking is also important, since chemicals in tobacco get into the bloodstream and promote clotting," Dr. Ginsburg says.

These nutritional approaches may also help prevent phlebitis and its worst consequences.

B Vitamins May Help Stop Clots

Several years ago researchers discovered that people with high blood levels of an amino acid called homocysteine had a high risk of developing damage to endothelial cells, the cells lining artery walls. Once these cells are damaged, cholesterol deposits can build up fast. These people frequently suffered from severe heart disease, experiencing heart attacks in their twenties and thirties.

Dutch researchers discovered a second problem connected with homocysteine. They found elevated blood levels of this substance in people who had recurring blood clots in their veins. As the blood levels of homocysteine increased, so did people's risk of forming clots. Even moderately elevated levels of homocysteine were linked to two to three times the normal risk of recurrent blood clots.

What do B vitamins have to do with all of this? Researchers now know that three B vitamins—folate (the naturally occurring form of folic acid), vitamin B_6, and vitamin B_{12}—help break down and clear homocysteine from the blood. "Deficiency of any one could lead to high levels of homocysteine," explains Jacques Genest Jr., M.D., director of the cardiovascular genetics laboratory at the Clinical Research Institute of Montreal, a research center that has done pioneering work on homocysteine and heart disease.

Dr. Genest usually measures blood levels of folate and vitamin B_6 in people found to have high blood levels of homocysteine. (He has found that the people he studies, mostly middle-aged men with coronary heart disease, aren't usually low in vitamin B_{12}.) Then he provides supplements as necessary.

"We've found that 2.5 milligrams (2,500 micrograms) of folic acid or 25 milligrams of vitamin B_6 reduces homocysteine levels to normal in most people," he says. Some people may need to take both, he says, and people at risk for vitamin B_{12} deficiency (older people, strict vegetarians, and those with absorption problems) also need to make sure that their blood levels of B_{12} are adequate. Dr. Genest recommends taking 2 micrograms of B_{12} a day.

The high amounts of folic acid and vitamin B_6 that Dr. Genest recommends are available only through supplements and, in the case of folic acid, should be taken only under medical supervision. Folic acid can actually mask signs of a vitamin B_{12} deficiency. Even those eating a healthy diet, with two to three servings of fruits and three to four servings of vegetables a day, get only about 190 micrograms of folate a day. As for B_6, men get about 1.9 milligrams and women get about 1.2 milligrams a day through foods such as chicken, fish, pork, and eggs.

Dietary vitamin B_{12} is less of a problem. Most

people do get enough from meats, dairy products, and eggs, with men getting almost 8 micrograms and women getting about 5 micrograms a day. People with absorption problems, however, usually need to get injections of this vitamin.

Vitamin E May Improve the Flow

Evidence is mounting that vitamin E helps protect against cardiovascular disease by helping to block the chemical processes that lead to atherosclerosis, or hardening of the arteries.

Vitamin E plays an additional role, one that's particularly important to people with phlebitis. Several studies indicate that vitamin E can help protect against potentially life-threatening blood clots. Specifically, vitamin E helps prevent platelets, components involved in blood clotting, from sticking to each other and to blood vessel walls.

"Sticky platelets can cause blood clots to build up fast," explains Joseph Pizzorno Jr., N.D., a naturopathic physician and president of Bastyr University in Seattle. Studies suggest that reducing platelet stickiness with vitamin E could have a role in the treatment of "thromboembolic events," or traveling blood clots, especially in people with Type I (insulin-dependent) diabetes, who are at particularly high risk for blood-clotting problems.

If you're going to take vitamin E, Dr. Pizzorno suggests that 200 to 600 international units (IU) daily should do the trick. Some research suggests that 200 IU is enough to reduce platelet adhesion.

Medical Alert

Consult your doctor before supplementing your diet with B vitamins. Blood tests need to be done to determine your exact deficiencies before a doctor can prescribe the best combination and amounts. In addition, folic acid in doses exceeding 400 micrograms daily can mask symptoms of vitamin B_{12} deficiency.

If you are taking anticoagulant drugs, you should not take vitamin E supplements.

Premenstrual Syndrome

Putting an End to Monthly Discomfort

Ask 10 women what premenstrual syndrome feels like, and you'll probably get 10 different answers. A few of those answers will be pretty predictable: bloated, sore, headachy. Other women feel okay physically but ride an emotional roller coaster of anxiety and depression.

And—something you probably don't want to hear if you have premenstrual syndrome—some women don't experience any premenstrual symptoms at all.

Experts estimate that as many as 50 percent of menstruating women in the United States have some degree of premenstrual syndrome, or PMS. Whether you're one of them depends on a variety of factors, including your genetic inheritance, how much stress you're under, whether you drink alcohol or caffeine, and how much you exercise. Age is also a factor: Women in their thirties and forties are more likely to get PMS than younger women.

And finally, some researchers believe that nutrition exerts a powerful influence on how a woman feels both before and during her period. PMS researcher Guy Abraham, M.D., became so convinced of the importance of nutrition that he left his teaching position at the University of California, Los Angeles, UCLA School of Medicine to found Optimox, a Torrance, California, company that manufactures nutritional supplements. "Nutrition is the single most important factor in whether or not a woman will have PMS," says Dr. Abraham. "This is why we see so much PMS among women in their thirties. Most of them have been pregnant, which has depleted their bodies of nutrients, so they're more likely to be deficient in the B vitamins and magnesium."

Here's what researchers have learned about the nutrition connection.

Calcium: Woman's Best Friend

If you've picked up a health book or magazine lately, you know all about calcium's role in preventing osteoporosis, the brittle-bone disease that incapacitates thousands of women (and men) each year. But if scientific studies are any indication, there may be another, more immediate reason to add a calcium supplement to your medicine chest.

A study conducted at Metropolitan Hospital in New York City found that a daily supplement of 1,000 milligrams of calcium reduced premenstrual symptoms in 73 percent of the women who took it. The women, who normally experienced premenstrual symptoms every month, reported less breast tenderness and swelling and fewer headaches and abdominal cramps when they took the calcium supplements every day during the preceding month. They also reported less discomfort during their periods.

It isn't clear exactly why calcium relieves PMS, but the researchers suspect that it eases the muscular contractions that lead to cramping.

And this isn't the only study to find a connection between calcium and PMS. A small study at the U.S. Department of Agriculture Grand Forks Human Nutrition Research Center in North Dakota found an intriguing connection between a diet low in both calcium and the trace mineral manganese and PMS. Women who experienced PMS on a low-calcium, low-manganese diet had fewer symptoms when their diet was supplemented with the two minerals.

What's interesting, says James G. Penland, Ph.D., head researcher at the Grand Forks Human Nutrition Research Center and one of the authors of the study, is that the diet that produced the worst premenstrual symptoms is actually closest to the way most American women eat. Dr. Penland's studies show that most women get about 587 milligrams of calcium a day, nowhere near the 1,000 milligrams they're supposed to get to build healthy bones and prevent osteoporosis.

Manganese intake among American women is only about 2.2 milligrams a day. That's a little more than the Daily Value for this mineral.

While researchers continue studying the connection between calcium and manganese and PMS, a daily supplement that includes both minerals can't hurt and might help if you're prone to PMS, says Dr. Penland. Check to see if your multivitamin/mineral formula provides 2 to 5 milligrams of manganese. As for calcium, "I would recommend increasing your intake of low-fat, calcium-rich foods such as low-fat yogurt and milk. If that is difficult, then I suggest taking 500 to 1,000 milligrams of supplemental calcium a day," he says.

Mellow Out with Magnesium

Magnesium is another mineral that seems to have a beneficial effect on women with PMS. A few studies have found lower magnesium levels in women with PMS than in women without symptoms. Other studies suggest that increasing magnesium levels might reduce or eliminate premenstrual discomfort, especially emotional symptoms such as tension and anxiety.

Magnesium deficiency causes a shortage of dopamine, a chemical found in the brain that regulates mood, according to Dr. Abraham. This shortage may have something to do with the premenstrual tension and irritability that many women experience.

In one Italian study of 28 women with PMS, a magnesium supplement of 360 milligrams was associated with fewer cramps, less water retention and an overall improvement in premenstrual symptoms.

The Daily Value for magnesium is 400 milligrams. The best sources of magnesium are nuts, legumes, whole grains, and green vegetables, all of the staples of a low-fat, high-fiber diet. But if your diet leans more toward white bread, white rice, meats, and dairy products, your body is probably coming up short on magnesium.

To help even things up, Dr. Abraham recommends a magnesium supplement of 300 to 400 milligrams.

"Your body will tell you exactly how much magnesium you need within that range. Too much will cause diarrhea, so I tell women to take magnesium to bowel tolerance." If you have heart or kidney problems, be sure to talk to your doctor before taking magnesium supplements.

Vitamin E Smoothes Out Rough Edges

Vitamin E also seems to lessen the severity of premenstrual symptoms. In two separate studies, a team of Baltimore scientists examined the effect of vitamin E supplements on women prone to PMS. The women received vitamin E in the form of d-alpha-tocopherol every day for two consecutive menstrual cycles. The supplement made a substantial difference in premenstrual symptoms such as mood swings, cravings, bloating, and depression.

The women in the study, like most women with PMS, had normal dietary intakes of vitamin E. But the amount of vitamin E in the typical diet apparently isn't enough to treat some PMS, according to Robert S. London, M.D., assistant professor of obstetrics and gynecology at Johns Hopkins University School of Medicine in Baltimore and one of the authors of the study.

"The average person consumes a small amount of vitamin E in foods such as vegetable oils, but this certainly isn't enough to have any effect on PMS," says Dr. London. "The effect was clearly dose-responsive: 400 international units (IU) was much more effective than 200 IU. It's impossible for a woman to get these levels of vitamin E through diet alone."

It isn't clear why vitamin E has an effect on PMS.

Some experts have suggested that it works by slowing the production of prostaglandins, hormonelike substances thought to play a role in premenstrual symptoms.

If you'd like to try vitamin E for PMS, experts generally advise a dosage of 400 IU daily. Take it for at least six weeks to give it a chance to work, advises Dr. London. "It usually takes about that long," he says. The d-alpha-tocopherol form of vitamin E used in the study is readily available; just be sure to check the label before you buy. (Other forms of the vitamin haven't been studied for PMS.)

Beat PMS with B$_6$

Finally, if you're bothered by premenstrual weight gain and emotional symptoms, vitamin B$_6$ can help control them, says Dr. Abraham. In a study of 25 women with PMS, Dr. Abraham found that a high-dose supplement of B$_6$ reduced premenstrual weight gain and lessened the severity of other premenstrual symptoms.

The women in the study were given high doses of vitamin B$_6$: 500 milligrams a day for three months (the Daily Value is only 2 milligrams). B$_6$ at this level eases PMS by changing blood levels of two female hormones, estrogen and progesterone, according to Dr. Abraham. But high doses of the vitamin can be dangerous, so supplementation should be used only under the supervision of your doctor.

If you'd like to try vitamin B$_6$ for premenstrual symptoms, Dr. Abraham recommends taking it as part of a B-complex supplement. "B$_6$ taken by itself can cause deficiencies of other nutrients, so it's important to balance it with the other B vitamins," he says.

You should also make sure that you're getting enough magnesium, he adds. "I generally recommend taking twice as much magnesium as vitamin B_6. So if you're taking 300 to 400 milligrams of magnesium, you need 150 to 200 milligrams of B_6."

Medical Alert

If you have heart or kidney problems, you should talk to your doctor before taking magnesium supplements.

High doses of B_6 can cause side effects and should be used only under the supervision of your doctor.

If you are taking anticoagulant drugs, you should not take vitamin E supplements.

Prostate Cancer

Surprising Findings Offer New Hope

For an organ the size of a walnut, the prostate can cause huge health problems. Although prostate cancer targets mainly men over age 50, it's never too early to start thinking about how to reduce your chances of developing the disease. Caught early, prostate cancer can be stopped cold 91 percent of the time. Because it shows no symptoms until it's serious, the American Cancer Society recommends that all men over age 40 get yearly checks.

First, get a yearly digital rectal exam, in which a doctor feels the prostate with a gloved finger to detect irregularities. This should begin at age 40. Second, get a blood test that measures prostate-specific antigen (PSA), a prostate-produced protein whose levels rise when the gland has a problem. For men over 50, the American Cancer Society recommends this blood test annually. High-risk men such as African-Americans and men who have a family history of prostate cancer should start both types of annual testing at age 40.

While testing is certainly important, scientists have uncovered intriguing evidence that certain nutrients may play a role in preventing prostate cancer.

Passing the Folic Acid Test

By age 50 or so, a man's prostate will most likely develop 10 to 1,000 cancerous cells, says Warren Heston, Ph.D., director of the George M. O'Brien Urology Center at Memorial Sloan-Kettering Cancer Center in New York City. It's like a breeding ground for cancer. If this microscopic area does not expand or spread, then prostate cancer as a disease will not develop. If, for whatever reason, the lesion does grow, full-blown prostate cancer develops.

It now appears that folic acid may play a key role in determining whether cancer develops. This B vitamin—known as folate when it comes naturally from food—can diffuse into healthy prostate membrane cells. The trouble comes when there is a lot of the enzyme folate hydrolase in the prostate. Folate hydrolase may block folic acid from being glutamylated. Glutamylation prevents folic acid from being able to leak back out of a cell. This puts the prostate at substantial risk to develop "localized folate deficiency," which acts in concert with cancer-causing agents to develop cancers. Folate-deficient cells are more susceptible to cancer mutations, Dr. Heston says.

"Is prostate tissue at risk for folate deficiency due to an excess of folate hydrolase? That's what we need to find out," says Dr. Heston.

Because the prostate has too much folate hydrolase, Dr. Heston thinks that obtaining higher amounts of folic acid in the diet might turn out to be useful in controlling the onset of prostate cancer. "However, that might be a two-edged sword, because even though the prostate develops malignant cells, prostate cancers are often very slow growing. It is not certain whether high folic acid supplementation would increase the rate of tumor growth, and it is one of the reasons why I'm cautious of recommending very high supplementation of folic acid to anybody," he says.

Dr. Heston consciously tries to get more folate in his daily diet, and he takes a multivitamin/mineral supplement with 100 percent of the Daily Value for folic acid (400 micrograms). Foods that contain folate include vegetables, beans, fruits, whole grains, and fortified breakfast cereals.

And keep in mind that vitamins B_6 and B_{12} help folic acid do its job better. "It's like a car being tuned up: You want to make sure that everything, not just one part of the engine, is running smoothly," says Dr. Heston. A good multivitamin should help take care of this.

Scientists are looking at the potential of other vitamins and minerals to protect your prostate. Here are the most promising areas.

Vitamin E May Be Protective

In lung cancer studies examining the effects of beta-carotene and vitamin E, an unexpected discovery was made. "Interestingly, even though it wasn't protective against lung cancer, vitamin E given to patients—with and without beta-carotene—was associated with a 60 to 70 percent decrease in prostate cancer," Dr. Heston says. "Given as a supplement to those individuals, it did look like it was having an impact on the number of patients developing prostate cancer within the time frame of the trial."

It is not yet clear whether the nutrient exerts its effect on an unidentified receptor in the prostate or whether it is having these beneficial effects by its known antioxidant effects, Dr. Heston says.

The vitamin E dosages in those studies were many times higher than the current Daily Value of 30 international units (IU), says Dr. Heston. Ongoing trials are now focusing on giving about 800 IU of alpha-tocopherol (the compound in vitamin E that appears to have the greatest anti-cancer benefits) daily to men. "At this level, it's strong enough to act like a medication rather than a nutrient but still well below toxic amounts," Dr. Heston says. It's still too early to recommend taking vitamin E to all men, he notes. However, taking 400 IU daily—the same safe amount recommended by many doctors for heart disease prevention—may be beneficial for men with troublesome PSA readings, Dr. Heston says. If you are taking anticoagulant medications, talk to your doctor before supplementing with vitamin E.

Selenium: A Promising Nutrient

In a study led by Larry Clark, Ph.D., of the Arizona Cancer Center in Tucson, 1,312 people with a history of skin cancer were given either 200 micrograms of high-selenium yeast (a supplement) or a placebo (inactive substance) over the course of 10 years. While skin cancer did not seem to be influenced, a significant reduction in risk was seen for prostate cancer.

While he feels that further research needs to be done before selenium supplementation can be promoted for prostate cancer prevention, Dr. Heston says that taking a multivitamin that includes selenium is safe and acceptable. High doses—100 to 200 micrograms—can be toxic and should only be taken under medical supervision.

The Link with Lycopene

There's a chemical in fruits and vegetables—especially tomatoes—called lycopene that may offer prostate cancer protection. Actually, lycopene comes from a good anti-cancer family. It's a carotenoid, like beta-carotene, and one of a growing number of phytochemicals in produce that researchers think might help fight off cancer, says James Anderson, M.D., professor of medicine and clinical nutrition at the University of Kentucky in Lexington.

A study of 47,849 men has shown a link between eating a lot of tomatoes, especially tomato sauce cooked with a little olive oil, and lower risk of prostate cancer. Compared with men who ate no tomato sauce, men who ate even as little as two servings a week had a 34 percent reduction in risk for prostate cancer. Researchers theorize that the cooking process and the touch of olive oil in the sauce seem to enhance the absorption of lycopene.

Medical Alert

Doses of selenium that exceed 100 micrograms daily should be taken only under medical supervision.

If you are taking anticoagulant drugs, you should not take vitamin E supplements.

Smoking

Damage Control While Kicking the Habit

Unless you come from another planet, you know the evils of smoking. And if you're a smoker, you've likely tried to quit more than once. And you plan to try again. That's good.

While kicking the habit is your number one priority, there are measures you can take nutritionally to block smoking's path of destruction while you work on "butting out" once and for all. For a little motivation, it helps to first understand how cigarette smoke damages your body.

A Radical Habit

Though all of the harmful reactions caused by smoking are not completely understood, researchers agree that the lion's share of smokers' ailments are the result of free radicals. Free radicals are unstable molecules that are missing electrons. They pillage your body's healthy molecules for replacement electrons, leaving more free radicals and damaged cells and tissues in their wake. This process is called oxidation, and it's what makes iron rust and fruit turn brown. And scientists are beginning to believe that oxidation is what makes people age.

Though free radicals are formed during everyday functions such as breathing, environmental stress factors such as smoking dramatically accelerate their production. In fact, each puff on a cigarette generates millions of free radicals, making smokers much more susceptible than nonsmokers to the ravages of oxidative tissue damage.

To fight this free radical onslaught, you need a strong defense. And according to research, one of the best defenses consists of nutrients known as antioxidants, most notably vitamins C and E and beta-carotene. Antioxidants act as your body's kamikaze fighters, protecting your body's healthy molecules by sacrificing their own electrons to neutralize hostile free radical invaders.

Though antioxidants aren't miracle cures and certainly shouldn't lure you into a false sense of security about smoking, these nutrients can help stave off smoking-related damage while you're kicking the habit. Here's what experts recommend.

E Is Essential for Smokers

When it comes to protecting your body from smoking's nasty side effects, vitamin E, an antioxidant found in sunflower seeds, sweet potatoes, and kale, is a top performer.

One of vitamin E's most important functions for smokers is slowing the progression of atherosclerosis, a condition in which the coronary arteries harden from deposits of cholesterol, calcium, and scar tissue, gradually restricting blood flow and leading to heart disease. Studies show that before atherosclerosis can occur, LDL cholesterol, the "bad" kind, has to undergo oxidation-related changes that allow it to deposit on artery walls. Vitamin E helps prevent those changes.

"Our data from two separate studies of men and women suggest that both smokers and nonsmokers taking vitamin E supplements reduce their risk of heart disease by 30 to 40 percent," says Eric Rimm, Sc.D., assistant professor in the department of epidemiology at Harvard School of Public Health.

Additionally, investigators believe that vitamin E's ability to scavenge free radicals can protect tissues from smoke irritation and discourage the cell mutation that marks cancer and other tobacco-associated chronic diseases.

For optimum effects, experts recommend getting 100 to 200 international units (IU) of vitamin E every day. Since you would have to eat between 10 and 20 cups of foods such as chopped kale and diced sweet potatoes to reach that amount, supplements are generally called·for.

Beta-Carotene Protection

Ever notice how Popeye is able to puff away on that pipe, yet never suffer from the smoking-related ailments typically seen in a man his age? That may be the result of his penchant for spinach, a vegetable rich in beta-carotene, which appears to have protective, immunity-building effects against cancer.

But before you start popping beta-carotene, you should know that although supplementation is considered okay by most experts, doctors say that it's even better to eat beta-carotene–rich foods such as spinach and other dark green leafy vegetables as well as cantaloupe, carrots, and other orange and yellow fruits and vegetables. Why? Because studies show that beta-carotene is good, but it's probably not the whole story.

On the one hand, myriad small studies have found positive results from beta-carotene supplementation in smokers. Canadian researchers, for example, found that 25 smokers experienced significant reductions in oxidation-related damage after receiving 20 milligrams (about 33,000 IU) of beta-carotene daily for just four weeks.

But in one large study from Finland of 29,133 male heavy smokers between 50 and 69 years of age, those who received 20 milligrams (about 33,000 IU) of beta-carotene for five to eight years not only didn't reap any benefits but actually experienced a higher incidence of lung cancer.

Which study should we believe? Both, says Jeffrey Blumberg, Ph.D., associate director and chief of the antioxidants research laboratory at the Jean Mayer USDA Human Nutrition Research Center on Aging at Tufts University in Boston. Dr. Blumberg contends that the Finnish study represents what we already know: "You can't undo a lifetime of damage by taking a vitamin pill for five years.

"That population was at extraordinarily high risk," says Dr. Blumberg. "They smoked an average of a pack a day for 35 years. Most of them were overweight. They had high cholesterol. They had moderate to high alcohol consumption. It would have been a public health nightmare if the study had worked, because it would have said 'Smoke and drink and eat all you want. This pill can turn around all of the damage.'"

Actually, the group in the Finnish study that did not receive supplements also taught us something, says Dr. Blumberg. "Among the people who weren't supplemented, those who had the highest blood levels of beta-carotene had the lowest risk of lung cancer," he says.

The bottom line? Dr. Blumberg recommends that everyone, smokers and nonsmokers, get between 16,500 and 50,000 IU of beta-carotene daily.

Finally, it's important to remember that beta-carotene is just one of many related substances called carotenoids that protect the body from cell damage, says Dr. Rimm. "All of the carotenoids function a little differently, so getting beta-carotene from fruits and vegetables covers a lot more bases than just taking a supplement." It's best to strive for getting as much of your 16,500 to 50,000 IU a day as possible from foods. If you're having trouble meeting your needs in this way, then talk to your doctor about supplementation.

Vitamin C for Healthy Cells and Sperm

It's a joke among male smokers that they don't feel as bad about smoking when they buy packs with the "Do not smoke while pregnant" warning on the side panel. Well, according to researchers, it may be time for male smokers to get a warning of their own.

Studies have found a connection linking smoking, low levels of ascorbic acid (vitamin C), and sperm abnormalities. These abnormalities could play roles not only in infertility in men but also in birth defects and childhood cancer in their offspring, the studies show.

"We've known that many gene mutations come through the male line, but since women carry the babies, most of the birth defect studies are done on women," says Bruce Ames, Ph.D., professor of biochemistry and molecular biology and director of the National Institute of Environmental Health Sciences Center at the University of California, Berkeley. "We're looking into the effects of paternal smoking on sperm damage, and the effects of antioxidant depletion are significant."

Smokers must ingest two to three times the daily intake of vitamin C recommended for nonsmokers, or about 180 milligrams, just to maintain comparable levels of ascorbic acid, says Dr. Ames. He has also found that as a group, smokers tend to make their deficiencies worse by not eating enough vitamin C–rich foods.

While studying the vitamin C consumption of 22 smokers and 27 nonsmokers, Dr. Ames and his colleagues found that the smokers consumed less vitamin C than the nonsmokers. In addition, the level of oxidative damage in the sperm was 52 percent higher in the smokers than in the nonsmokers.

Of course, sperm are not alone in their need for vitamin C. The rest of your body, whether you're male or female, needs it, too. And because smokers have too little vitamin C in their bodies and need more vitamin C to fight free radical damage, experts suggest that they take much more than nonsmokers: up to 2,000 milligrams a day, if they are older and smoke heavily. Just keep in mind that the Daily Value for vitamin C is only 60 milligrams. Higher amounts are considered safe but may cause diarrhea in some people.

Calcium May Help Prevent Bone Loss

Research shows that people, especially women, who smoke accelerate the bone loss that occurs naturally with age, putting them at greater risk for osteoporosis, a condition of brittle, easily fractured bones.

In fact, a study done at the University of Melbourne in Australia looked at 41 pairs of female twins between 27 and 73 years of age in which one of the twins smoked and the other did not. The researchers reported that by the time women reach menopause, those who smoke a pack a day throughout adulthood have an average bone density deficit of 5 to 10 percent compared with those who are smoke-free.

Though the only surefire way to stem this bone deterioration is to snuff your cigarette habit, some doctors recommend stepping up your calcium intake in the meantime to nourish your bones. And while it will help to increase your intake of calcium-filled foods, including low-fat dairy products and certain vegetables such as broccoli, the best way to get the 1,500 milligrams that experts recommend is through supplements.

Better Body Function with B Complex

Because the B vitamins are essential for maintaining physical and mental fitness and healthy skin, eyes, nerves, and tissues—things that are deteriorated by smoking—many experts also recommend taking supplements of the B-complex vitamins.

Especially important, say researchers, is folic acid, a nutrient that is often deficient in smokers and one that your lungs love. Studies have shown that increased folic acid intake can lessen symptoms of bronchitis as well as reduce the number of abnormal or precancerous bronchial cells in smokers. Plus inadequate folic acid intake has been linked to increased susceptibility to cancerous changes in the lungs of smokers.

"Not only does smoking deplete the B vitamins, but smokers' diets often aren't as good as those of nonsmokers, so smokers don't get enough of these nutrients to begin with," says nutritionist James Scala, Ph.D., author of *If You Can't/Won't Stop Smoking*. Dr. Scala recommends that smokers take a B-complex supplement that contains the Daily Values of all of the B vitamins.

Finish Off with a Multivitamin

"Because smoking depletes the body of all vitamins, smokers absolutely need to take a multivitamin/mineral supplement on top of their specific nutritional supplements," says Dr. Scala.

He also stresses the importance of smokers' adding more fruits and vegetables to their diets. "Smokers generally eat poor diets, which contributes to their nutritional deficiencies," he says.

Medical Alert

Some people may experience diarrhea when taking vitamin C in doses that exceed 1,500 milligrams daily.

If you are taking anticoagulant drugs, you should not take vitamin E supplements.

Surgery

Minding Your Mending

No doubt about it: Surgery is a major insult to your body. Even though it's done with the best of intentions and in a clean environment, your body needs to put out extra effort to mend from even minor surgery. And while you're recuperating, you're more vulnerable than usual to pneumonia, bedsores, urinary tract infections, and other kinds of infections.

That's why good nutrition is vital both before and after surgery. "It gives your body the building blocks to fight off infection, replenish lost blood, and mend tissues, all things that can help you heal as quickly as possible with the least pain and discomfort," explains Ray C. Wunderlich Jr., M.D., a doctor in St. Petersburg, Florida, who practices nutritional/preventive medicine and health promotion and author of *Natural Alternatives to Antibiotics*.

Medical experts are well aware that every single nutrient that your body normally needs is also needed when you're facing surgery, including everything from calories and protein to copper and vitamin B_6. "Keep in mind that every person's condition when undergoing surgery is different, so the types of vitamins and minerals that your doctor prescribes for you, if any, will depend on your own particular case," says Joanne Curran-Celentano, R.D., Ph.D., associate professor of nutrition and food sciences at the University of New Hampshire in Durham. "Because of the wide range of problems and conditions surrounding surgery, it is recommended that anyone who is about to undergo surgery check with his doctor before taking any kind of supplementation."

Not all doctors have the same approach to nutritional therapy and surgery. If you are facing surgery and want to pay special attention to nutrients that might be helpful, you'll have to find a doctor who uses methods that you feel most comfortable with.

Here are a few key nutrients that some doctors believe are important for getting your body on the high road to healing.

Vitamin C Speeds Healing

Doctors know that any kind of trauma, including surgery, can pull the plug on your vitamin C stores. After surgery, blood levels of vitamin C drop rapidly. And it's no secret that a vitamin C deficiency makes wounds heal slower. Delayed healing was noted hundreds of years ago in sailors with scurvy, a mystery disease at the time that turned out to be nothing more than severe vitamin C deficiency. "Today, it's more likely that people simply won't be getting enough vitamin C for optimum healing," Dr. Wunderlich says.

Many studies have shown that vitamin C is essential for the body to produce wound-healing collagen, which provides the basic structure for many tissues, including skin, bone, and blood vessels. Vitamin C is also needed for the skin to produce elastin, a tissue that lets wounds stretch without breaking.

Vitamin C also helps maintain a healthy immune system, vital for anyone who's undergoing surgery, Dr. Wunderlich says.

One study, by Russian researchers, found that

people who had gallbladder surgery who received 200 to 250 milligrams of supplemental vitamin C a day were able to leave the hospital one or two days earlier compared with people who simply got their vitamin C from foods.

At most hospitals, you're expected to get your vitamin C from foods such as citrus juices and fruits. Eight ounces of orange juice, for instance, offers about 124 milligrams, while one orange has about 70 milligrams.

Some doctors, however, recommend amounts of vitamin C that are much higher than you normally obtain from foods alone. Dr. Wunderlich believes this to be especially important when you're recovering from surgery.

He tells his patients that "if you can take 1,000 milligrams of buffered or esterified vitamin C every eight hours for two weeks before and several weeks after surgery, you'll most likely be able to keep the vitamin C in your blood at a level that promotes optimum healing." Some people experience diarrhea and other digestive discomforts from such high levels of vitamin C. Buffered vitamin C and esterified vitamin C (a slow-release form) are easier on the stomach, says Dr. Wunderlich. Vitamin C can interfere with the results of certain diagnostic blood and urine tests, however, so it's important that you discuss supplementation with your doctor.

Dr. Wunderlich also recommends 1,000 milligrams of bioflavonoids a day to some of his patients. These chemical compounds are related to vitamin C and are often found in the same foods as the vitamin, especially citrus fruits. He maintains that bioflavonoids can help maintain blood vessel strength and control inflammation.

Vitamin A Mends Skin

Vitamin A has been called the skin vitamin, and with good reason. At burn centers such as Shriners Burns Institute in Cincinnati, large amounts of vitamin A are added to liquid formulas designed to help prevent infection and promote the growth of new skin.

In studies with laboratory animals, vitamin A enhances healing that has been retarded by steroid drugs, immune suppression, diabetes, or radiation, reports Thomas K. Hunt, M.D., professor of surgery at the University of California, San Francisco.

"Vitamin A works in many different ways," Dr. Hunt says. "It's required for cell growth and differentiation, or the ability of a cell to mature into its final form. This is important for the generation of new tissues." Vitamin A also seems to activate the production of connective tissue, including collagen, and to promote the growth of new blood vessels, he explains. That's important for nourishing newly forming tissues.

"Adequate vitamin A really is essential for anyone undergoing surgery," Dr. Wunderlich agrees. He recommends up to 25,000 international units (IU) of water-soluble vitamin A (available in health food stores) for certain patients undergoing surgery. Vitamin A can be toxic in doses exceeding 15,000 IU daily and has been found to cause birth defects in doses of 10,000 IU daily when taken during early pregnancy. For this reason, the dosage of vitamin A recommended here should be taken only under medical supervision, especially if you are a woman of childbearing age. And you should not use this therapy if you are pregnant.

Studies show that most people get about 5,000 IU

a day from foods such as carrots, eggs, and vitamin A–fortified milk.

Zinc Zeros In on Tissue Repair

Medical research shows that in people who are low in zinc, supplements can dramatically speed up the healing of surgical incisions. In a study by researchers at Wright-Patterson Air Force Base in Ohio, people taking 220 milligrams of zinc sulfate three times a day were completely healed in roughly 46 days, while a group taking no zinc required about 80 days to heal.

Zinc, like vitamins A and C, is needed in the body for many things, Dr. Wunderlich says. It's necessary for the production of collagen, the connective tissue that allows scars to form. It interacts with vitamin A, making the vitamin available for use. And it plays a vital role in immune function.

The people most likely to be short on zinc include those who've lost lots of fluid, those who've lost weight because of loss of appetite, those who've experienced loss of taste, and those who've been getting lots of colds and infections, says Keith Watson, D.O., professor of surgery and associate dean for clinical affairs at the University of Osteopathic Medicine and Health Sciences in Des Moines, Iowa. "In addition to slow healing," he says, "bedsores, skin changes, and depression can also be signs of zinc deficiency."

It's hard to determine if someone is actually short on zinc, Dr. Watson says. "So we may give a patient zinc and other nutrients, since an isolated deficiency is rare," he says. "Then if he doesn't soon start improving, we'll check his zinc status to see if the amount we are giving is bringing the patient's blood level back to normal."

Dr. Wunderlich recommends 15 milligrams of zinc citrate (an easily absorbed form) twice daily to a number of his patients undergoing surgery. It's best to take this much zinc only under your doctor's care, as amounts exceeding 15 milligrams daily can be toxic.

Vitamin E: For Healing Hearts

Some doctors add vitamin E to their on-the-mend menus, especially for people who've had heart surgery. There's some evidence that vitamin E helps stop the process of atherosclerosis, or the buildup of fatty deposits in arteries. And one study, by researchers at the University of Toronto, suggests that it can also help limit tissue damage during coronary bypass surgery.

In this study, half of a group of people undergoing bypass surgery took vitamin E before their operations. The other half took placebos (blank pills). After the surgery, the people taking 300 IU of vitamin E for two weeks prior to surgery had "small but significant" improvement in heart function compared with the people taking the placebos.

"Heart cells can be damaged when their blood supply is cut off and then restarted, a condition called reperfusion injury," says Donald Mickle, M.D., professor of clinical biochemistry at the University of Toronto and one of the study's authors. When oxygenated blood circulates through the oxygen-deprived heart, free radicals can form and can injure the heart cells, he says. (Free radicals are unstable molecules that steal electrons from your body's healthy molecules to balance themselves.)

Vitamin E is known as an antioxidant. In the right place at the right time, it neutralizes harmful free radicals by giving up its own electrons, sparing healthy molecules from harm.

"Our study suggests that for people at high risk—those with unstable angina, for instance—treatment with vitamin E prior to bypass surgery may be of benefit," Dr. Mickle says. (For people who require immediate surgery, a water-soluble form of vitamin E that can be given intravenously just prior to or during surgery is being developed, he says.)

Doctors who recommend vitamin E to their surgery patients often prescribe about 400 IU of vitamin E daily. Don't take more than 600 IU without your doctor's okay, especially if you've had a stroke or bleeding problems in the past. "In large amounts, I'd say more than 800 IU, vitamin E can enhance bleeding problems," Dr. Wunderlich says. If you're taking anticoagulants, it's best not to take vitamin E supplements.

In fact, when you're going into surgery, it's a good idea to be aware of any and all nutritional therapy you are taking that might interfere with blood clotting, Dr. Wunderlich advises. "Some of my heart patients take garlic for their conditions, and since garlic can cause bleeding problems, I recommend stopping the garlic for a few weeks prior to surgery," he says.

"Remember, taking any kind of supplementation may interfere with your surgical procedure and recovery," says Dr. Curran-Celentano. "To be safe, take supplements only under medical supervision." A few weeks prior to surgery, you might want to discuss any supplements you've been taking with your doctor.

The most commonly offered bit of advice, from doctors and dietitians alike? Ask your doctor about taking a multivitamin/mineral supplement that provides the Daily Value of every essential nutrient. And if necessary, get enough protein and calories by adding nutritional liquids to your menu.

Medical Alert

Some people experience diarrhea and other digestive discomforts from such high levels of vitamin C. Also, vitamin C can interfere with the results of certain diagnostic blood and urine tests, so it's important that you discuss supplementation with your doctor.

Vitamin A can be toxic in doses exceeding 15,000 IU daily and has been found to cause birth defects in doses of 10,000 IU daily when taken during early pregnancy.

Amounts exceeding 15 milligrams of zinc daily can be toxic and should be taken only under medical supervision.

If you're taking anticoagulants, it's best not to take vitamin E supplements.

Tinnitus

Silencing the Ring

Susan J. Seidel, an otologist (hearing specialist) at the Greater Baltimore Medical Center, knows exactly how she developed the cicada-like chirp in her left ear.

"I was standing outside an airport, waiting to get on a plane, when a jet taxied toward our line," she recalls. "When it got close, it revved one of its engines to make a turn. The sound was so intense, I remember, that I clenched my teeth and thought 'Good grief, that's loud.'"

The blast lasted only a few seconds, but it set off the buzz that has pretty much stayed with her for more than 20 years. "I've gotten used to it, and lucky for me, it's in only one ear. But it has made me more interested in helping other people who have the same problem," she says.

Like Seidel, most of us have noticed that our ears can play their own tune for a time after being blasted by loud music or machinery, firecrackers, or gunshots. Usually, the sound is barely noticeable, lasting anywhere from a few minutes to a couple of days.

For people with a condition called tinnitus, though, the ringing, hissing, or buzzing becomes a persistent presence. *Tinnitus*, which in Latin means "tinkling like a bell," has been reported to reach volumes as high as 70 decibels. That's equivalent to having a vacuum cleaner in your head.

Tinnitus occurs when nerve cells in the cochlea, the tiny, snail shell–shaped inner ear, are damaged, explains Michael Seidman, M.D., director of the Tinnitus Center at the Henry Ford Hospital in Detroit. These nerves project hairlike endings into the cochlea, which is filled with fluid that moves in waves in response to sounds traveling through the ear. When a sound sends waves through the cochlea, the hairlike endings send a signal to the brain that gets interpreted as sound. When the sounds are too loud and the waves through the cochlea are too intense, the tiny nerve endings become damaged and may send abnormal signals that can cause hissing or buzzing.

Noise-induced spasms of the tiny arteries feeding

the inner ears can also damage the tiny hairlike cells by cutting off their blood supply. The nerve cells can also be damaged by viruses, high blood pressure, high blood cholesterol, and high insulin levels as well as by drugs, particularly aspirin and the -*mycin* antibiotics. Aminoglycosides such as gentamicin, which are often used to treat pneumonia, are probably the number one offenders, says Dr. Seidman. Tinnitus is often one symptom of Ménière's disease, a condition that is caused by excess fluid pressure in the inner ear.

Finally, degeneration of the aging ear, usually because of poor circulation, accounts for a large percentage of cases.

If you develop tinnitus, it's important to see a doctor to make sure that you don't have a tumor on an ear nerve or a damaged ear membrane, Dr. Seidman says. Both are treatable conditions.

While most doctors don't yet use nutrition to treat tinnitus, there is some intriguing new research, mostly from Israel, that holds promise for some people with this condition. Here's what doctors say may help.

Vitamin B$_{12}$ Sheathes Ear Nerves

When it comes to nerves, vitamin B$_{12}$ plays a special role. The body needs this nutrient to manufacture myelin, the fatty sheath that wraps around nerve fibers, insulating them and allowing them to conduct their electrical impulses normally.

A vitamin B$_{12}$ deficiency can raise blood levels of homocysteine, an amino acid that is thought to be toxic to nerves. Low levels of B$_{12}$ have been linked to a number of nervous system disorders, including memory loss, decreased reflexes, impaired touch, or pain perception, and, apparently, tinnitus and noise-induced hearing loss.

Researchers from the Institute for Noise Hazards Research and Evoked Potentials Laboratory at Chaim-Sheba Medical Center in Ramat Gan and from Tel Aviv University, both in Israel, looked at a group of 385 people with tinnitus and found that 36 to 47 percent had vitamin B_{12} deficiency. All of the people low in B_{12} received injections of 1,000 micrograms weekly for four to six months. At the end of that time, their hearing and tinnitus were evaluated. Fifty-four percent reported improvement in their tinnitus, and approximately one-fourth reported reductions in the measured loudness of their tinnitus, according to Joseph Attias, D.Sc., head of the institute and one of the study's main researchers.

"Vitamin B_{12} deficiency is somehow associated with chronic tinnitus," says Dr. Attias. "Long-term exposure to noise may deplete body levels of B_{12} and so make the ears more vulnerable to noise-induced damage."

Most of the people in this study had tinnitus for six years or longer. "It's possible that people who are treated earlier for vitamin B_{12} deficiency may have more improvement in their tinnitus than occurred in this study," says Dr. Attias.

If you have tinnitus, and especially if you also have memory problems, ask your doctor to check your blood level of vitamin B_{12}, he suggests.

Although most people get enough vitamin B_{12} from foods, absorption problems can cause shortages, especially in older people. Strict vegetarians, who eat no meats, dairy products, or eggs, are also at risk for deficiency, since B_{12} comes only from animal foods.

If your doctor determines that you have absorption problems, you'll need vitamin B_{12} shots for the rest of your life. If you don't have absorption problems, experts say that it's safe to take about 1,000 micrograms of B_{12} a day.

Magnesium May Shield Sensitive Ears

It's true that you won't find laboratory animals handling heavy artillery or using chain saws. But you can thank these creatures for another dietary recommendation for protecting ears: magnesium.

Magnesium-deficient lab animals exposed to noise have much more damage to the nerve cells in their cochleas than animals fed a diet adequate in magnesium, Dr. Attias says. What happens to these cells when the noise level gets too high? "The tiny hairs on these cells fuse or disappear, and they and their supporting cells eventually disintegrate, along with the nerve fibers going to these cells," explains Dr. Attias. Low levels of magnesium combined with noise exposure eventually deplete the cells' energy stores, leading to exhaustion, damage, and death of the inner ear cells, he explains.

Low magnesium levels can also cause blood vessels, including the tiny arteries going to the inner ears, to constrict. (Remember, noise-induced vasospasm is thought to play a role in tinnitus.)

Human ears, even young, healthy, normal-hearing ones, can benefit from extra magnesium, Dr. Attias says. He found that Israeli soldiers who got an additional 167 milligrams of supplemental magnesium daily had less inner ear damage than soldiers getting placebos (blank look-alike pills). According to Dr. Attias, a more recent study showed that supplemental intake has this same protective effect against long-term noise exposure.

If you're faced with a noisy environment, you'll want to make sure that you're getting the Daily Value of magnesium, which is 400 milligrams, Dr. Attias says. Most people fall short in that regard, with men getting about 329 milligrams a day and women averaging 207 milligrams a day. Green vegetables, whole grains, nuts, and beans are packed with magnesium. (If you're considering taking magnesium supplements, be sure to talk to your doctor first if you have heart or kidney problems.)

If your tinnitus includes a sensation of fullness in your ear and balance problems, experts recommend that you get adequate amounts of calcium and potassium as well. These additional symptoms could be a sign of Ménière's disease.

Antioxidants May Help Spare Ears

Tinnitus is sometimes caused by impaired blood flow to the ears, which can happen in two ways, Dr. Seidman says. First, the tiny artery leading to the inner ear can get clogged with cholesterol, causing a kind of stroke in the ear, he explains. Second, loud noises can send this artery into spasm, reducing blood supply to the cochlea. In either case, an interrupted blood supply can lead to hearing problems.

That's where the antioxidant nutrients—vitamin C, vitamin E, beta-carotene, and others—come in. "Antioxidants work by helping to prevent oxygen-caused damage to cell membranes," Dr. Seidman explains. Antioxidants also help keep arteries open and free of plaque buildup, experts say.

Dr. Seidman and some other ear doctors suggest that you consider a smorgasbord of antioxidant nutrients: 400 international units (IU) of vitamin E daily, 250 milligrams of vitamin C twice daily, 50 to 200 micrograms of the mineral selenium daily, and about 50,000 IU of beta-carotene twice daily. Doses of selenium exceeding 100 micrograms daily can be toxic and should be taken only under medical supervision.

Zinc Can Make a Difference

Some parts of the body have much higher concentrations of certain vitamins and minerals than other parts. That's the case with the inner ear, which, like the retina of the eye, has a high concentration of zinc. That finding has led some doctors to speculate that zinc deficiency may play a role in inner ear problems such as tinnitus.

"We don't know much about how zinc works in the inner ear, but it's evident that the cochlea needs zinc to function properly," explains George E. Shambaugh Jr., M.D., professor emeritus of otolaryngology and head and neck surgery at Northwestern University Medical School in Chicago. "Animals fed a diet low in zinc partially lose the ability to hear, and apparently, even the kind of marginal zinc deficiency often seen in older people worsens the hearing loss associated with ear damage from noise or aging." Zinc is involved in a wide array of functions, including helping to maintain healthy cell membranes and protecting cells from oxygen-related damage.

Dr. Shambaugh estimates that about 25 percent of the people he sees with severe tinnitus are zinc-deficient. Sometimes they also have poor appetite, hair loss, diminished taste or smell, or skin problems. All of these symptoms are related to zinc deficiency. For these people, he recommends supplemental zinc, along with a potent multivitamin/mineral that supplies other nutrients.

Although Dr. Shambaugh and other ear, nose, and throat specialists may initially give large doses of zinc—up to 150 milligrams a day—it's important to take no more than about 15 milligrams a day without medical supervision. Doctors monitor blood levels of zinc when they prescribe higher amounts. That's because zinc can be toxic in large doses. Zinc also interferes with copper absorption, so if you're taking high doses of zinc, you may need to take supplemental copper (the ratio that's generally recommended is 1 milligram of copper for every 10 milligrams of zinc). Copper, too, can be toxic, so follow your doctor's advice on this.

The Daily Value for zinc is 15 milligrams. According to Dr. Shambaugh, few people get 10 to 15 milligrams a day in their diets, while people over age 75 rarely get as much as 7 milligrams a day. Look to meats and shellfish for zinc; cooked oysters, beef, crab, and lamb all offer good amounts.

Vitamin A May Aid Hearing

Like zinc, vitamin A is found in high concentrations in the cochlea. "All special sensory receptor cells, including the retina of the eye and the hair cells of the inner ear, depend upon vitamin A and zinc to function properly," Dr. Shambaugh says.

In one study, low blood levels of vitamin A were associated with decreased ability to hear. And in several studies, from 24 to 74 percent of people with tinnitus reported at least partial relief with vitamin A supplements.

"I recommend beta-carotene, which you can take

without worrying about toxicity," Dr. Shambaugh says. (The body can use beta-carotene to make vitamin A.) He recommends taking 30 milligrams (about 50,000 IU) of beta-carotene twice a day.

Medical Alert

If you have heart or kidney problems, be sure to talk to your doctor before beginning magnesium supplementation.

Doses of selenium exceeding 100 micrograms daily can be toxic and should be taken only under medical supervision.

If you are taking anticoagulant drugs, you should not take vitamin E supplements.

Varicose Veins

Winning an Uphill Battle

That marbled look might work well on a fireplace mantel or a coffee table, but when it's on your legs—no way! You'd prefer them without those blue squiggles, thank you very much.

Why is it that some people have those squiggles and others don't?

To understand that, it helps to look at how the veins function. The heart pumps blood to the lungs to pick up oxygen. Then the blood travels back to the heart to be pumped out through arteries, thus delivering oxygen throughout the body. The heart pushes blood out through the arteries with a great deal of force. And when blood is making its return trip to the heart from various parts of the body, it moves through veins.

"Veins can't rely on the same forceful pressure that arteries have to move blood," explains Robert Ginsburg, M.D., director of the cardiovascular intervention unit at the University of Colorado Health Sciences Center in Denver. "Instead, they use valves that open in one direction only, toward the heart, to keep blood from flowing backward. And they rely on muscle contractions to squeeze blood in the right direction." Inefficient? Well, send your complaints to Mother Nature.

Varicose veins, those blue bulges, develop when veins can't return blood to the heart efficiently. Blood pools in the veins, making them dilate. That hinders the valves' ability to close tightly and stop backward blood flow. Eventually, veins may become permanently dilated and scarred and take on a torturous configuration similar to a road map of West Virginia.

Varicose veins are not just a cosmetic problem. They can contribute to swollen, tired legs and muscle cramps.

Some people develop varicose veins because they have inherited structural problems with the valves in the upper parts of their legs, says Joseph Pizzorno Jr., N.D., a naturopathic physician and president of Bastyr University in Seattle. "Even if just one or two valves fail, that can put enough pressure on the lower part of a vein so that it, too, has problems," Dr. Pizzorno says.

Other people have leaky valves because their veins are simply too weak to withstand the pressure of backflowing blood.

Most doctors' nutritional advice for varicose veins is limited to "Lose weight, eat more fiber." Both of these dietary measures help reduce pressure in veins. The few doctors who go beyond this advice to recommend nutritional supplements say that they're focusing on nutrients that help maintain the structural integrity of the vein wall and help reduce the possibility of blood clots in veins. Here's what these doctors recommend.

Vitamin C Helps Fragile Veins

Keeping vein walls strong is important when it comes to preventing varicose veins or keeping them from getting worse, according to medical experts. Strong vein walls can resist more pressure without dilating, which allows the veins' valves to work better.

That's where vitamin C comes in. The body needs it to manufacture two important connective tissues: collagen and elastin. Both of these fibers are used to repair and maintain veins to keep them strong and flexible, explains Dr. Pizzorno. Vitamin C, he says, may be especially important for you if you bruise easily or have broken capillaries, which may show up on your skin as tiny "spider veins."

Even more important to keeping veins and capillaries in tip-top shape may be vitamin C's first cousin, bioflavonoids. Bioflavonoids are chemical compounds often found in the same foods as vitamin C.

Dr. Pizzorno recommends 500 to 3,000 milligrams of vitamin C and 100 to 1,000 milligrams of bioflavonoids daily. These high amounts are easily obtained only with supplements. Some people experience diarrhea with as little as 1,200 milligrams of vitamin C a day, so you should discuss taking this much with your doctor.

Vitamin E Keeps Blood Flowing

While there are no studies to show that vitamin E heals varicose veins, people with varicose veins apparently do use it, hoping that it will help prevent the biggest potential complication: blood clots.

"Vitamin E helps keep platelets—blood components involved in clotting—from sticking together and from adhering to the sides of blood vessel walls," Dr. Pizzorno explains. Research shows that reducing platelet stickiness with vitamin E could help people at particularly high risk for blood-clotting problems, such as those with diabetes.

If you're going to take vitamin E, aim for 200 to 600 international units (IU) daily, suggests Dr. Pizzorno. Some research suggests that 200 IU a day is enough to reduce platelet adhesion. If you've had bleeding problems or a stroke, it's important that you talk to your doctor before starting vitamin E supplementation. If you are taking anticoagulants, you should not take vitamin E supplements.

A Trace Mineral Helps Keep Veins Strong

We all know that minerals help keep bones strong. Studies show that some minerals do the same for blood vessels, helping to build and maintain the layers of tissues that form blood vessel walls.

Copper, which we all need in small amounts, is used in the body to knit together collagen and elastin, the same connective tissues that require vitamin C.

"Copper is involved in the cross-linking between the molecules that make up these tissues," explains

Leslie Klevay, M.D., Sc.D., of the U.S. Department of Agriculture Grand Forks Human Nutrition Research Center in North Dakota. Research has shown that copper-deficient animals have weakened arteries and capillaries, two of the three types of blood vessels in our bodies (the third is veins), that can bulge out under pressure.

According to Dr. Klevay, little research has been done on copper's effect on veins. But because arteries and veins have similar structures, it is quite possible that the strength of veins depends on adequate copper levels, too. This is why everyone, including people with varicose veins, should make sure that they're getting adequate amounts of this trace mineral, Dr. Klevay says.

Copper is also needed to build and repair endothelial cells, the smooth protective cells lining the insides of blood vessels, Dr. Klevay explains. Getting adequate copper appears to help protect blood vessels against microscopic tears and rough spots, caused by high blood pressure and smoking, that can lead to the buildup of cholesterol-laden plaque and to blood clots.

The Daily Value for copper is 2 milligrams. Your best bet for getting enough is to include whole grains, nuts, and seeds, along with shellfish (especially cooked oysters) and lean red meat in your diet, recommends Dr. Klevay.

B Vitamins May Help Stop Clots

Endothelial cells are also damaged by high blood levels of an amino acid called homocysteine. The damage has been linked to early heart disease and, more recently, to increased risk of recurrent blood clots in veins.

That's where the three Bs come in. Researchers now know that folate (the naturally occurring form of folic acid) and vitamins B_6 and B_{12} help break down and clear homocysteine from the blood. "Deficiency of any one could lead to a high level of homocysteine," explains Jacques Genest Jr., M.D., director of the cardiovascular genetics laboratory at the Clinical Research Institute of Montreal, a research center that has done pioneering work on homocysteine and heart disease. "We've found that 2.5 milligrams (2,500 micrograms) of folic acid or 25 milligrams of vitamin B_6 reduces homocysteine levels to normal in most people," he says.

These high amounts of folic acid and vitamin B_6 are well above the Daily Values (400 micrograms and 2 milligrams, respectively) and are available only through supplements. This much folic acid should be taken only under medical supervision, as amounts exceeding the Daily Value can mask symptoms of pernicious anemia, a vitamin B_{12}–deficiency disease.

Even those eating healthy diets, with two or three servings of fruits and three or four servings of vegetables a day, get only about 190 micrograms of folate daily. As for vitamin B_6, men get about 1.9 milligrams a day and women average 1.2 milligrams a day through foods such as chicken, fish, pork, and eggs. Some people may need to take both, and older people and strict vegetarians may also need extra vitamin B_{12}, Dr. Genest adds. He recommends taking 2 micrograms of B_{12} a day.

Medical Alert

Folic acid in doses exceeding 400 micrograms daily can mask symptoms of pernicious anemia, a vitamin B_{12}–deficiency disease, and should be taken only under medical supervision.

Some people may experience diarrhea when taking vitamin C in doses of more than 1,500 milligrams daily.

If you've had bleeding problems or a stroke, it's important that you talk to your doctor before starting vitamin E supplementation. If you are taking anticoagulants, you should not take vitamin E supplements.

Water Retention

Beating the Bloat

Forget that "ashes to ashes, dust to dust" stuff. Water to water is more like it. Our aquatic ancestors brought the sea with them when they crawled on land, and human beings remain mostly fluid. We're 56 percent fluid, to be exact—but sometimes more, sometimes less, depending on the degree of bloat.

People who retain fluid know just how easy it is to swell up like a sponge. "Weight fluctuations of as much as four to five pounds in a single day are not uncommon in women with fluid retention problems," says Marilynn Pratt, M.D., a physician in private practice in Playa del Rey, California, who specializes in women's health.

Bloating occurs when fluid that normally flows through the body in blood vessels, lymph ducts, and tissues gets trapped in tissues in the interstitial spaces, the tiny channels between cells. The fluid flows through the membranes of tiny blood capillaries into the tissue cells because of osmotic pressure (cell wall pressure), which is controlled by electrolytes such as sodium. A high sodium level attracts more fluid from the blood into the cells, where the fluid gets trapped and the cells become overhydrated. This occurs more readily in women, because their tissues are designed to fluctuate or expand for pregnancy.

Lots of things can cause waterlogged tissues: allergic reactions to foods, heart and kidney problems, and prescription drugs such as hormones. In women, hormonal changes often cause bloating beginning 7 to 10 days prior to menstruation, as higher levels of estrogen and progesterone during that part of the cycle cause the body to retain salt (sodium) and therefore to retain fluid in tissues. "Replacement hormones (especially estrogen alone) can also cause substantial bloating and weight gain," says Dr. Pratt.

Usually, fluid retention is uncomfortable but not health-threatening. People who retain fluid because of heart or kidney problems, however, or who are taking diuretics (water pills) need to be under a doctor's care for their problems, says Dr. Pratt.

Nutritional changes for fluid retention are meant to counteract hormonal changes, balance the minerals that influence body fluid, and eliminate foods that trigger bloating in some people. Here's what doctors say helps.

The Salt Connection

Most of us know that too much salt in our bodies can lead to temporary swelling. An evening's overload on movie popcorn or ballpark franks can leave us puffy-eyed and headachy, with stiff, swollen hands and feet, the next morning. "That's because our kidneys retain fluid in our bodies so that the excess salt can be diluted," explains David McCarron, M.D., professor of medicine and head of the division of nephrology, hypertension, and clinical pharmacology at Oregon Health Sciences University in Portland. And, contrary to what you might think, drinking more water will not worsen fluid retention and may even help.

And some researchers believe that too little salt in the diet can also cause fluid retention, Dr. McCarron says. "We speculate that too little salt may trigger the kidneys to secrete more of a hormone that conserves salt, in part by reducing urinary output," Dr. McCarron says. He recommends keeping sodium intake at 2,400 milligrams (a little more than one teaspoon of salt) a day, an amount thought to maintain optimum blood pressure.

For most people, this still means cutting back by about 1,000 milligrams (about a half-teaspoon) a day. Since most of our salt comes from processed foods, not from the shaker, the best way to cut back is to look for sodium-free or low-sodium versions of cheeses, nuts, crackers, lunchmeats, canned soups, and vegetables.

"And women who are dieting may be eating a lot of celery, which has a higher level of sodium than any other vegetable," Dr. Pratt says. Munch on carrot sticks instead, she suggests.

Mix-and-Match Minerals

Getting too little potassium, calcium, or magnesium in your diet can also contribute to fluid retention, Dr. McCarron says. "These minerals all play important roles in the fluid balance in your body—your body's ability to move fluid into and out of cells and from the bloodstream or lymphatic system into tissues and back again," he says.

He recommends getting about 3,500 milligrams of potassium a day (the Daily Value), an amount you can obtain by eating at least five servings of fruits and vegetables. (Potassium is lost in cooking water, though, so don't depend on boiled potatoes or greens for this mineral unless you consume the water that they are cooked in.)

For magnesium, aim for the Daily Value of 400 milligrams, Dr. McCarron suggests. Most people fall short of this amount, with men getting about 329 milligrams a day and women averaging 207 milligrams a day. Nuts, legumes, and whole grains supply the most magnesium; other good food sources are green vegetables and bananas.

And for calcium, doctors recommend striving for 1,000 to 1,500 milligrams a day. One quart of skim milk contains about 1,400 milligrams of calcium. On average, men between ages 30 and 70 get close to 1,000 milligrams a day, while women in the same age group consume only about 700 milligrams daily, at least 300 milligrams less than they need.

If you have heart, kidney, or liver problems or diabetes or if you're taking a diuretic to relieve fluid retention or high blood pressure, you should supplement these minerals only under medical supervision to make sure that you don't develop dangerously high blood levels, says Dr. McCarron. People who are taking nonsteroidal anti-inflammatory drugs, potassium-sparing diuretics, ACE inhibitors, or heart medications such as heparin should also check with their doctors before supplementing potassium.

Vitamin B₆ May Aid Hormone-Related Bloating

Most women don't need a calendar to tell them when that time of the month is imminent. Their tender breasts, swollen hands and feet, and tightening blue jeans from abdominal swelling—all signs of fluid retention—mark time as well as any calendar.

In addition to the changes in mineral intake outlined above, some doctors recommend increases in the B vitamins, B_6 in particular. "Vitamin B_6 plays a role in the body's use of several hormones associated with fluid retention, including estrogen and progesterone," says Dr. Pratt. "By helping the body metabolize these hormones, B_6 may help the liver metabolize excess amounts, which may be present during the premenstrual period."

In one study, in fact, 500 milligrams of vitamin B_6 daily relieved the breast tenderness, headaches, and weight gain associated with water retention in 215 women.

If you'd like to try vitamin B_6 for hormone-related fluid retention, Dr. Pratt recommends taking 200 milligrams a day (50 milligrams four times a day) for the five days before your period begins. Take a B_6 supplement along with a supplement containing the rest of the B-complex vitamins. "These nutrients interact, so they work better when adequate amounts of all are available," Dr. Pratt says.

Vitamin B_6 can be toxic and can cause serious nerve damage in excessive amounts. For these reasons, it's best not to take more than 100 milligrams a day without checking with your doctor. You may, however, safely take up to 200 milligrams daily for five days to relieve premenstrual bloating, Dr. Pratt says. If your hands or feet start to feel numb or clumsy, stop taking B_6 and tell your doctor.

Medical Alert

Doctors recommend limiting your sodium intake to no more than 2,400 milligrams a day.

Some doctors advise against supplementing calcium, magnesium, or potassium without medical supervision if you have diabetes or heart, kidney, or liver problems or if you are taking diuretics.

People who are taking nonsteroidal anti-inflammatory drugs, potassium-sparing diuretics, ACE inhibitors, or heart medications such as heparin should also check with their doctors before supplementing potassium.

Vitamin B_6 can be toxic in large amounts. Do not take more than 100 milligrams a day without medical supervision.

Yeast Infections

Ditch the Itch

Have itchy palms? Some would say that money is coming your way. A seven-year itch? Better have a heartfelt chat with your mate. An itch where . . . well, you'd rather not discuss it? Welcome to one of the most common of feminine struggles: woman versus the beast called yeast.

In fact, at some point during their childbearing years, three in four women will wonder what they did to deserve the itching, burning, odor, and unpleasant discharge that accompany vaginal yeast infections. They'll also want to know exactly what they can do to stop it from ever happening again.

The Nature of the Yeast

Fortunately, there are steps that women can take to prevent these itchy episodes. But first, it helps to understand why a yeast infection happens at all.

The most likely culprit behind this maddening malady is a generally mild-mannered fungus known as *Candida albicans* that lives in the vagina, mouth, and intestines. Normally, candida is kept to its small, harmless colonies by the immune system and by *Lactobacillus acidophilus*, bacteria commonly found in the vagina that create an acidic environment that candida doesn't like. When something throws this ecosystem off balance, however, candida runs rampant, and yeast infections can result.

The most common offenders, things that upset this delicate ecosystem, include wet bathing suits, panty hose, skintight jeans, and leotards. All of these things foster a warm, moist environment that candida loves. Women are also prone to yeast infections during pregnancy, just before they get their periods, and during menopause. Candida also multiplies when women are taking antibiotics, because such medications often kill too many good bacteria, such as lactobacillus, along with the bad, leaving candida unchecked.

Be a Bad Host with Good Nutrition

Once candida has become a flaming yeast infection, doctors commonly recommend over-the-counter medications such as miconazole (Monistat) and clotrimazole (Gyne-Lotrimin) or the one-dose, prescription-only fluconazole (Diflucan), all of which can have you sitting comfortably again in less than a week. But since these medications won't kick candida out for good and since yeast infection recurrence is common, doctors say that you have to be a bad host if you want to stay yeast-free.

"Treating the vagina alone is often a waste of time and money," says William Crook, M.D., a physician in Jackson, Tennessee, and author of *The Yeast Connection and the Woman*. "Although vaginal suppositories may help, we also need to concentrate on putting the right things in your body to take care of the source of the problem."

According to the experts, that means boosting your immunity through good diet and nutritional supplements such as vitamins A, C, and E and the mineral zinc. Here's what they recommend.

Note: Although *Candida albicans* is the most common cause of vaginal infections, it isn't the only cause. So if you've never had a yeast infection before, see your doctor for a proper diagnosis before starting any treatment on your own.

Keep Yeast from Rising with Zinc

When it comes to fighting disease, the mineral zinc is often a heavyweight contender. It stimulates the production of T lymphocytes, the cells in your immune system that are responsible for cleaning up cells that have been invaded by infection. According to medical research, this makes zinc a prize-fighter against *Candida albicans*.

In fact, zinc supplements are likely beneficial even if your body's zinc levels are normal, according to a study done in India. Researchers there worked with laboratory animals that were not deficient in zinc. They gave these animals high-dose zinc supplements and found that they were significantly more resistant to infection from *Candida albicans* than those not supplemented with zinc.

"Zinc is essential in preventing infection," agrees Dr. Crook. "And though it's best to get your vitamins and minerals through a healthy diet, supplementation is probably a good idea, given how many essential nutrients our food loses by the time it's processed, packaged, shipped, and bought."

To fight candida, Tori Hudson, M.D., professor at the National College of Naturopathic Medicine in Portland, Oregon, suggests taking the Daily Value of zinc, which is 15 milligrams. And to get more zinc through your diet, try cooked oysters. They contain about 76 milligrams of zinc per half dozen.

Acidify with Vitamin C

When it comes to fighting *Candida albicans*, vitamin C does double duty.

First, research has shown that vitamin C boosts immunity by keeping disease-fighting white blood cells up and running, so the body is better able to stave off infections, especially opportunistic ones such as candida that take advantage of a weak immune system. As a bonus, vitamin C adds acidic zip to your vaginal environment. "Candida-fighting lactobacillus grows in acid," explains Roy M. Pitkin, M.D., professor of obstetrics and gynecology at the University of California, Los Angeles.

"So taking vitamin C may help, though it isn't likely to be completely effective by itself."

For optimum results, Dr. Hudson recommends 4,000 milligrams of vitamin C a day, divided into two 2,000-milligram doses and taken once in the morning and once in the evening for better absorption. This amount is considerably higher than the Daily Value, which is only 60 milligrams. Although such high amounts of vitamin C are considered safe, some people experience diarrhea from taking just 1,500 milligrams daily. If you want to try this higher dose to prevent yeast infections, discuss it with your doctor.

Think fruits and vegetables to boost the vitamin C in your diet. One cup of broccoli, orange juice, or Brussels sprouts provides about 100 milligrams.

Build Immunity with A and E

For women who are having ongoing battles with candida, Dr. Hudson recommends adding two more immunity-boosting nutrients to the mix: vitamins A and E.

"Vitamin A can be used either of two ways," says Dr. Hudson. Women can take vitamin A supplements of 25,000 international units (IU) a day, an amount that is five times the Daily Value and that should be taken only under medical supervision. This is especially important for women of childbearing age, since daily doses of 10,000 IU of vitamin A during early pregnancy have been linked to birth defects. It's for this reason that women who are pregnant should not use this therapy. If a woman prefers not to take such a high amount orally, she can insert the vitamin into the vagina instead.

"Inserting vitamin A stimulates the immune system right in the vagina," says Dr. Hudson. "You can simply insert a vitamin A gelatin capsule, although they are less potent than the vitamin A suppositories made by several companies."

As a final precautionary measure, she recommends taking 400 IU of vitamin E.

If you are a frequent victim of the yeast beast and would like to increase these nutrients in your diet, try cooking with vegetable oils and eating whole-grain cereals for more vitamin E, drinking fortified skim milk for a burst of vitamin A, and upping your intake of bright orange and yellow vegetables to increase beta-carotene (a substance that turns to vitamin A in the body).

Medical Alert

If you've never had a yeast infection before, be sure to see a doctor for proper diagnosis before starting treatment on your own.

Vitamin A can be toxic in doses exceeding 15,000 international units daily and has been found to cause birth defects in doses of 10,000 international units daily when taken in early pregnancy.

Some people experience diarrhea from taking more than 1,500 milligrams of vitamin C daily. So check with your doctor before trying this higher dose.

If you are taking anticoagulants, you should not take vitamin E supplements.

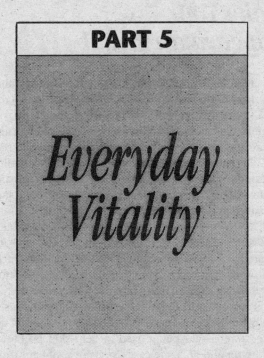

PART 5

*Everyday
Vitality*

Looking Great

Make Your Appearance Healthy

An old-time Western explorer didn't look anything like Clint Eastwood, no matter how much he squinted. Living off dry rations all winter, he was woefully deficient in vitamins and minerals come spring. As a result, his skin was dry and rough, covered in reddish-blue spots. His swollen gums were bleeding, his lips and tongue inflamed. There were cracks on his lips and a flaky skin rash on parts of his body exposed to the sun. He was nothing to set Miss Kitty's heart aflutter.

All this says that vitamins and minerals are absolutely necessary for healthy skin and appearance. But all that's required to achieve this is getting the Daily Values, which, by now, you know are not that hard to get. The question is, can taking extra vitamins improve how you look?

Probably not. But some vitamins and minerals—mostly those that are part of your body's antioxidant defense system—are being used to help skin problems heal better and, in some cases, prevent problems from occurring.

The Ravages of Sunshine

The sun is responsible for the majority of changes that your skin undergoes as you age, according to Karen E. Burke, M.D., Ph.D., a dermatologic surgeon and dermatologist in private practice in New York City. Ultraviolet

514

radiation from the sun produces droves of free radicals at the same time that it compromises your skin's antioxidant defenses. Prolonged exposure damages the elastic collagen fibers that make your skin resilient. When those fibers break down, wrinkles form. Sun damage also starts the process that can lead to skin cancer.

You can repair the ravages of the sun with tretinoin, a derivative of vitamin A, says Melvin L. Elson, M.D., medical director of the Dermatology Center in Nashville. The prescription topical medication Renova—which is tretinoin in a moisturizing base—has been approved by the Food and Drug Administration to treat fine lines and wrinkles and fade brown spots. It works by enhancing the production of collagen and forming thicker, moister epidermis, the top layer of your skin. The result is smoother skin.

Here are other ways to use vitamins to deflect the sun's harm.

Soothe with selenium. While all the antioxidant vitamins help protect the skin from sun damage, the mineral selenium appears to shine brightest. "If you have enough selenium, you won't get as many blistering sunburns," Dr. Burke says. "Because you get fewer sunburns, you have less aging of the skin and fewer skin cancers." Depending on the soil levels of selenium where you live, Dr. Burke recommends 50 to 200 micrograms of selenium in the more biologically available form, l-selenomethionine. Doses above 100 micrograms should only be taken under medical supervision. Good food sources of selenium include grains (tabbouleh is high on Dr. Burke's list) and saltwater fish, especially salmon.

Apply C at the sea. Topical vitamin C may allow the skin to withstand more ultraviolet exposure without getting as damaged, says Thomas N. Helm, M.D., assistant clinical professor of dermatology at the State University of New York at Buffalo School of Medicine and Biomedical Sciences. In studies at Duke University Medical Center, skin pretreated with vitamin C had less severe sunburns than untreated skin.

Heal burns with E. If you do get a sunburn, "take 400 international units (IU) of vitamin E every 4 hours starting immediately after the burn and continuing for one or two days," suggests Dr. Burke. "The d-alpha-tocopherol form is best." (You may want to check with your doctor first, especially if you are on certain blood-thinning medications).

Battle cancer with A. Vitamin A and vitamin A derivatives like tretinoin may also play an important role in preventing skin cancer. In one study, people with a high risk for skin cancer because of earlier sun damage were given 25,000 IU of vitamin A each day. "The people who got vitamin A developed fewer squamous cell cancers than those who didn't get vitamin A," says Norman Levine, M.D., chief of dermatology at the University of Arizona Health Sciences Center in Tucson. "The dosage we used was fairly high, but our patients didn't get many reactions. Still, at this level it is no longer a vitamin; it is a drug." Dosages above 15,000 IU should be taken only under medical supervision.

Healing the Skin

Oral and topical vitamins can also help restore your skin to normal if it has been injured or if you suffer from psoriasis. "If I had a serious burn or surgery, I would carefully watch my nutrition intake and take a multivitamin with minerals," says Dr. Helm. "You want to cover the whole spectrum."

Dr. Burke suggests taking 400 IU of vitamin E. "It

helps wound healing and is excellent for preventing raised scars or keloids. Just don't take it right before surgery, since it is a mild anticoagulant."

A synthetic form of prescription topical vitamin D, called calcipotriene (Dovonex), has proven effective in reducing red, itchy, scaly raised patches on knees and elbows that are the hallmarks of psoriasis. "If we use it on 100 patients, four-fifths of them show some improvement. For 15 percent, it is almost a home run hit," says Dr. Helm. For severe psoriasis, prescription etretinate (Tegison), a superpotent form of vitamin A, is given orally and only under a doctor's strict supervision.

The Happy Head

Want to use vitamins to achieve healthy hair and a happy smile? Here's what works.

Nourish the living. The hair you see is dead, so fancy vitamins in shampoos aren't going to help any. You need to nourish the living follicle inside your skin. "I recommend 1,000 milligrams of L-cysteine, an essential amino acid, plus 3,000 milligrams of vitamin C and 400 IU of vitamin E," says Dr. Burke. "I give this to anyone with hair problems. And a B-complex vitamin can't hurt either." One caution: Taking more than 1,500 milligrams of vitamin C may cause diarrhea in some people. Check with your doctor before supplementing at high levels.

Build a firm foundation. By now, your teeth have finished forming, but the bone supporting your teeth is continually broken down and rebuilt. It needs a continual supply of calcium and vitamin D to stay strong. Too little of these nutrients and the bone supporting your teeth could weaken, says Heidi K. Hausauer, D.D.S., spokesperson for the Academy of General Dentistry and assistant clinical professor at the

University of the Pacific Dental School's department of operative dentistry in San Francisco. In extreme cases you could even lose some teeth. In the healthy periodontal disease–free person, the Daily Value of calcium is enough. Some people with osteoporosis may need more, says Dr. Hausauer.

Attack gum disease with C. "A vitamin C deficiency alone does not cause gingivitis," says Dr. Hausauer. "You have to have a local irritant like plaque or tartar to get it. But people with a vitamin C deficiency have worse symptoms, such as bone loss, bleeding gums, and tooth loosening and loss." So prevent gum disease two ways: through smart mouth maintenance (brushing, flossing, and regular professional dental visits) and by getting enough vitamin C in your diet. Make sure that you get at least the Daily Value of vitamin C.

Losing Weight

Eat Your Way to a Slender Frame

Remember crash diets? They were fine if you were a crash-test dummy. But for flesh-and-blood people, they didn't work.

The pattern went like this: You'd eat nothing but the occasional grapefruit or dollop of cottage cheese.

You'd walk around for a few days feeling weak, deprived, and crabby. Then you'd quit the diet in frustration and dive into a three-day pizza and ice cream binge. In the long run, you didn't lose weight . . . you lost friends.

Even if you had the willpower to stick to a deprivation diet long enough to lose a few pounds, you'd be making a big mistake. Your bodily systems will not function without the nutrients that come with regular, sensible eating, nutrition experts say. This leads us to a weight-loss rule you'll love: Make sure that you get enough to eat.

Very low calorie diets are out—way out. Eating moderately, in a nutritionally balanced way, is the key to successful weight loss, says Gail Frank, R.D., Dr. P.H., professor of nutrition at California State University, Long Beach, and nutritional epidemiologist. If you eat enough food to prevent feeling deprived, it will be easier to keep up your healthier eating habits over the long haul.

Here are some tips to help you lose the pounds you want without losing vital nutrients.

Make every calorie count. Vitamins and minerals do not help you lose weight faster, but they are important in your weight-loss program. "Vitamins and minerals help in the metabolism of fat, carbohydrate, and protein. If you aren't getting enough of these nutrients because of your weight-loss plan, you run the very real risk of interfering with these functions," says Dr. Frank. Many vitamins and minerals help each other get absorbed better, too. So to make every calorie count, don't just fill your stomach—choose foods that are packed with these nutrients.

Diversify your assets. Make variety your dietary motto. "There are so many low-fat and fat-free choices of vegetables, fruits, and grains available in today's supermarkets, it's easier than ever to keep your vitamin and mineral sources interesting and diverse," says Leslie Bonci, R.D., nutritionist at the University of Pittsburgh Medical Center. If getting variety into your regular meals is hard for you to arrange, eat lots of different fruits and vegetables as snacks throughout the day. Then you can eat smaller portions of your usual fare at mealtime.

Ponder a multi. If you're restricting the calories you consume to lose weight, you may want to consider taking a multivitamin/mineral supplement, but only as an addition to a nutritious diet. "They are called supplements and not substitutes for a reason. Relying on supplements to take care of your micronutrient needs is like putting an adhesive bandage on a gaping wound," says Bonci. It won't replace eating the complex arrangements of nutrients found in healthy foods. A supplement can, however, act as nutritional insurance in case you accidentally fall short of any of your essential nutrients from one day to the next.

Accelerate the process. It all seems like a frustrating catch-22: You want to lose weight, but to prevent wrecking your body in the process, you have to keep up your nutrient consumption, which means eating. This means more calories, which get stored as body fat if they aren't burned up.

If you want to accelerate the weight-loss process, shave off those excess calories by stepping up your physical activity. "You can achieve your weight-loss goals and nutritional goals at the same time and obtain other health benefits by incorporating exercise into your moderate-calorie weight-management plan," says Dr. Frank. Exercising will increase the amount of calories your body burns throughout the day, not just when you are working out. A very low calorie diet won't do that for you.

No Substitute for Good Eating

Processed nonfat and low-fat snack foods might help you shave some fat out of your diet. But the trouble is that most of these products contain refined carbohydrates—basically sugar—and they offer zip for vitamins or minerals. Check the label. Steer clear of snacks low in fat but having less than 10 percent of Daily Values for vitamins and minerals or you will be eating truly empty calories, says Gail Frank, R.D., Dr. P.H., professor of nutrition at California State University in Long Beach and a nutritional epidemiologist. Some better choices include a banana, an orange, a bagel with apple butter, carrot sticks with salsa, or some other naturally low-fat food that provides nutrients along with its calories.

"Fat-soluble vitamins are forfeited when a person restricts all dietary fat for these fat-substitute products," says Anne Dubner, R.D., a dietitian in Houston who is a spokesperson for the American Dietetic Association. Vitamins A, D, E, and K all need a little fat in order to be absorbed by the body. "I tell my patients to aim for 20 percent of total calories from fat because, that way, if they underestimate the fat in foods or cheat on this plan a little, they will still be able to lose weight and maintain proper fat-soluble vitamin absorption," she says.

Don't assume that a multivitamin/mineral supplement will help offset the excessive use of processed snack foods. A pill could never replicate the vast combinations of known and unknown nutrients locked inside fruits, vegetables, whole grains, and other naturally low-fat foods, says Dr. Frank.

Contrary to one popular myth, exercise has no effect on vitamin or mineral absorption. "Exercise does affect how the body uses fat, protein, and carbohydrate; but it does not affect the body's use of vitamins and minerals," says Anne Dubner, R.D., a dietitian in Houston who is a spokesperson for the American Dietetic Association.

Eating a Vegetarian Diet

Be a B$_{12}$ Booster

Okay, we're going to play a little visualization game. Picture a typical serving plate at a typical American restaurant. What does it look like? Big slab of meat. A heaping spoonful of potatoes, rice, or noodles. And over in the corner, a small pile of vegetables that you could count individually. Now, take away the meat. What do you fill the plate with?

Vegetarians face that choice daily. Whatever their personal reasons for eschewing meat, vegetarians gain a distinct advantage over their meat-eating brethren in getting the upper levels of the recommended servings of fruit and vegetables each day. Their diets also are likely to be lower in saturated fats and higher in vitamins, minerals, and fiber, calorie per calorie.

But when you take away the meat, you may be taking away something else, something very important: vitamin B_{12}. Also called cobalamin, this nutrient is vital to the production of myelin, which insulates nerve fibers and helps keep electrical impulses moving through the body.

Vitamin B_{12} is also important in the production of red blood cells. In its natural form, vitamin B_{12} is found exclusively in animal products, such as red meat, dairy products, fish, and eggs. The Daily Value for vitamin B_{12} is only 6 micrograms, but this scant amount is essential.

"Long-term deficiencies in B_{12} can result in irreversible nerve damage. This can be a concern, depending on the type of vegetarian diet a person subscribes to," says Anne Dubner, R.D., a dietitian in Houston who is a spokesperson for the American Dietetic Association.

Getting Enough

Vegetarian diets that include animal products, but not meat, can generally offer enough vitamin B_{12} to ward off deficiency, says Dubner. Lacto vegetarians (those who eat dairy products like cheeses and milk) and lacto-ovo vegetarians (those who eat dairy products and eggs), for example, can usually get plenty of B_{12} without too much effort by incorporating dairy products and fortified cereals and breads into their diets. Vegetarians who also eat seafood have it even easier, since foods such as clams, tuna, and salmon are good sources of B_{12}.

Vegans, who do not eat any animal-based foods whatsoever, are the vegetarians who need to really think hard about where they can get their B_{12}. "True vegans have to supplement their vitamin B_{12} supply somehow; there's no way around it," Dubner says. "Luckily, there are simple ways to do this."

For starters, vegetarians who are concerned about their B_{12} consumption should eat breakfast cereals and breads that are fortified with vitamin B_{12}, Dubner says. Use the B_{12} information on the nutrition label to help you select these products. A daily multivitamin/mineral supplement also can provide your daily supply of the essential vitamin.

Because excessive amounts of B_{12} are excreted in the urine, supplementing this vitamin is considered extremely safe, even in large doses.

You may have heard about vitamin-B_{12} shots for senior citizens whose bodies no longer properly absorb the nutrient. "That's really unnecessary for a vegetarian because there are so many easier ways to get adequate amounts of vitamin B_{12}," Dubner says.

Other Needs

Here are some other pointers that vegetarians should keep in mind.

Iron out your problems. Vegetarians can sometimes shortchange themselves when it comes to iron. That's because the heme iron found in meat is easily absorbed by the body, while the nonheme iron found in plant foods is less absorbable.

"Vegetarians can easily make up for the amount of readily absorbable iron found in meat by consuming vitamin C and iron together," says Leslie Bonci, R.D., nutritionist at the University of Pittsburgh Medical Center. Vitamin C consumed with iron increases the mineral's absorption. Plant foods that contain a good supply of iron include dark green leafy vegetables (such as spinach), hot breakfast cereals (such as Cream of Wheat), dried beans, dried fruit, and soybean products. When you eat these foods, increase their effectiveness by also having vitamin

The Pseudo Solution

If you're like a lot of people, you just can't go cold turkey when it comes to meat. But if you're tempted by the health benefits of vegetarianism, you don't have to go whole hog. It may actually be to your advantage to cut back rather than cut out meat. Join the ranks of the pseudo-vegetarians.

Instead of giving up all meat all the time, do the next best thing and give up all meat (that is, beef, pork, and poultry) most of the time. "You'll get all the B_{12} and iron you'll need, without feeling deprived of the taste of meat," says Anne Dubner, R.D., a dietitian in Houston who is a spokesperson for the American Dietetic Association.

Cut down your meat consumption to one 3-ounce portion (about the size of a deck of playing cards) a day. Save it for the meal where it would give you the most satisfaction, Dubner recommends. Fill the rest of your meals and snacks with other types of foods, such as whole grains, fruits, and vegetables. After a few weeks, you may even want to cut back to having meat only a few days a week, says Dubner.

"One way to make sure that you stick with a pseudo-vegetarian program is to indulge yourself with the freshest or most flavorful varieties of produce and grains," Dubner says. "Spoil yourself with the meat alternatives." Use part of the money that you'd normally spend on several large cuts of lesser-quality meat on one good 3-ounce cut, then spend the rest on the best quality of fruits and vegetables you can find, Dubner recommends.

C-rich foods, such as a glass of orange juice, red bell pepper slices, or maybe some tomato wedges.

Bone up. By not eating meat, vegetarians may protect their bones from future fractures and deformities. Several studies have shown that excessive consumption of animal protein is linked to an increased calcium loss through the urine. This may increase a person's risk of developing osteoporosis, a debilitating bone-thinning disease.

Since this has not been found to be the case with vegetable-protein sources, vegetarians may actually have a lower risk for osteoporosis than meat-eaters. "Lacto vegetarians have been shown to have good bone density," Bonci says.

Strategies for Vegetable-Haters

11 Ways to Get What You Need

You know that you're supposed to eat three to five servings of vegetables a day. You know that vegetables are loaded with disease-fighting and health-promoting vitamins and minerals. You know that they contain other mysterious nutrients that scientists haven't even pinpointed yet. And you know that you can't get the same nutritional boost from some pill.

There's just one problem: You hate vegetables.

"Ask yourself, 'What do I hate about vegetables?' If it's the way you were served them as a kid, that can be changed," says Anne Dubner, R.D., a dietitian in Houston who is a spokesperson for the American Dietetic Association.

The Energizing Eleven

Let's be honest: There are some vegetables that you're just not going to eat, regardless of how they're prepared. That's fine. But there are a lot of others that may surprise you. All it takes is a dash of creativity and an open mind.

Here are 11 expert tips that you can use to painlessly—perhaps even deliciously—increase the number and variety of vegetables in your daily diet.

Eat 'em raw. Cooking can cause vegetables to lose some of their nutrients. If you aren't getting many vegetables to begin with, stick to uncooked ones to get the maximum nutritional benefits. "Some people just can't stand the sight, smell, texture, or taste of cooked spinach. But they will gladly eat a spinach salad," Dubner says. Raw vegetables tend to be brighter, fresher-smelling, and crisper than ones that have been cooked, especially in boiling water. Raw vegetables can often taste more lively, too. "If all you've ever had are mushy, overcooked vegetables, try the raw versions and you won't believe how much better they taste," Dubner says.

Flash them. When cooking vegetables in water, let the pot reach a rolling boil first. Then drop in the vegetables, count to 10, and drain them. This method of cooking, called flash-boiling, retains more vitamins in vegetables than longer methods of cooking, says Dubner. Other cooking methods that limit nutrient loss are steaming, stir-frying, and microwaving.

Sneak them in. "Try adding vegetables to recipes with so much stuff going on that you won't notice anything has been added," says Leslie Bonci, R.D., nutritionist at the University of Pittsburgh Medical Center. Bulk up your favorite casserole, soup, lasagna, or chili with chopped or shredded vegetables. The added ingredients will take on the flavorings of the dish, making them painlessly disappear from your plate.

Add spice. If you think that plain vegetables taste boring, spice them with your favorite seasonings, herbs, hot sauce, or soy sauce. Dubner recommends throwing dill on steamed carrots or oregano on flash-boiled green beans. You also can glaze your vegetables with a small amount of honey or sugar if they need sweetening.

Enjoy your salad days. "A lot of people who hate vegetables will still eat salads," Dubner says. "If you can agree to at least eat some salad with your meals, you're doing a lot of good." Salads can be a great diet-enhancing tool. Salads made from a wide assortment of produce give you variety as well as nutrients, says Dubner. Every cup of salad equals one serving of vegetables, as long as it's not a quarter head of iceberg lettuce thrown in a bowl with some dressing.

If you don't mind eating salads but can't seem to find the time or patience to prepare your own, supermarket salad bars take away the hassle of preparation, says Dubner. Buy ready-to-eat packages of greens so that you don't have to wash and chop them at home. When you eat out, order a salad whenever it comes with your entrée, and consider ordering one if it doesn't come

The Big Chill

Frozen and canned vegetables are equally convenient but are not always equally nutritious. "Frozen vegetables are flash-frozen not long after they are ripe so that the nutritional value stays quite high, naturally. Nothing is depleted from them," says Leslie Bonci, R.D., nutritionist at the University of Pittsburgh Medical Center. However, when vegetables are canned, the B-vitamin levels drop during heating. That's because B vitamins aren't heat-stable.

"Of course, canned vegetables are better than none," says Bonci. So if nothing else is available, grab a can opener.

with your meal. And yes, that includes fast-food restaurants, too—a side salad instead of a side order of fries can make a huge nutritional difference. Specify that the dressing be served on the side. That way *you* decide how much you eat.

Be a big dipper. Pass on the chips and grab hold of some crisp vegetables when you crack open the onion dip, cheese spread, salsa, or some other enticing concoction. Have a bag of washed and cut vegetables ready in the refrigerator for when the mood hits you. Sugar snap peas, carrot sticks, and bell pepper wedges have excellent dip-scooping abilities. When the cupboard is bare, salad dressing makes a good veggie dip in a pinch, says Dubner.

Be extravagant. Some rich accompaniments can be used sparingly to make vegetables more appealing. "It's better to have some fat and get the vegetables in than it is to forfeit the produce all together," says Bonci. Try adding a bit of cheese or creamy sauce to your vegetables. If you are counting calories and fat for health or weight-loss reasons, use low-fat cheeses or condiments. Or consider having smaller portions or low-fat varieties of meats or desserts in order to allow yourself a more satisfying vegetable dish, says Bonci.

Batter up. Mild-tasting vegetables, such as zucchini, mushrooms, and squashes, can be coated with light or nonfat mayonnaise and bread crumbs, then baked in the oven to make them more palatable, says Bonci.

Get juiced. Drinking a vegetable beverage, such as V-8 or carrot juice, is one way to get the vitamins and minerals of vegetables, although you lose out on the fiber, Dubner says. If you are eating whole-grain foods and fresh fruit, this shouldn't be a huge concern.

Get yelled at. "When you go shopping, look for the produce that has eye-catching color. Let the vegetables scream at you in the aisle," Dubner says. Bright colors are usually signs that the vegetables are rich in vitamins—just look at tomatoes, bell peppers, and carrots. Choose romaine lettuce over iceberg; the washed-out color of iceberg lettuce is a hint that it contains few nutrients, she says. Other vegetables, such as cucumbers and celery, have pale inside flesh that show they are also low in nutritional value.

When all else fails, eat fruit. Until you have gotten into the swing of eating vegetables, pad your diet with the other star of the produce aisle. "Fruit will provide most of the same vitamins and minerals. So if you like more of them, count some fruit as part of your three to five servings of vegetables each day," says Bonci.

Index